Geriatric Rehabilitation
A Textbook for the
Physical Therapist Assistant

Geriatric Rehabilitation
A Textbook for the
Physical Therapist Assistant

Jennifer M. Bottomley PT, MS, PhD[2]

Geriatric Rehabilitation Consultant & Educator

Boston, Massachusetts

PTA Advisors:

Peggy DeCelle Newman PT, MHR

Karen Ryan PTA

Stacy Potvin PTA

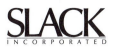

www.slackbooks.com

ISBN: 978-1-55642-816-6

The procedures and practices described in this book should be implemented in a manner consistent with the professional standards set for the circumstances that apply in each specific situation. Every effort has been made to confirm the accuracy of the information presented and to correctly relate generally accepted practices. The authors, editor, and publisher cannot accept responsibility for errors or exclusions or for the outcome of the material presented herein. There is no expressed or implied warranty of this book or information imparted by it. Care has been taken to ensure that drug selection and dosages are in accordance with currently accepted/recommended practice. Due to continuing research, changes in government policy and regulations, and various effects of drug reactions and interactions, it is recommended that the reader carefully review all materials and literature provided for each drug, especially those that are new or not frequently used. Any review or mention of specific companies or products is not intended as an endorsement by the author or publisher.

SLACK Incorporated uses a review process to evaluate submitted material. Prior to publication, educators or clinicians provide important feedback on the content that we publish. We welcome feedback on this work.

Published by: SLACK Incorporated
                  6900 Grove Road
                  Thorofare, NJ 08086 USA
                  Telephone: 856-848-1000
                  Fax: 856-848-6091
                  www.slackbooks.com

Contact SLACK Incorporated for more information about other books in this field or about the availability of our books from distributors outside the United States.

Library of Congress Cataloging-in-Publication Data

Bottomley, Jennifer M.
  Geriatric rehabilitation : a textbook for the physical therapist assistant / Jennifer Bottomley.
    p. ; cm.
  Includes bibliographical references and index.
  ISBN 978-1-55642-816-6 (alk. paper)
  1. Physical therapy for older people. 2. Older people–Rehabilitation. I. Title.
  [DNLM: 1. Physical Therapy Modalities. 2. Aged. 3. Aging–physiology. 4. Allied Health Personnel. 5. Geriatric Assessment–methods.
  6. Rehabilitation–methods. WB 460 B751g 2010]
  RC953.8.P58B68 2010
  615.8'20846–dc22
                          2010005295

Last digit is print number: 10 9 8 7 6 5 4 3 2 1

DEDICATION

To Senator Ted Kennedy (1932–2009), whose inspiring life and service in the US Senate has made the path for aging Americans so much easier. What happens to the people you touch and never really know? Thanks to your work, Senator Kennedy, you've touched and inspired many lives. If there are only 5 people for each of us to meet in heaven, I will hope that one of them will be you.

- 1965: supported the creation of Medicare and Medicaid, programs he fought to strengthen and expand for decades
- 1966: expanding the Economic Opportunity Act of 1964 to create a national health centered system
- 1972: Women, Infants and Children program, providing nutrition assistance to low-income mothers and their children
- 1975: Education for All Handicapped Children Act, guaranteeing free and equal public education for disabled children
- 1977: offered his first National Healthcare Plan, meant to cover all Americans
- 1985: Consolidated Omnibus Budget Reconciliation Act (COBRA), the Kennedy-sponsored law that allows workers to get stop-gap health insurance while between jobs
- 1992: Mammography Quality Standards Act, improving the safety and accuracy of mammograms
- 1994: Family and Medical Leave Act, guaranteeing employees unpaid time off for illness and to care for a family member
- 1996: Health Insurance Portability and Accountability Act, installing privacy standards for health information and protecting workers from losing their health insurance when they change or lose their jobs
- 1997: State Children's Health Insurance Program, helping states provide health coverage to low-income uninsured children
- 2000: Minority Health and Health Disparities Research and Education Act, increasing research and data collection on minority health
- 2006: Family Opportunity Act, expanding Medicaid to include funds to children with special needs
- 2010: Health care reform passed the House and Senate in March

Note: This only includes the bills Senator Kennedy inspired and help to write in the area of health. Of the more than 2,500 bills written in his 46-year career in the US Senate, these highlights do not touch foreign affairs, civil rights, or education, to name a few. These highlights are only some of the measures Senator Kennedy sponsored, cosponsored, or negotiated in the area of health.

CONTENTS

ACKNOWLEDGMENTS

From conception to completion of *Geriatric Rehabilitation: A Textbook for the Physical Therapist Assistant* it has been a long, long journey. The path toward completion has been easy at times, and at others, many obstacles were encountered. Through it all, Carrie Kotlar, John Bond, and Brien Cummings have helped to keep the flame burning and the path well lit. I thank each of them for their patience, perseverance, and guidance, as well as encouragement along the way.

My work has been made enjoyable and educational by the dependable and able assistance of my colleagues, Stacy Potvin, PTA, Peggy DeCelle, Newman PT, MHR, and Karen Ryan, PTA, who have reviewed and edited every chapter, often more than once, and have provided the "Pearls" for each chapter, which I know each reader will appreciate. They have provided the tender loving care in the provision of top-quality information, and each chapter has been fostered and enhanced by their many contributions.

Though way too many to name, I also thank my interprofessional family and faculty colleagues, especially those from the Massachusetts Institute of Health Care Professionals, Brigham & Women's Hospital, and Beth Israel Hospital, who have read and improved many of the following chapters with their clinical and professional expertise and skill. You each know who you are, and I thank you for your creative and scholarly input and suggestions along the way.

On a personal note, I thank my life partner (in the state of Massachusetts, my wife), Jennifer M. Buchwald, for her neverending love, energy, and inspiration. Without her patience and gentle pushing, you would not be holding this textbook in your hands. I thank "the other Jennifer" for sharing and enriching my life so completely.

My Gratitude to All,
Jennifer M. Bottomley

ABOUT THE AUTHOR

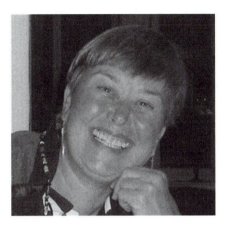

Jennifer M. Bottomley, PT, MS, PhD[2], has a bachelor's degree in Physical Therapy from the University of Wisconsin–Madison and an advanced master's degree in Physical Therapy from the MGH Institute of Health Professionals in Boston, MA. She also has a combined intercollegiate doctoral degree in Gerontology (University of Massachusetts) and Health Science and Service Administration (Union Institute), as well as a second doctoral degree in Health Service Administration, Legislation, and Policy Management with a specialty in Gerontology (Union Institute).

Dr. Bottomley has been clinically practicing since 1974 in acute care, home care, outpatient clinics, nursing homes and long-term care facilities. Currently, she serves as an academic and clinical educator in Geriatric Physical Therapy internationally and throughout the United States in numerous university programs. In addition to teaching, Dr. Bottomley is a rehabilitation consultant for Amedisys Home Health and Hospice, Inc. She practices clinically in the Boston area in homeless shelters and has orchestrated free screening and intervention projects for the homeless elderly of Massachusetts, obtaining federal grants to provide free screening and care for low-income elders in 14 central Massachusetts cities and towns.

Dr. Bottomley has served on advisory boards for the Office of the Surgeon General and the Office of Women's Health for the Department of Health and Human Services, and was appointed to a White House Interdisciplinary Medicare Reform Advisory Panel for rehabilitation in home care and long-term care settings. She continues to serve in that capacity.

Dr. Bottomley is a nationally renowned speaker, author, and educator. She has contributed chapters to many texts, published numerous articles and co-authored a geriatric text, now in its 3rd edition, with Carole B. Lewis entitled *Geriatric Rehabilitation: A Clinical Approach* published in 2008. She has also edited the *Quick Reference Dictionary for Physical Therapy*, now in its 2nd edition, published by SLACK Incorporated in 2004.

In 2006, MGH Institute of Health Professions recognized Dr. Bottomley with the 2nd annual Most Distinguished Alumni Award. The Massachusetts chapter of the APTA also awarded her the Mary MacDonald Distinguished Service Award in 2008.

About the PT & PTA Advisors

Peggy DeCelle, Newman PT, MHR has practiced as a physical therapist for 27 years in a variety of settings including acute care, outpatient orthopedics, institutional long-term care, and home health. Additionally, she has managed allied health professionals in all of these settings. Currently, she continues to work with patients in an outpatient setting, 2 afternoons per week.

Ms. Newman served as PTA Program Director at the Oklahoma City Community College from 1995-2006. She also served as Academic Coordinator of Clinical Education (ACCE) at the University of Oklahoma from 1988-1993. After leaving OCCC, she practiced clinically for a year, in a variety of settings, and returned to the University of Oklahoma's Department of Rehabilitation Sciences in 2007. She is currently serving as the Director of Clinical Education, in addition to Director of the Faculty Continuing Education Program and Assistant Professor.

Ms. Newman has served the OPTA in many roles including Chapter President and Chief Delegate, and she currently serves as Chief Delegate and Membership Committee Co-Chair. She was appointed to the Oversight Panel for the Analysis of Practice for the PT and PTA licensure examination by the Federation of State Boards of Physical Therapy from 2005-2007.

She has presented locally and nationally on topics including "Vision 2020," "Using Support Personnel Effectively," "The Guide to PT Practice: An Introduction," "Let's Talk Ethics," and "Ethical and Legal Challenges for Therapists in Today's Health Care Environment." She presented "Enhancing the Therapist: Therapist Assistant Partnership" at the APTA Annual Conference in Boston in 2010.

Ms. Newman is the co-author of *The PTA Handbook: Keys to Success in School and Career for the Physical Therapist Assistant*, published by SLACK in 2005. She recently authored the chapter "Standards of Practice" in the *Study Guide for the Physical Therapist Assistant's Examination*.

Karen Ryan, PTA has been an educator, author and physical therapist assistant clinician for over 20 years. She received her associate in applied science degree as a PTA from St. Catherine's College in Minneapolis, MN and is currently completing her bachelor's degree in Health Administration and Public Education at Metro State College in Denver, CO. As a clinician, Ms. Ryan has worked in a multitude of practice settings and is currently the administrator for a private physical therapy clinic, Back to Motion Physical Therapy, in Denver, where she continues to keep her hand in direct client care every week. Ms. Ryan is also the editor and contributing author for a national PTA licensure review and study guide, and teaches courses for PTA graduates preparing for their licensure examination. In her spare time she takes full advantage of living in Colorado, snowshoeing and hiking as often as possible.

Stacy Potvin, PTA, BA, BS received a bachelor of arts degree in English from Niagara University in 1986, and a bachelor of science degree in Physical Education in 1990 from Canisius College. She worked as a physical education teacher and athletic director before beginning her career as a physical therapist assistant. She received an associate of science degree in Physical Therapy from Bay State College in 1996 and has been working as a physical therapist assistant in the outpatient rehabilitation department at Beth Israel Deaconess Medical Center since graduating. She is a PTA III, the senior PTA on staff, and treats patients with a wide range of musculoskeletal problems, with a special interest in aquatic therapy, geriatrics, and sports medicine. Ms. Potvin has been very involved in clinical education for physical therapist assistants, and is an APTA credentialed clinical instructor who supervises students from Bay State College, North Shore College, and Hesser College. She has also served on the advisory board for the clinical education program at Bay State College.

ABOUT THE COVER

The cover portrait, "Newton," by artist Deborah L. Bottomley, is of the author's and artist's grandfather. Ms. Bottomley has captured the essence of Grandpa Newton in this beautifully detailed drawing, one in a series of drawings of elders' faces, reflecting life's many challenges and joys in lines that go from the face right to the heart.

Artist Info: Deborah L. Bottomley
www.dlbottomley.com

PREFACE

Geriatric Rehabilitation: A Textbook for the Physical Therapist Assistant is a comprehensive guide for the physical therapist assistant (PTA) student or clinician who has an interest in or is currently working in geriatric-based settings. Assessing and treating the medically complex older patient presents a unique challenge and opportunity for the PTA to expand his or her knowledge base and stretch his or her clinical skills to the maximum. Older patients present a complicated clinical puzzle: they are referred to the PTA with many diagnoses and are therefore medically complex; they are often taking multiple medications; and they likely have nutritional problems and socioeconomic issues that will broaden and test the skills of any clinician. Clinical expertise will be rapidly honed when the PTA is working in geriatric care settings. It is hoped that this text will guide and facilitate success in this endeavor.

Geriatric Rehabilitation is a comprehensive look at the practical and clinically applicable components needed in the special care of the elderly across the spectrum of care for the PTA. The book's focus is the clinically relevant assessment, treatment, and management of the geriatric population and it spotlights attention on primary, secondary, and tertiary prevention and a return to maximal level of functional capabilities. Pathological manifestations commonly seen in the elderly patient are addressed from a systems perspective and attention is paid to what is seen clinically and how it affects function. Each pathological area is inclusive of screening/assessment/evaluation, treatment prescription, goal setting, modification of treatment, and anticipated outcomes. Important psychosocial, pharmacological, and nutritional elements are also addressed to enhance the PTA's knowledge of factors that affect an older person throughout the course of intervention.

Geriatric Rehabilitation puts an emphasis on how the PTA should use a balance of theory, clinical application of knowledge, and clinical skills in assessing and treating the geriatric patient. The unifying element of the book is the special needs of the elderly in all health care settings. The conceptual framework for the organization and presentation of the material focuses on practical, hands-on components of intervention, assessment and decision-making skills needed for comprehensive geriatric care at each point along the continuum of care. This book addresses and incorporates aspects of prevention, fitness, and wellness in addition to the rehabilitative model of care for elders with pathological conditions resulting in functional losses.

This text provides many resources and tools for the assessment and treatment of geriatric patients and encourages PTAs to extend their knowledge, make informed choices about intervention and progression of therapy, and facilitate the success of physical therapy in obtaining an older person's own goals, his or her maximal functional abilities, and improving his or her quality of life.

I welcome your feedback and ideas on how this journey into geriatrics can be more successful and more fulfilling. The future of geriatric physical therapy is in the hands of those students, new graduates, and practicing PTAs who choose to practice geriatric rehabilitation in our current and ever-changing health care environment. I wish you all the best and hope that in some small way this book will make your journey more rewarding.

Section I

Fundamental Concepts in Geriatric Rehabilitation

Introduction to Geriatric Rehabilitation: Principles of Practice

1

The face of aging in the United States is changing dramatically and rapidly.[1] Today's older Americans are very different from their predecessors. They are living longer and have lower disability rates, allowing them to be more active; they are achieving higher levels of education and are living in poverty less often. Baby boomers promise to further redefine what it means to grow old in America.

As a result, the scope of physical therapy practice is shifting to meet the needs of our aging population. A greater number of older people will require physical therapy simply because of their sheer numbers; however, there will be a shift in clinical focus that includes preventive interventions, treatment of sports and leisure-related injuries, more home and community-based care, and more attention to health and fitness. That's not to say that the treatment of conditions more traditionally associated with aging (such as stroke, Parkinson's disease, and Alzheimer's) will decrease, but more so that people over 65 years of age are a more heterogeneous group that will require physical therapy interventions across a spectrum of health care and wellness issues.

As the number of older adults increases, the physical therapist (PT) will have greater demands on his or her time for screening, assessment, examination, and evaluation. This will result in a greater need for the physical therapist assistant (PTA) to perform more of the treatments, as prescribed by the PT. The PTA will play a key role in the provision of rehabilitative care as the population ages.

This chapter is intended to introduce the PTA to the unique practice of geriatrics. A comprehensive look at principles and practices will be presented in this stand-alone chapter to acquaint the PTA student to the multi-faceted aspects of geriatric care in rehabilitation. Subsequent chapters will then provide greater depth to each area of geriatrics discussed here.

DEFINING GERIATRICS

Geriatrics is the branch of medicine that focuses on the specialized care of aging populations, healthy living, and the prevention and treatment of disease and disability in later life. A geriatric PT treats older patients to prevent and manage multiple disease symptoms, and develops comprehensive care plans that address their specific health care needs. Older persons may react to illness and disease differently than younger adults. As a result, the study of geriatrics is unique to other areas of rehabilitation.

PTAs play an important role in treating the impairments or functional limitations that lead to the development of many of the pathologies associated with the aging process. Normal aging is not necessarily burdened with disability; however, almost all conditions that cause disability are more frequently seen in the older population.[2] As a result, the aged are more likely to require assessment for rehabilitative services. Functional assessment for needed rehabilitative services should be an essential part of routine evaluation

Bottomley J. *Geriatric Rehabilitation: A Textbook for the Physical Therapist Assistant* (pp 3-28).

by all health care disciplines working with the aged population. Geriatrics teaches that *maximal functional capabilities* can be attained; therefore, it can be argued that rehabilitation is the foundation of geriatric care.

The basis of geriatric rehabilitation is to assist the disabled aged in recovering lost physical, psychological, or social skills so that they may become more independent, live in personally satisfying environments, and maintain meaningful social interactions. This may be done in any number of settings including acute and subacute care settings, rehabilitation centers, assisted living environments, home and office settings, community settings, or in long-term care facilities such as nursing homes (see Chapter 8).

INTERDISCIPLINARY CARE: AN IMPORTANT ELEMENT IN GERIATRICS

Because of the complexity of the interventions needed in dealing with the aged, an interdisciplinary team approach is required. The geriatrics team is made up of skilled health professionals who contribute valuable expertise in the proper assessment and care of an older patient, and may include any or all of the following professionals: physician, nurse, social worker, nutritionist, PT, PTA, occupational therapist, occupational therapist assistant, consultant pharmacist, and geriatric psychiatrist. Each team member plays an important role in coordinating care and providing the most comprehensive, holistic care available and evaluating the social support (ie, spouse, children, friends, living and community resources) available to a patient. The geriatric PT on the team often serves as the "point person" for functional and physical aspects of care.

Because rehabilitation is key to recovery, patients and their families must be educated toward the best steps and methods in their therapies and the importance in following them correctly. Rehabilitation is more than a medical intervention: it is a philosophical approach that recognizes that diagnoses and chronological age are poor predictors of functional abilities, that interventions directed at enhancing function are important, and that the "team" should always include patients and their families.

THE ROLE OF THE PHYSICAL THERAPIST ASSISTANT

The PTA is an integral part of the geriatric team. Working in a geriatric setting offers a rewarding opportunity to make a positive difference in the quality of older people's lives. The PTA role requires a personal and direct approach to meeting an individual's health needs. The services of PTAs are utilized throughout the country in a variety of geriatric care settings.

PTAs work under the supervision of a PT, with duties including assisting the PT in implementing treatment programs according to the plan of care, training patients in exercises and activities of daily living (ADL), conducting treatments using special equipment, administering modalities and other treatment procedures, and reporting to the therapist on the patient's responses. Both the PT and PTA are critical to the optimal delivery of therapy to older adults in need. Although the patient population encompasses older individuals who have medically complex situations, the process of delineation and delegation of responsibilities is not specific to geriatric rehabilitation. PTs are responsible for the evaluation and design of the treatment plan and intervention program.[3] PTAs use their skills to participate in the subsequent assessment process and carry out many aspects of the treatment plan designed by the PT. The PTA plays a critical role by interacting and observing the patient and his or her progress while moving through rehabilitation, and subsequently corresponds with the PT in a collaborative manner to determine any necessary changes to the treatment approach based on the patient's status.

The role of the PTA working in a patient's home varies greatly from working in a care facility. Each state has its own defined state practice acts, in which supervision requirements are defined and regulations as to whom the PTA may make recommendations are specified. Some states require that the PT be in the same physical location as a PTA, which then may preclude a PTA from working independently in a patient's home. Some state practice acts allow a PTA to make recommendations only to a PT, thereby limiting the PTA's ability to provide input to other health care professionals or family members involved in the care of a patient. The role of the PTA in a home environment during a visit, therefore, would be information and data collection, which is then provided to the PT to assess and make recommendations to the patient, other health care providers, and family caregivers. State practice acts also specify requirements for supervision in other health care facilities. The requirements on to whom the PTA can report and why they can recommend usually applies in either setting. Nonetheless, it is recommended that practice acts be reviewed and applied as required by state law.

THE AGING PROCESS

As we age, our bodies change in many ways that affect the function of both individual cells and organ systems. These changes occur and progress over time in subtle ways.[4] Research in aging is starting to establish a fairly clear picture that components (eg, genetics, nutrition, lifestyle behaviors, exercise, sleep, and environmental factors) may influence the way a person ages.

The aging process depends on a combination of genetic, lifestyle, and environmental factors.[5] Recognizing that every individual has his or her own unique makeup and environment, which interact with each other, helps us understand why the aging process can occur at such different rates in different people. Overall, genetic factors seem to be more powerful than lifestyle or environmental factors in determining the large differences among people in healthy aging and lifespan.[6] The theories related to genetic factors in aging will be discussed in greater detail in Chapter 2.

Many environmental conditions, such as the quality of health care that one receives, the amount of water one drinks and of sleep one gets, and one's outlook on life, have substantial effects on the aging process.[7] A healthy lifestyle certainly gives one an advantage toward a healthy and long life. Preventive behavioral factors for a healthy lifestyle are listed in Box 1-1.

Greater detail of aging changes will be provided in Chapter 3; subsequent sections of this chapter will briefly introduce aging changes as they relate to the principles and practices of geriatric rehabilitation.

Box 1-1: Behaviors of a Healthy Lifestyle

- Not smoking
- Drinking alcohol in moderation
- Having a positive outlook
- Exercising regularly
- Getting adequate rest/sleep
- Drinking enough water
- Eating a balanced diet, high in fruits and vegetables
- Coping with stress
- Healthy relationships with others
- Being financially stable

DEMOGRAPHICS OF AGING

The size and character of the elderly population in the United States is rapidly changing. These major demographic shifts have prompted numerous concerns in US social and health policy. Aging "baby boomers" (the generation born between 1946 and 1964) are expected to have major effects on our health and social systems.

The number of senior citizens in the United States is rapidly increasing. During the 20th century, the US population under age 65 tripled, but those 65 and older increased by a factor of 11. By the year 2030, about 1 out of every 5 Americans, or 20% of the population, will be a senior citizen. This is a global phenomenon.[8] In many other developed countries, including Japan, Italy, Sweden, and the United Kingdom, the proportion of seniors to the rest of the population is even greater.

Half of the people ages 65 or older live in 9 states. Figure 1-1 shows the distribution of elders throughout the United States.[9] Currently, the senior US population is mostly White, but the fraction from other races is growing rapidly. Within the next 50 years, the number of elderly Black Americans is expected to triple. The elderly Hispanic American population is growing at an even faster rate and may exceed that of the elderly Black American population within 30 years.

MAXIMAL ACHIEVABLE LIFESPAN

Length of life is an important demographic. The maximum lifespan is the theoretical, longest length of life, excluding premature "unnatural" death. It is a measure of the maximum amount of time one or more members of a group has been observed to survive between birth and death. Life expectancy is defined as the average number of additional years of life that is expected for a member of a population, as determined by mortality rates in a specific geographic region. It can be a useful predictor of actual lifespan for a given individual. People almost always die of disease or accident before they reach their biologic limit.[10]

On average, women live longer than men, and White Americans live longer than Black Americans. Based on recent statistics, women who live until age 65 can, on average, expect to live to age 84; those who live to age 85 can expect to live to age 92. Men who live to age 65 can expect to live to age 79, and those who live to age 80 are very likely to live to at least age 90. The number of individuals living to age 100 in the United States is difficult to estimate, but their numbers are certainly growing. For people

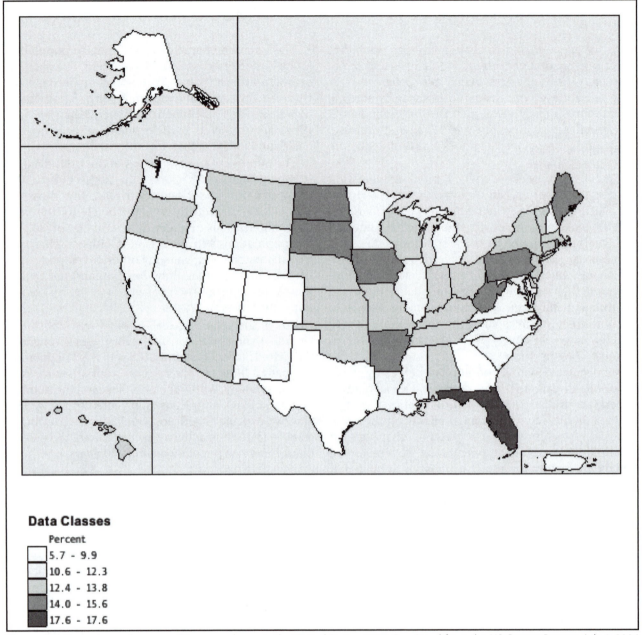

Data Classes

Percent

☐	5.7 - 9.9
☐	10.6 - 12.3
☐	12.4 - 13.8
■	14.0 - 15.6
■	17.6 - 17.6

Figure 1-1. Percentage of persons 65 years and over in the United States, 2000. Reprinted from the US Census Bureau. July 1, 2006 Population Estimates from the 2000 Census Summary.[9]

born in 1899, the odds of living to 100 were 400 to 1. However, for people born in 1980, the odds improved substantially to an overwhelming 87 to 1.[10]

Many studies assess the aging process by measuring clinical and functional variables.[11] However, recent research supports the fact that, beyond genetics, attitude and quality of life play a very important role in successful aging. Such components as perceptions of health, well being, valued abilities, activities, relationships, social support, control, sense of coherence, and personal outlook comprise variables in a model of healthy aging.[12] Older people age better when certain psychosocial elements are

in place. In other words, older people define health as being active and engaged, and includes 4 factors: having something worthwhile to do, having a balance between abilities and challenges, having appropriate external resources, and having personal attitudinal characteristics (eg, a positive attitude vs a pessimistic one).[13] What this implies for rehabilitation professionals is that—by reframing healthy aging in older people's terms—an interdisciplinary support of desired goals and outcomes is necessary, rather than success into older age being reliant on a purely medical approach to expected deficits, functional limitations, and challenges.

Causes of Death

Nearly 75% of deaths in the United States are those of elderly people.[14] For many decades, heart disease, cancer, and stroke have been the leading causes of death among the elderly, accounting for 70% of all deaths in this age group. The next most common causes of death are chronic lung disease, pneumonia, influenza, diabetes, accidental injuries, Alzheimer's disease, kidney disease, blood infections, and suicide.

Trends in Health and Functioning

Disease and disability is much more common in the elderly population than in people younger than 65. Some illnesses and diseases, such as hip fractures or Parkinson's disease, are prominent in the later stages of life. Other diseases, such as cardiovascular disease, malignant cancer, malnutrition, thyroid gland problems, and tuberculosis, can be seen at any age, but are more common among the elderly.

In the United States, 79% of people ages 70 and older have 1 or more of 7 chronic conditions.[15] The most common pathologies among older adults include:

- Arthritis
- High blood pressure
- Heart disease
- Diabetes
- Lung disease
- Stroke
- Cancer.

MEDICALLY COMPLEX ELDERS

The likelihood of having more than 1 disease increases with age. Among people ages 65 and older, 30% have 3 or more chronic diseases. Having more than 1 disease complicates care in several ways. Sudden change or illness in one body system may stress another body system, making the interpretation of symptoms more complex. For example, it is more difficult to evaluate mental confusion in someone who also has a fever caused by pneumonia.

Sometimes, the symptoms of one disease may hide those of another. Someone who has arthritis may never be physically active enough to show symptoms of heart disease, making the heart disease difficult to recognize. This is why it is crucial that the PT must perform a comprehensive examination and evaluation to establish a physical therapy diagnosis.

DEFINING DISABILITY

The meaning of disability is central to an understanding of rehabilitation. When referring to alterations in people's function, 3 terms are often used interchangeably: *impairment*, *disability*, and *handicap*. A more distinct understanding of these concepts is useful in geriatric rehabilitation, and a *systems approach* is most useful. In the systems approach, a problem at the organ level (eg, an infarct in the right cerebral hemisphere) must be viewed not only in terms of its effects on the brain, but also its effects on the person, the family, the society, and, ultimately, the nation.

In the elderly, rehabilitation interventions are most often oriented toward adaptation to or recovery from disabilities. Impairments such as a limp when walking, or pain in a joint following an activity, are treated to prevent disability and eliminate the impairment's restriction on function. Given the proper training or adaptive equipment, older people with disabilities can pursue independent lives. Obstructions in the pursuit of independence can arise, however, when people with disabilities confront inaccessible buildings or situations that limit safety and independence, such as low toilet seats, buttons on an elevator that are too high, or signs that are not readable. In these cases, a disability becomes a handicap—created by society's environment.

DEFINING FRAILTY

Although it is difficult to concisely define the term *frailty*, the concept of frailty is well understood in geriatric rehabilitation, and the use of the word conjures up a clear mental image for most clinicians; a picture of brittleness, fragility, infirmity, and weakness. Frailty makes one think of susceptibility to physical and medical insults, and brings to mind the need for assistance. Compromises in cognition, sensorimotor input and integration,[16] the use of many medications, dehydration, and malnutrition are components of frailty. The decline in muscle strength and mass,[17] respiratory reserve and cardiovascular functioning, kyphotic postural changes, poorer eyesight, poor hydration and marginal nutritional intake, as well as many other physiological and physical changes associated with inactivity and aging, lead to frailty. Any of these conditions, in isolation or in combination, can create frailty. The presence of multi-diagnostic situations in the elderly leads to multiple drug and nutrient interactions and complex medical management with the resulting side effects of progressive loss in functional reserve and physiological homeostasis. Concomitant diseases such as congestive heart failure, renal disease, osteoporosis, diabetes, chronic lung disease, and arthritis (to name a few), all add to the level of frailty.

FUNCTIONAL ASSESSMENT OF THE AGED

The word *function*, as used in the health field, refers to the ability to manage a daily routine. Physical ability is closely associated with the ability to live independently. Function reflects the skills necessary to perform basic ADL and is helpful in making decisions related to what type of assistance may be needed. An evaluation of functional abilities is useful in defining disability and need for assistance.[18]

Functional capacity is defined by 3 levels of ADL: (1) basic ADL, including self-care activities such as bathing, dressing, using the toilet, continence, and feeding; (2) instrumental ADL (IADL), such as using the telephone, driving, shopping, housekeeping, cooking, laundry, managing money, and managing medications; and (3) mobility, described as a more complicated combination of ADL and IADL, such as leaving one's residence and moving from one location to another via public transportation. Mobility and IADL are more complex and are concerned with a person's ability to cope with his or her environment.[19,20] This classification of ADL, IADL, and mobility has become standard in most functional assessment tools.

The assessment of functional capabilities is a primary tool used in geriatric rehabilitation.[21] The ability to walk, to transfer (eg, move from bed to chair or chair to toilet), and manage basic ADL independently is often the determinant of whether hospitalized aged patients will be discharged to their home or to an extended care facility. Functional assessment tools are necessary to assist all interdisciplinary team members in determining the need for rehabilitation or long-term care services.[22] In the home care setting, precise assessment of a patient's function can detect early deterioration and allow for immediate intervention.

Each domain of function, such as dressing, eating, bathing, walking, transfers, and mobility, includes a set of activities that can be ordered along a continuum from simple to complex activities (eg, the simple task of picking up the telephone receiver vs the more complex task of picking up the telephone receiver and dialing a number). ADL that cover more than one domain of self-maintenance are utilized within a broader set of functions. For instance, mobility and ambulation (or locomotion) are basic self-maintenance functions that enable an aged individual to adjust and adapt within his or her environment. The ability to ambulate one block, and ascend and descend stairs, would enable the aged person to walk to the bus stop and board a bus.

FUNCTIONAL ABILITIES OF THE CAREGIVER

Elderly people who need assistance with routine ADL rely first and foremost on family. Most people who help community-dwelling elderly are unpaid or informal caregivers. Spouses and adult children make up the bulk of unpaid caregivers, and the use of paid helpers is consistently higher among older adults living alone. The need for assistance from others increases linearly with age.[23]

Aged individuals, given a choice, would prefer to stay at home rather than recuperate and rehabilitate in an institutional setting. Home care by professionals can protect the health of informal caregivers and maximize the patient's ability to perform ADL by including an assessment of the caregiver and the living environment as a part of care planning.

Many caregivers (often aged themselves) have some decrease in physical ability, and this needs to be considered as it relates to caring for disabled relatives. It has been demonstrated that more than 90% of persons ages 75 to 84 can manage to perform such tasks as grooming, bathing, dressing, and eating on their own.[24] However, the more complicated skills of transferring and ambulation are compromised, with over 50% of persons ages 75 to 84 displaying limitations in their capabilities of performing these activities without assistance. These ADL require greater assistive skills on the part of the caregiver.

Assessment of the home environment needs to incorporate the abilities (or disabilities) of the individuals providing care. Adaptive equipment, such as a sliding board for transfers or a rolling walker for ambulation, is available to assist the caregiver. Attention to the abilities of the caregiver can facilitate the ease of care and decrease the burden placed on the caregiver.

PRINCIPLES OF GERIATRIC REHABILITATION

Three major principles are important in the rehabilitation of the aged. First, the *variability* of the aged must be considered. Variability of capabilities within an aged population is much more pronounced than that of younger cohorts. What one 80 year old can do physically, cognitively, or motivationally, another may not be able to accomplish. Second, the concept of *inactivity,* or sedentary lifestyle, is central to rehabilitation of the aged; many changes in lifestyle and physical ability over time are attributable to disuse. Finally, *optimum health* and overall well being is directly related to optimum functional ability.[25]

In acute situations, rehabilitation must be directed toward (1) stabilizing the primary problems; (2) preventing secondary complications such as bedsores, pneumonias, and contractures; and (3) restoring lost functions. In chronic situations, rehabilitation is directed primarily toward restoring lost functions. This can best be accomplished by promoting maximum health so that the aged are able to adapt to their care environment and their disabilities. Each of these principles—variability, inactivity, and optimum health—will be discussed in greater detail in the following sections.

Chronological Age and the Variability of the Older Adult

Unlike any other age group, the aged are more variable in their level of functional capabilities. This can been seen in, for example, a 65-year-old individual who is severely physically disabled, sitting right alongside another 65-year-old individual who is still capable of home repairs and hiking with grandchildren. Even in the old-old, variability in physical and cognitive functioning is remarkable. Chronological age is a poor indicator of physical or cognitive function.

The impact of this variability is an important consideration in defining rehabilitation principles and practices of the aged. A wide range of rehabilitative services needs to be provided to address the diverse needs of the aged population in different care settings. Awareness of this heterogeneity helps to combat the myths and stereotypes of aging and presents a foundation for developing creative rehabilitation programs. Older persons tend to be more different from themselves (as a collective group) than other segments of the population.

Reaction time is good example of variability in the aged. In general, reaction time tends to slow with age,[26] but this does not necessarily mean a decline in functioning of the nervous system. Research indicates that those aged who are more physically active are capable of performing as well as, and in some cases better than, younger subjects on reaction time performance tasks, while those who are sedentary tend to have poor reaction time.[27]

Vision is another example of variability in any older age group. Reaction time and the ability to function safely in a given environment can be related to how well one sees. A decline in visual acuity may result in a decrease in function. Research indicates that visual capabilities do not normally decline as part of aging. Instead, like so many other systems, the eyes are affected by nutritional deficits and environmental hazards (eg, intense sunlight, poor lighting, and airborne contaminants).[28,29]

Strength is another variable that directly affects an aged individual's ability to function at his or her maximum capability. One study compared strength measures in a group of 70+ year olds to a group of 40 to 50 year olds (both male and female subjects), and showed a greater range in strength values in the 70+ group.[30] Part of the variability is a result of the difficulty in separating age-dependent muscle changes from other factors that influence muscle strength, such as physical activity, disease, cardiovascular condition, and hormonal and neural influences. The younger group in this study had fewer confounding factors. This variability in strength leads to different levels of functioning within an aged population.

Mental ability is another example of an area that varies greatly within an aged population and directly affects the rehabilitation potential of an older individual. Cognitive problems can severely influence an individual's ability to safely function within his or her environment. In the absence of pathology, however, an elderly individual's cognitive abilities have been shown to undergo little or no change.[31]

The principle of variability in geriatric rehabilitation is important in providing therapeutic interventions that address the range of physical, physiological, and mental capabilities in aged individuals. Although changes are bound to occur in many physical and cognitive variables in the rehabilitative setting, it is possible that healthy aged individuals who maintain an active life, with good hydration and nutrition, and adequate rest and sleep, will show little or no loss of abilities even into their 80s and beyond.[32]

ACTIVITY VS SEDENTARY LIFESTYLE AND BED REST

Inactivity is the most common reason for losses in functional capabilities. *Acute immobilization* often accompanies acute illnesses, such as a hip fracture, pneumonia, or stroke. Activity level is severely curtailed until acute illnesses become medically stable. *Chronic immobilization* may result from chronic problems such as cerebrovascular accidents (strokes), amputations, arthritis, Parkinson's disease, cardiac disease, pulmonary disease, or low back pain. *Accidental immobilization* may occur due to environmental barriers in both the acute and chronic care settings; these include bed rails, the height of the bed, physical restraints, an inappropriate chair, no physical assistance available, fall precautions imposed by medical staff, no orders in the chart for mobilization, social isolation, and environmental obstacles such as stairs or doorway thresholds.

Cognitive impairments, central nervous system (CNS) disorders (such as cerebrovascular accidents, Parkinson's disease, and multiple sclerosis), peripheral neuropathies resulting from diabetes, and pain with movement can also severely reduce mobility. Affective disorders such as depression, anxiety, or fear of falling may also lead to accidental immobilization.

Deconditioning involves changes in multiple organ systems, including the neurological, cardiovascular, and musculoskeletal systems to varying degrees. The degree of deconditioning depends on the degree of superimposed inactivity and the prior level of the person's physical fitness. The phrase "use it or lose it" has tremendous ramifications for aging individuals, especially in geriatric rehabilitation. Exercise is beneficial for both the primary and secondary prevention of disease.[33]

The challenge of understanding the relationship between physiologic decline and functional loss is important in geriatric rehabilitation.[34] The inability to climb stairs in an 85 year old may be because of cardiovascular deconditioning, muscle weakness, impaired balance secondary to sensory losses, or a sedentary lifestyle. Changes in functional ability could reflect a new illness evolving. An understanding of the consequences of inactivity is particularly important in addressing rehabilitation needs of the aged individual. Table 1-1 summarizes the complications of bed rest.

The consequences of inactivity on all systems may be particularly extreme and occur more rapidly in the older adult.[35] Inactivity has been shown to decrease muscle and tendon flexibility and full immobilization in bed has been shown to result in a loss of approximately 3% per day of strength.[36] Increased time spent sitting significantly affects the body's flexor muscles, as adhesions are more likely to develop if the flexors of the body are maintained in a shortened position for extended periods of time.

A mnemonic representation of the effects of bed rest is helpful for remembering the overall effects of inactivity on functional capabilities:

B—*bladder and bowel incontinence and retention; bedsores*

E—*emotional trauma; electrolyte imbalances*

D—*deconditioning of muscles and nerves; depression; demineralization of bones; decubiti*

R—*range of motion loss and contractures; restlessness; renal dysfunction*

E—*energy depletion; EEG activity decreases*

S—*sensory deprivation; sleep disorders; skin problems*

T—*trouble in all systems*

The elderly are especially susceptible to the complications of bed rest. Aging-related changes and common chronic diseases result in a decrease in physiologic reserve and a decreased ability to tolerate the changes with bed rest. Some common problems that often are associated with aging can also occur because of prolonged bed rest; some complications include osteoporosis, decreased endurance, impaired mobility, and an increase in predisposition to falls, deep venous thrombosis, sensory deprivation, and pressure sores.[37]

With the numerous adverse effects of bed rest, clearly it should be prescribed judiciously and with full awareness of its potential complications and need for preventive exercise. Any elderly patient on bed rest should be on a physical therapy program. When full activity is not possible, limited activity such as movement in bed, ADL, intermittent sitting, and standing will reduce the frequency of some complications of bed rest. Prolonged bed rest causes significant cardiovascular, respiratory, musculoskeletal, and neuropsychological changes. Complications of bed rest are often irreversible. Complete bed rest should be avoided at all costs.

The Concept of Well-Being: Optimal Health

The last principle in geriatric rehabilitation is that of *optimal health*. The World Health Organization (WHO) defines health as a state of complete physical, mental, and social well-being, not merely the absence of disease or infirmity.[38] The existence of complete physical health refers to the absence of pathology, impairment, or disability. Physical health is quite achievable. Mental and social well-being are closely related. Mental health as defined by WHO would include cognitive and intellectual intactness as well as emotional well-being. The social components of health would include living situation, social roles (ie, mother, daughter, vocation, etc), and economic status.

It is reasonable to assume that the health status of an individual in his or her 70s, and subsequent decades

Table 1-1

SYSTEMIC COMPLICATIONS WITH BED REST

Neurosensory
- Sensory deprivation
- ↓ EEG activity
- ↓ Thermoregulation
- ↓ Cognition
- ↓ In reaction time
- ↓ Balance
- ↑ Postural sway

Musculoskeletal
- Muscle atrophy
- Bone loss (osteoporosis)
- Joint contractures
- Osteoarthritis
- ↓ Glycoproteins
- ↓ Hyaluronic acid
- ↓ Muscle oxidative capacity
- ↓ Aerobic capacity
- ↓ Muscle strength

Cardiovascular
- Delayed post-activity recovery time
- Orthostatic hypotension
- ↓ Total blood volume
- ↓ Aerobic capacity
- ↑ Heart rate and blood pressure with activity
- ↓ Cardiac output
- ↑ Resting heart rate
- ↓ Oxygen uptake

Gastrointestinal
- Constipation

Genitourinary
- Renal calculi
- Urinary incontinence
- Urinary tract infection

Skin
- Pressure sores

Respiratory
- Atelectasis
- Impaired gas exchange
- Relative hypoxemia
- ↑ Alveolar-arterial oxygen gradient
- ↑ Risk of pneumonia
- ↓ Peripheral perfusion
- ↓ Chest wall compliance
- ↓ Intercostal muscle strength
- ↓ Vital capacity
- ↓ Resting arterial oxygen tension

Functional
- Impaired ambulation
- ↓ Activities of daily living
- ↑ Risk of falls

Psychological
- Sensory deprivation
- Anxiety, fear, depression
- Hallucinations
- Perceptual disturbances
- Sleep disturbances
- Mood changes

of life, are in a suboptimal range. When considering less than optimal health, the goal of geriatric rehabilitation should be to strive for *relative optimal health* (ie, the maximal functional and physical capabilities of the aged individual considering his or her current health status).

An example of an aged woman with a hip fracture may help to demonstrate this principle. The woman, who is in suboptimal health and suffering from osteoporosis, should be screened for balance abilities and the risk of falls. In today's health care system, where screening is not a reimbursable intervention, this woman is not treated until she falls and fractures her hip. She may face resulting complications such as pneumonia, decubiti (ulcers caused from pressure) from bed rest, all of the changes noted in

Table 1-1 related to inactivity, and the possibility of death. Recognizing that osteoporosis is a risk for future fractures, preventive intervention could have reduced the chances or circumstances that caused the fall; such measures could have included weight-bearing exercises to enhance the strength of the bone, strengthening exercises of the lower extremities to provide adequate stability and endurance, balance and postural exercises to facilitate effective balance reactions and safety, education in nutrition, and modification of her living environment to ensure added safety in hopes of avoiding the kind of fall that results in a hip fracture. Intervention at the suboptimal level was needed here rather than waiting for an illness or disability to occur. This is preventative care.

The principle of obtaining relative optimal health in geriatric rehabilitation is not only cost effective, but clearly would lead to an overall improvement in the quality of life.[39] Encouraging healthy behaviors, such as decreasing obesity, stress, smoking, and increasing activity, could be the elements necessary in maintaining health and striving for optimal health as defined by WHO.[40]

Health care professionals involved in geriatric rehabilitation need to utilize exceptional observational skills to provide appropriate *assessment*, *examination, evaluation,* and *screening.* Good assessment skills could detect a minor problem that has the potential of developing into a major problem. Careful monitoring of physical, cognitive, and social needs on a regular basis could help to modify rehabilitation programs accordingly and to truly improve the health, functional ability, and well-being of aged clients.

REHABILITATION: TREATMENT APPROACHES FOCUSING ON FUNCTION

Rehabilitation should be directed at preventing premature disability. A deconditioned aged individual is less capable of performing activities than a conditioned aged individual. For example, the speed of walking is positively correlated to the level of physical fitness in an aged person.[41] When cardiovascular capabilities are diminished (ie, maximum aerobic capacity), walking speeds are adjusted by the aged person to levels of comfort. Exercise programs geared for improving cardiovascular fitness improve the speed of walking.[41] The faster the walking pace, the smoother the momentum, thus decreasing the likelihood of falling. The better conditioned elder is

more agile and has better reaction times when balance is perturbed. As a result, he or she is less likely to injure him- or herself when compared to an unfit older individual.

Pain may also lead to deconditioning. For instance, the pain experienced by an aged individual with an acute exacerbation of an osteoarthritic knee, accompanied by inflammation of the knee capsule, may reflexively inhibit quadricep contraction. While quadricep strength may have been poor in the first place due to inactivity, the absence of pain still permitted him or her to rise from a chair or ascend shallow steps. Now, with the presence of acute pain, these activities cause severe discomfort and threaten the ability of maintaining an independent lifestyle. In this situation, rehabilitation efforts should focus medically on:

- Reducing the inflammation through drugs or ice (physician, nurse)
- Maintaining joint mobility during the acute phases (with both physical and occupational therapy)
- Providing joint protection (with both physical and occupational therapy)
- Creating provisions for maintaining proper nutrition in light of medications/nutrients (pharmacist, dietician)
- Having social and psychological support (eg, social worker, psychologist, religious personnel) to provide emotional and motivational support.

Rehabilitation of the aged individual should emphasize functional activity to *maintain functional mobility* and capability, improvement of balance through exercise and functional activity programs (ie, weight-shifting exercises, ambulation with direction and elevation changes, and reaching activities, to name a few), good nutrition and good general care (including hygiene, hydration, bowel and bladder considerations, appropriate rest and sleep), as well as social and emotional support. The more an individual does, the more he or she is capable of doing independently. The more that is done for an aged individual, the less capable he or she becomes of functioning at an optimal independent level, therefore increasing the likely progression of a disability.[42]

Perceived Health Status

Advancing stages of disability increase the individual's vulnerability to illness, emotional stress, and injury. A person's subjective appraisal of his or her health status influences how he or she will react to symptoms, such as shortness of breath or pain. Often an aged person's self-appraisal of his or her health is a good predictor to the rehabilitation clinician's evaluation of health and functional status. It is important to keep in mind that an aged individual's perception of his or her health status is an important motivator in compliance with a rehabilitation program. The use of standardized tools for self-assessment will be discussed in Chapter 9.

One interesting study showed that even when age, sex, and health status (as evaluated by physicians) were controlled for, perceived health and mortality from heart disease were strongly related.[43] Those who rated their health as poor were 2 to 3 times as likely to die as those who rated their health as excellent.

The aged are known to fail to report serious symptoms and wait longer than younger persons to seek help. Rehabilitation professionals need to listen carefully to their aged clients with this in mind. It appears that, contrary to the popular view that older individuals are somewhat hypochondriacal, the aged generally deserve serious attention when they bring complaints to their caregivers. Rosillo and Fagel[44] found that improvement in rehabilitation tasks correlated well with the patient's own appraisal of his or her potential for recovery but not very well with others' appraisal. Stoedefalke[45] reported that positive reinforcement (frequent positive feedback) for older persons in rehabilitation greatly improved their performance and feelings of success. This indicates that aged persons can improve in their physical functioning when modifications in therapeutic interventions provide feedback more often, and allow for success and a level of functioning comparable with the patients' abilities.

Some research indicates that older persons with chronic illness have low initial aspirations with regard to their ability to perform various tasks. As situations in which they succeeded or failed occurred, their aspirations changed to more closely reflect their abilities.[46] Aged individuals may have a higher anxiety level in rehabilitation situations because they fear failure or are afraid of looking bad to their family or therapist. These are important motivational components to keep in mind when working with an aged client. The therapeutic approach of the clinician may have the greatest impact on the successful functional outcomes in a geriatric rehabilitation setting.

Exercise in the Elderly

Exercise programs have potential for improving physical fitness, agility, and speed of response. They also serve to improve muscle strength, flexibility, bone health, cardiovascular and respiratory response, and tolerance to activity.[47] Evidence suggests that reaction time is better in elders who engage in physical exercise than in those who are sedentary. There is a positive correlation between an individual's ability to maintain balance when stressed and his or her level of fitness.[48] Initial test scores on reaction time were significantly improved following a 6-week stretching and calisthenics program in individuals 65 years of age and older. This has great clinical significance when considering the increasing incidence of falls with age.

In addition, exercise has been shown to provide social and psychological benefits affecting the quality of life and the sense of well-being in the elderly. Exercise provides a higher level of independence and a resulting improvement in an elder's perceived quality of life. The risks of encouraging physical activity are small and can be minimized through careful evaluation. Table 1-2 summarizes therapies for various conditions seen most frequently in geriatric rehabilitation settings.

Exercise Prescription Principles

One therapeutic principle that can be used successfully in motivating elderly individuals is to not give them instructions that include specific times or numbers of repetitions. For instance, "do this exercise for as long as you feel comfortable and then stop and rest" or, "lift this weight as many times as you feel comfortable lifting it and then stop and rest." This omits the potential for failing by not connecting to a prescribed time or number of repetitions. Once a specific number or target is not looming in front of the older exerciser as a measure of success, fatigue does not set in as readily. They no longer have markers (ie, "I'm halfway there") by which to measure, so the task becomes less ominous and never results in failure.

Another principle that works well with the older adult exerciser is the communication rule of exercise. Rather than having the individual focus on vital sign monitoring (which the clinician can do during assessment and evaluation), the level of exercise is based on the ease of speaking. Mild exercise that is not aerobic results in the individual's ability to carry on a fluid conversation without shortness of breath. Moderate exercise, or exercise in the submaximal aerobic range, results in more shortened, faltering (staccato) sentences with frequent pauses for breath. In other words, the individual can speak but would rather not. The maximal exercise range results in the inability to speak (eg, imagine mountain climbers in low oxygen environments). In the maximal range, all air inhaled is needed for the provision of oxygen to the working muscles.

What should be the prescribed level of exercise in an older adult? This will be based on the elder's overall physical, physiological, emotional, and cognitive condition. However, a good rule of thumb in activity and exercise in the elderly is *anything above rest works*.

Table 1-2

REHABILITATION THERAPIES FOR COMMON CONDITIONS

CEREBROVASCULAR ACCIDENT (STROKE)

PHYSICAL THERAPY

- Pre-gait activities (if individual is not ambulatory)
- Positioning and posturing (chair, feeding needs)
- Gait/balance training (if individual is ambulatory)
- Provision of assistive ambulatory devices (quad cane, hemi-walker)
- Ambulation on different types of surfaces (stairs, ramps)
- Provision of appropriate shoe gear and orthotics
- Sensory integration
- Education and provision of appropriate bracing
- Joint mobilization techniques (when appropriate)
- Proprioceptive neuromuscular facilitation
- Bobath techniques to modify tone
- Functional electrical stimulation (when appropriate)
- Family and patient education for home management including environmental modifications
- Range of motion, strengthening, coordination exercises
- Alternative interventions—Qigong, T'ai Chi, Yoga, Feldenkrais

OCCUPATIONAL THERAPY

- Training in activities of daily living (grooming, dressing, cooking, etc)
- Transfer training (toilet, bathtub, car, etc)
- Activities and exercise to enhance function of upper extremities
- Training to compensate for visual-perceptual problems
- Provision of adaptive devices (reachers, special eating utensils)

SPEECH THERAPY

- Reading, writing, and math retraining
- Oral muscular strengthening
- Therapy for swallowing disorders
- Functional skills practice (checkbook balancing, making change)
- Language production work

PARKINSON'S DISEASE

PHYSICAL THERAPY

- Gait training
- Provision for appropriate shoe gear and orthotics
- Training in position changes
- General conditioning, strengthening, coordination, and range-of-motion exercises
- Breathing exercises
- Alternative interventions—Qigong, T'ai Chi, Feldenkrais, aquatic therapy
- Proprioceptive neuromuscular facilitation/sensory integration
- Training in functional instrumental activities of daily living

OCCUPATIONAL THERAPY

- Fine/gross motor coordination of upper extremities
- Provision of adaptive equipment
- Basic self-care activity training
- Transfer training

SPEECH THERAPY

- Improving respiratory control
- Improving control of rate of speech
- Improving coordination between speech and respiration
- Use of voice amplifiers and/or alternate communication devices

(Continued)

Table 1-2 continued

REHABILITATION THERAPIES FOR COMMON CONDITIONS

ARTHRITIS

PHYSICAL THERAPY

- Joint protection techniques
- Joint mobilization for pain control and mobility
- Conditioning, strengthening, and range-of-motion exercises
- Gait training
- Alternative interventions—Qigong, T'ai Chi, Yoga, Feldenkrais, aquatics
- Modalities to decrease pain and edema, and break up adhesions
- Provision of assistive ambulatory devices (when appropriate)
- Provision of proper shoe gear and orthotics
- Refer for nutritional counseling

OCCUPATIONAL THERAPY

- Provision of adaptive devices to promote independence and avoid undue stress on involved joints
- Splinting to protect involved joints, decrease inflammation, and prevent deformity
- Joint protection techniques
- Range-of-motion and strengthening exercise of upper extremities

AMPUTEES

PHYSICAL THERAPY

- Balance activities
- Teaching donning and doffing of prostheses
- Progressive ambulation
- Training in residual limb care
- Wound care (when appropriate)
- Provision of shoe gear and protective orthotics for uninvolved extremity
- Instruction in range-of-motion strengthening and endurance activities for both involved and uninvolved extremities
- Fitting and provision of temporary and permanent prosthetic devices
- Transfer training
- Patient education in skin care and monitoring
- Alternative interventions—Qigong, Yoga, Feldenkrais
- Refer for nutritional counseling

OCCUPATIONAL THERAPY

- Teaching donning and doffing of prostheses
- Training in stump care
- Transfer training
- Training in activities of daily living

(Continued)

Table 1-2 continued

REHABILITATION THERAPIES FOR COMMON CONDITIONS

CARDIAC DISEASE

PHYSICAL THERAPY

- Patient education
- Conditioning and endurance exercises (walking, biking, etc)
- Breathing and relaxation exercises
- Strengthening and flexibility exercises
- Monitoring of patients' vital signs during exercise
- Stress management techniques
- Alternative interventions—Qigong, T'ai Chi, Yoga
- Refer for nutritional counseling

OCCUPATIONAL THERAPY

- Labor-saving techniques
- Improving overall endurance for participation in activities of daily living
- Monitoring patients' participation in activities of daily living

PULMONARY DISEASE

PHYSICAL THERAPY

- Patient education
- Breathing control exercises
- Alternative interventions that incorporate controlled breathing patterns—Qigong, T'ai Chi, Yoga, Feldenkrais
- Conditioning exercises
- Joint mobilization of rib cage
- Relaxation and stress management techniques
- Chest physical therapy

OCCUPATIONAL THERAPY

- Training in labor-saving techniques
- Improving endurance of upper extremities
- Monitoring of participation in activities of daily living

HIP FRACTURES

PHYSICAL THERAPY

- Positioning and transfer training
- Range-of-motion, strengthening, and conditioning exercises
- Provision of proper shoe gear, lift on the involved side, and orthotics for shock absorption
- Provision of assistive ambulation devices
- Balance activities
- Referral to nutritionist in presence of osteoporosis
- Patient and caregiver instruction and education
- Progressive weight bearing and gait training

OCCUPATIONAL THERAPY

- Sensory integration techniques
- Activities of daily living (grooming, feeding, dressing, etc)
- Standing balance and endurance for functional activities
- Patient and caregiver education

(Continued)

Table 1-2 continued

REHABILITATION THERAPIES FOR COMMON CONDITIONS

LOWER BACK PAIN

PHYSICAL THERAPY

- Joint mobilization/stabilization
- Modalities to decrease pain and improve tissue mobility
- Instruction in proper body mechanics for lifting, sitting, and sleeping
- Strengthening and flexibility exercises
- Provision of proper shoe gear and shock absorbing orthotics
- Correction of leg length discrepancy (when appropriate)
- Postural training for positioning
- Relaxation and stress management techniques
- Alternative interventions—Qigong, T'ai Chi, Yoga, Feldenkrais
- Aquatic therapy for strengthening and conditioning
- Environmental modifications

OCCUPATIONAL THERAPY

- Training in ergonomic techniques
- Training in energy conservation and positioning at rest

ALZHEIMER'S DISEASE

PHYSICAL THERAPY

- Sensory integration techniques
- Gait training (when appropriate)
- Balance activities
- General conditioning exercises
- Provision of proper shoe gear and orthotics
- Family/caregiver instructions for environmental modifications for self-preservation
- Nutritional program addressing feeding/oral skills, swallowing, position
- Reality orientation activities and/or validation techniques
- Alternative interventions—Qigong, T'ai Chi, dancing, hammock

OCCUPATIONAL THERAPY

- Sensory integration techniques
- Activities of daily living (grooming, feeding, etc)
- Reality orientation activities and/or validation techniques
- Feeding program and provision of adaptive utensils
- Family/caregiver instructions for environmental modifications for self-preservation

SPEECH THERAPY

- Cognitive therapy
- Oral and feeding skills
- Reality orientation activities and validation techniques
- Language skills and object identification

Note: Specific treatment approaches, including alternative approaches, are covered in Chapter 10.

In providing activity and exercise programs for the aged, normal aging changes in the musculoskeletal, neuromuscular, cardiovascular, and pulmonary systems will affect functional capacity. In addition, confusion, decreased sensory awareness, postural changes, cardiovascular limitations resulting from deconditioning, motivation, and perceived level of fatigue all affect the potential for rehabilitation and need to be assessed prior to implementing activity or exercise programs.

The Neurosensory System in Exercise in the Elderly

Changes in the sensory system with age provide less information to the CNS, which results from a decrease in sensory perception during movement.[49] With loss of sensory input, in combination with any cognitive changes, the aged individual is less able to assess his or her environment accurately. This leads to incorrect choices.[50] Sensory losses and cognitive impairments, in addition to physical changes associated with aging, need to be given special consideration in geriatric rehabilitation (see Chapter 3).

The effects of the aging process on the neuromuscular system are seen clinically in deterioration of strength, speed, motor coordination, and gait. Muscle strength is defined by the rate of motor unit firing, the number and frequency of motor unit recruitment, and the cross-sectional diameter of the muscle.[51] Muscular atrophy may be attributed to a decrease in the number of muscle fibers (as described in Chapter 3). Despite the obvious relationship between neuromuscular changes and loss of strength, disuse appears to play a very important role. Changes in lifestyle as one ages apparently contribute to disuse of the muscles.

Bone Mass and Function in the Elderly

A decrease in total bone mass is a characteristic change with age. Osteoporosis is the result of progression of this loss past the threshold of what is considered normal. Although often asymptomatic, osteoporosis can be a major cause of pain, fractures, and postural changes in the musculoskeletal system.[52] Functional mobility is often curtailed as a result of the fragility of bone mass. The risk of pathological fractures may prohibit functional independence in the elderly. Functional rolling, rotation, flexion, and bending could lead to bony fracture and needs to be considered when prescribing activity and exercise in the older adult.

Balance, Flexibility, Strength, Posture, and Gait in Function

Balance, flexibility, and strength provide the posture necessary to ensure efficient ambulation. In aging, poor posture results from a decline in flexibility and strength and from bony changes in the vertebral spine, resulting in less safe gait patterns. *Gait* is the functional application of motion. Changes in the gait cycle seen in the aged include:

- Mild rigidity (greater proximally than distally), producing less body movement
- Fewer automatic movements with a decreased amplitude and speed (such as arm swing)
- Less accuracy of foot placement
- Shorter steps due to changes in kinesthetic sense and slower rate of motor unit firing
- Wider stride width (broad based gait) in the attempt to enhance safety
- Decrease in swing-to-stance ratio, which improves safety by allowing more time in the double support phase (ie, both feet in contact with the ground at the same time)
- Decrease in vertical displacement, which is the up and down movement created by pushing off from the toes for forward propulsion and the alternate heel strike, usually secondary to stiffness (a distinct push-off and heel strike are not observed in the aged)
- Decrease in toe-to-floor clearance
- Decrease in excursion of the leg (arc of movement) during the swing phase
- Decrease in the heel-to-floor angle (usually due to the lack of flexibility of the plantar flexor muscles and weakness of dorsiflexors)
- Slower cadence (step rate per minute) as another safety mechanism
- Decrease in velocity of limb motions during gait—which costs more in energy demands and fatigue.

The Cardiovascular and Cardiopulmonary Systems in Function of the Elderly

Exercise is a physical stimulus, which produces an increase above the resting levels of vital signs. In a healthy, young individual, the cardiovascular system responds quickly to increase the metabolic rate by increasing heart rate, stroke volume (the amount of blood delivered to the system with each heartbeat), and peripheral blood flow to deliver oxygen and nutrients to the working muscles. In the aged, response time of the cardiovascular system is delayed in restoring homeostasis (balance) when the level of physical activity has been increased. The aged have a lower resting cardiac output and basal metabolic rate primarily due to age-related loss of lean body mass and inactivity. Heart rate and stroke volume decrease and as exercise levels increase, this manifests as reduced oxygen uptake.

In respiration there is a 50% decrease in the maximum volume of ventilation and 40% decrease in the vital capacity by the age of 85. These limitations in oxygen transport capability translate directly into a reduced physical work capacity.[53] An elderly patient may feel that he or she is working at an extreme level during relatively simple tasks. For example, when transferring from sitting to standing, an elder may become short of breath and feel fatigued. The PTA needs to pay close attention to the elderly patient's response to movement, allow frequent rest periods, and progress only as tolerated.

Understanding and managing a patient's perception of fatigue is essential in any geriatric rehabilitation program. Fatigue can occur in several forms and include muscle fatigue from prolonged use of a muscle group, circulatory fatigue associated with elevated blood lactate levels during prolonged activity, and metabolic fatigue in which exercise depletes glycogen (energy) stores. General fatigue is related to more subtle factors like interest, reward, and motivation.

Activities of Daily Living

A general measure to ensure the highest functional capacity should encourage early resumption of basic daily activities following trauma or acute illness. ADL are wonderful exercises for gaining functional independence for an older individual. *Functional* exercise often makes more sense to the older individual than standard exercises do. For instance, standing up from the chair, which strengthens the knee and hip extensors, seems more practical to the older adult than strengthening the quad with resistance.

Pain Management

Pain management is a very important factor in geriatric rehabilitation.[54] Treatment of acute or chronic pain may include medications to reduce inflammation, ice, heat, compression (also to reduce edema when warranted), rest, and gentle mobility exercises (low-grade oscillation techniques of joint mobilization are very helpful in pain relief and maintenance of joint mobility).

Assistive Devices

Assistive devices, such as a cane, a quad cane, or a walker, can also be prescribed to improve stability during ambulation and reduce the stresses on painful joints.

Wheelchair prescription may be necessary for longer distances (eg, outside the home) or when ambulation is no longer possible (eg, in the case of a bilateral amputation or severe diabetic neuropathy). Wheelchairs should be prescribed to meet the specific needs of the aged individual. For instance, removable arms may be needed to enhance the ease of transfers, or elevating leg rests may be prescribed for lower extremity elevation when severe cardiac disease results in lower extremity edema. Likewise, if advanced rheumatoid arthritis or quadriplegia limits upper extremity capabilities, an electric wheelchair will greatly improve that individual's capabilities of locomotion. Other considerations may be a one-arm manual drive chair for a hemiplegic or a "weighted" chair to shift the center of gravity and improve the stability of the chair in transfers for the bilateral amputee. The use of golf carts or other motorized scooters for community-dwelling elders to enhance their ability to move around town or long corridors in senior housing environments is often recommended for conserving an individual's energy level. Although the older individual may ambulate independently within his or her home, the use of such a cart is a means of energy conservation when longer distances of locomotion are required.

Positioning and Seating

Proper positioning and seating for the aged individual who must sit for extended periods is required to decrease discomfort and keep pressure off of bony prominences, provide adequate postural support, facilitate feeding, and prevent progression of joint contractures and deformities. Many specialized chairs and adaptive positioning pads are on the market and address specific positioning needs. Armchairs that assist in rising from a seated position include higher chairs that decrease the work of the lower extremities for standing or electric "ejection" chairs that actually extend to bring the individual to a near standing position. Functional assessment of the aged person is vital in the prescription of these specialized devices.

Nutritional Considerations

Nutrition has a great impact on functional capabilities. A car needs gas in order to run; a human being needs adequate energy sources in order to function at an optimal level. Nutritional levels need close monitoring in relation to energy needs and functional activity levels. Increased feeding difficulties may be secondary to decreased appetite, poor oral status, visual or sensorimotor agnosia (loss of the ability to recognize sensory stimuli), cognitive declines (decreasing attentiveness), and physical limitations.

Specialized feeding programs may be necessary in geriatric rehabilitation. For example, if there is neuromuscular involvement such as those sustained in a cerebrovascular accident, the individual may have difficulty swallowing or closing the mouth. In these cases, specialized muscle facilitation techniques can be employed to promote swallowing and facilitate mouth closure. Physical therapy can comprehensively address the feeding needs of a neurologically involved individual in the geriatric rehabilitation setting. Ultimately, the goal is to permit independent feeding by the aged person. The PTA is often a part of a nutritional team in skilled nursing facilities, and despite the fact that nutrition may not be a part of a PTA's typical academic curriculum, information on nutritional programs will be a vital part of your clinical experiences (nutritional considerations will be dealt with in greater detail in Chapter 6).

Restraints

The use of physical restraints in an attempt to keep patients safe continues to be practiced despite evidence that restraints increase the incidence of falls.[55] Decreasing the use of physical restraints continues to be a challenge for the health care team. It is important to understand the law regarding restraints as well as the risks, benefits, and implications for their use. Regulations, types of restraints, documentation, and alternatives to the use of restraints are discussed.

The reasons given by long-term care team members for the use of physical restraints are numerous: to prevent injury to self and other patients, control of agitated or restless behavior, management of a patient's cognitive deficit and poor judgment, mobility impairments placing the patient at risk for falls, and resistance to medical treatment. Although these may seem to be noble support statements, there are a number of risks associated with physical restraints. A list of benefits and risks associated with the use of restraints is provided in Table 1-3.

In order for the long-term care team to reduce restraints, it is important to understand which devices are considered restraints and the implications of their use. The Centers for Medicare and Medicaid Services (CMS) interpretive guidelines define a physical restraint as "any manual method or physical or mechanical device, material or equipment attached to or adjacent to the resident's body, which the individual cannot remove easily, that restricts freedom of movement or normal access to one's body." Further, the guidelines state that physical restraints include using leg, arm, vest restraints, hand mitts, and soft ties; binding a patient who is bed-bound by tucking sheets in tightly; and using bed rails and chairs that prevent rising. "Devices on clothing that trigger electronic alarms to warn staff that a resident is leaving a room" are not necessarily considered restraints, according to the guidelines.[56]

Side rails are often utilized to deter attempts to get out of the bed and keep an individual from falling. A number of deleterious effects have been cited due to the use of side rails, such as increasing the distance one falls from the bed, obstructing the patient's vision, creating noise, creating trauma if the body strikes the side rails, creating a sense of being trapped, and dislodging/pulling tubes during raising and lowering. A thorough risk level assessment to determine necessity of side rail use should be done with each patient. Table 1-4 provides examples of a risk level assessment for the use of side rails as described by CMS.

Vest, waist, pelvic, and extremity tie-on devices are generally considered to be restraints. These types of restraints should rarely be used and only if other alternatives have failed. Furthermore, they should be used for only brief periods of time.

Reclining wheelchairs and Geri-chairs are considered restraints when they restrict a patient's normal mobility. Lap cushions or trays, wheelchair bars, and seat belts can be restraints if the patient is unable to remove these devices independently. Lap cushions and trays particularly are not restraints if they are used to provide support for patients who do not attempt to stand or lean forward. Wedge cushions that raise patients' feet off the floor, if they propel a wheelchair or limit the ability to stand, are considered a restraint. The use of any restraint requires a physician's order for use and state laws dictates the length of time between reassessment and updated orders. It is important that the PTA provide input—both by written documentation and verbal communication—to the PT regarding any changes in mobility, judgment, and safety awareness that might assist in reducing the level of restraint or possibly eliminating the need for restraints.

Table 1-3

BENEFITS AND RISKS OF PHYSICAL RESTRAINTS

BENEFITS

- Prevention and protection from falls and other accidents or injuries
- Protects other patients and staff from physical harm
- Maintenance of body alignment
- Increases patient's feeling of security and safety
- Allows medical treatment to proceed without patient interference

RISKS

- Injury from falls
- Disorganized behavior
- Accidental death by strangulation
- Skin abrasions and breakdown
- Decline in activities of daily life, functional mobility
- Cardiac stress
- Social and emotional isolation
- Dehydration, reduced appetite
- Increased mortality
- Immobilization sequelae (deconditioning, muscle atrophy, contractures, osteoporosis, orthostatic hypotension, deep vein thrombosis, pneumonia, incontinence)

SPECIAL GERIATRIC REHABILITATION CONSIDERATIONS

Balance Problems and Falls

Falls are not part of the normal aging process, but are due to an interaction of underlying physical dysfunction, medications, and environmental hazards. Poor health status, impaired mobility from inactivity or chronic illness, postural instability, and a history of previous falls are observable risk factors. The ultimate goals of rehabilitation are to combat the inactivity and loss of mobility that predisposes one to falls.[57]

Medical conditions are often a cause of falling and will be discussed in greater detail in Chapter 4. As examples, a pathological fracture due to severe osteoporosis may result in a fall (rather than the fracture resulting from the fall), or an arrhythmia may induce dizziness.

Certain drugs, such as digoxin used in treating an arrhythmia, may also induce dizziness or fatigue. (See Chapter 7 for tables listing drugs that cause adverse side effects that may result in falls in the elderly.)

Poor nutrition and hydration are also associated with falls and balance problems in older adults. Extreme hunger or thirst, for example, can result in fatigue, dizziness, muscle cramping, and poorer cognition and judgment. This topic is discussed in further detail in Chapter 6.

Fear of Falling

The fear of falling is often a cause for inactivity and is commonly seen in an individual who has sustained a previous fall. It must be noted here that older individuals may not have experienced a fall themselves, but may limit their activity because their neighbor fell and they are fearful of going through the same experience. The guarding patterns that aged individuals use as a result of this fear (ie, grabbing furniture that may not be stable or supportive) may lead to further danger.

Functional Limitations and Falls

Functionality, limitations of range of motion, decreased muscle strength and joint mobility, coordination problems, or gait deviations can predispose an aged individual to falling. Specific strengthening and gait training programs assist individuals in preventing falls by improving overall strength and coordination, balance responses and reaction time, and awareness of safe ambulation practices (eg, freeing one hand for use of a handrail when carrying packages up the stairs). Some individuals will have inadequate strength and balance to ambulate without an assistive device; for others, assistive ambulatory devices may provide a safer mode for locomotion. While walking aids, such as canes and walkers, are beneficial for prevention of falls in some cases, in others, they may actually contribute to the cause of the fall. The PTA serves an important

Table 1-4

RISK LEVEL ASSESSMENT FOR USE OF SIDE RAILS ON A BED

- **LEVEL I: LOW RISK**

Side rails are not necessary for patients in this group. They may be used because of the person's preference but are not considered restraints. Patients at this level are able to get into and out of bed safely without assistance, or do not move without staff assistance.

- **LEVEL II: MODERATE RISK**

These patients have the desire to get into and out of bed unassisted but lack the ability to do so safely. They need side rails or an alternative if side rails are not used. Side rails are then considered restraints and require a physician's order.

- **LEVEL III: HIGH RISK**

Side rails are used to restrict movement of these patients because there are no alternatives, alternatives have failed, or the benefit of using side rails outweighs the burden. Side rails are then considered restraints and require a physician's order.

Source: Centers for Medicare and Medicaid Web site http://www.cms.gov.

role in ensuring the appropriateness of an assistive device and that the aged individual is using it properly. With proper instruction and risk management, the aged person can usually function safely within his or her environment without falling.[58]

Gait assessment is an important component in fall prevention. Testing functional strength, balance, coordination, and safety during gait and turns provides information necessary for comprehensive rehabilitative intervention.[59]

Functional losses may predispose an older individual to an increased likelihood of falls. For instance, the inability to arise from a chair without the assistance of the hands is indicative of hip extensor, quadricep weakness, or both. If step symmetry is absent (ie, the individual is taking irregular steps), the cause of the fall can often be pinpointed just by observation. For example, there may be a leg length discrepancy or the hip abductors may be weak. Lower extremity pain may also result in nonrhythmical steps as the individual attempts to avoid the painful extremity. Tendencies to swerve and lose balance or hold on to surrounding objects may be indicative of dizziness, muscle weakness, or poor vision. A loss of balance while turning or a stiff disjointed turn may alert the clinician to the possibility of neurological disorders, such as Parkinson's disease, or drug-induced muscle rigidity (often seen in aged individuals on haloperidol or other psychotropic medications).[60]

With proper patient and family education and modification of the environment to reduce hazards, it is possible to prevent falls through methods that facilitate mobility and do not undermine autonomy.

PTs and PTAs have an important role in recommending interventions to prevent falls. When disease states, medications, and nutritional responses are stable, an individualized program of safety education, environmental adaptations, lower extremity strengthening exercises, balance exercises, and gait training can be implemented.

Education in Safety

Safety education is an important first step in the prevention of falls. Many older individuals are not aware that they are at risk for falling. Often, simple instructions about environmental adaptations and encouraging a person to allow plenty of time for functional activities are all that is needed to ensure safety. Many aged people feel the need to rush to answer a phone or doorbell. They should be discouraged from rushing because that could result in a fall. Caregivers and visitors should also be a part of the safety education process. They are often able to remind the person who is at risk for falling of the need for added precaution. Environmental evaluation and adaptation is needed for those aged individuals who have fallen or are at risk for falling. Table 1-5 presents a safety checklist for use in the home.[61]

A safety evaluation should address issues such as: if the carpeting is properly tacked down, if the pathway from the bed to the bathroom is obstacle free, and if there is ample nighttime lighting. Additional environmental suggestions include adaptive equipment for the shower or bathtub (ie, tub seat or hand-held showerhead can improve safety and independence

Table 1-5

HOME ASSESSMENT CHECKLIST—PREVENTION OF FALLS

EXTERIOR

- Are step surfaces nonslip?
- Are step edges visibly marked to avoid tripping?
- Are stairway handrails present? Are handrails secured?
- Are walkways covered with a nonslip surface and free of objects that could be tripped over?
- Is there sufficient outdoor lighting to provide safe ambulation at night?

INTERIOR

- Are lights bright enough to compensate for limited vision?
- Are light switches accessible before entering a room?
- Are lights glare free?
- Are handrails present on both sides of staircases?
- Are stairways adequately lit?
- Are handrails securely fastened to walls?
- Are step edges outlined with colored adhesive tape and nonslip?
- Are throw rugs secured with nonslip backing?
- Are carpet edges taped or tacked down?
- Are rooms uncluttered to permit unobstructed mobility?
- Are chairs throughout home strong enough to provide support during transfers? Are armrests present?
- Are tables (dining room, kitchen) strong enough to lean on?
- Do low-lying objects (coffee tables, stools) present a hazard?
- Are telephones accessible?

KITCHEN

- Are storage areas easily reached without standing on tiptoes or a chair?
- Are linoleum floors slippery?
- Is there a nonslip mat in front of sink to soak up spilled water?
- Are chairs wheel free, armrest equipped, and of the proper height to allow for safe transfers?
- If the pilot light goes out, is odor strong enough to alert the person?
- Are step stools strong enough to provide support?
- Are stool treads strong, in good repair, and slip resistant?

BATHROOM

- Are doors wide enough to accommodate assistive devices?
- Do door thresholds present tripping hazards?
- Are floors slippery, especially when wet?

(Continued)

Table 1-5 continued

HOME ASSESSMENT CHECKLIST—PREVENTION OF FALLS

- Are skid-proof strips or mats in place in tub or shower?
- Are tub and toilet bars available? Are they well secured?
- Are toilets low in height? Is an elevated toilet seat available?
- Is there sufficient, accessible, and glare-free light available?

BEDROOM

- Is there adequate, accessible lighting? Are there nightlights and/or bedside lamps available?
- Is the pathway from the bed to the bathroom unobstructed?
- Are beds of appropriate height for safe transfers on and off?
- Are floors covered with a nonslip surface and obstacle free?
- Can individual reach objects on closet shelves without standing on tiptoes or a chair?

Adapted from: Tideiksaar R. Fall prevention in the home. *Topics in Geriatric Rehabilitation.* 1987;3:57.

while bathing). Adaptations may also be necessary in order to avoid falls en route to the bathroom. Individuals with urinary urgency, evening fatigue, or disorientation in the middle of the night should be encouraged to use a bedside commode. No matter which approach is selected for rehabilitation, the following precautions are recommended:

- Many aged individuals are diagnosed with osteoporosis. Resistance and unilateral weight bearing may be excessive for them. It is possible to fracture an osteoporotic bone during strengthening exercises.

- Many aged individuals have osteoarthritis. Isometric exercise may be less painful for them. Increasing the amount of time that the contraction is held (eg, from the count of 3 to the count of 4) is an effective way to increase strength without adding external resistance.

- It is especially important for aged individuals to avoid holding their breath (Valsalva maneuver) during exercise. Counting out loud helps to avoid this problem.

- Aged individuals should be taught to monitor their heart rate during exercise or utilize perceived exertion scales (described in Chapter 9).

Therapeutic exercises designed to improve balance are an important part of fall prevention. Balance exercises address 3 areas of posture control: response to perturbation, weight shifting, and anticipatory adjustments to limb movements. Individuals must be able to

respond to an external perturbation, such as a push to the shoulder or sternum, with a postural adjustment that brings the center of gravity back over the base of support.[62]

Weight shifting of the entire body during standing involves muscular activity similar to that used in response to a perturbation; however, during weight shifting, muscle activation occurs voluntarily. Balance must also be controlled when a limb movement occurs, such as reaching with the upper extremity or swinging with the lower extremity. In this case, the postural adjustment actually occurs in anticipation of the limb movement, in order to prevent the center of gravity from moving outside of the base of support. For example, a forward movement of the arm should be preceded by ankle plantar flexion and hip extension. In this way, a small backward movement of the center of gravity counteracts the forward displacement caused by the moving arm. The PTA should include practicing each of these activities whenever a balance deficit has been determined by the PT. It is important to elicit a balance, response to perturbation, voluntary weight shifting, and postural adjustment in anticipation of limb movement in standing. These activities and supervised challenges to an elder's balance will help prepare the aged individual to use postural adjustment effectively during functional standing activities, such as cooking, self-care, transfers, and ambulation. These activities are directed toward improvement of the motor component of balance.[63]

Balance exercises can be incorporated into functional activities for the aged. Moving from sitting to standing, and from standing to sitting, are examples of controlled voluntary weight shifting. Shifting the trunk forward and back, and from side to side, while sitting are also examples of voluntary weight shifting. Voluntary weight shifting while standing with the individual's back to a wall is a safe way to facilitate control of balance. Dancing has also been recommended as a functional activity to improve balance for prevention of falls. T'ai Chi and Qigong exercises, because of their slow, controlled movements beyond the center of gravity, have also been shown to substantially improve balance and postural stability in the elderly.[64,65] Postural adjustments in anticipation of arm movements can be practiced during functional activities by standing and reaching for objects on the kitchen or closet shelves. Reaching should be practiced in a variety of directions.

Ambulation requires weight shifting. Manual guidance during ambulation helps organize the time and direction of weight shifting. Functional ambulation requires interaction with a variety of different support surfaces; therefore, it should be practiced on both smooth and uneven surfaces as well as on differing levels such as inclines, curbs, and stairs. Varying the amount of available light and background noise also stimulates realistic environmental conditions. If step lengths are irregular, footprints on the floor make good targets for foot placement; if posture is an issue, auditory feedback for foot placement is extremely helpful in keeping the older person from looking down.[66] Manual guidance is also useful for improving ambulation speed. A variety of ambulation speeds is necessary for function. Challenging activities, like crossing a busy street, can be made less threatening and should be practiced with the therapist or caregiver prior to discharge.

Difficulty rising from the floor after a fall is common in older adults and is associated with substantial morbidity. This tends to be an underappreciated problem, one that is rarely addressed when working with the elderly. The inability to get up after a fall is common and may not be a consequence of a fall-related injury, but of decreased strength, flexibility, and mobility.[67] Fear of falling appears to be increased in previous fallers, particularly in those with a history of difficulty rising alone after a fall.[68] Despite the high risk of difficulty for an elder when rising from the floor after a fall, few therapists teach older adults how to rise from the floor (see Chapter 10).

ADAPTING THE ENVIRONMENT

The process of adapting to the environment, or of adapting the environment to the aged person, is especially important in geriatric rehabilitation. The interaction between a person and the environment becomes potentially precarious as one gets older, and the physiologic reserves, underlying medical problems, affective states, and a host of other factors complicate the relationship between the aged individual and his or her environment.

The purpose of rehabilitation providers is to manipulate the environment to make it safer. Evaluation of the environment is more difficult than task analysis because the environment of concern is the one in which the individual actually lives and has to function, rather than a hospital or nursing home. Evaluation of physical space aims at ascertaining architectural barriers, safety and functional features, and the extent to which available equipment can be operated by the aged individual. Evaluation of the social context probes the availability of caregivers, their skills in rendering care and their need for training, their attitudes toward functional independence, and their experience of caregiver burden.

Furniture

Higher, reasonably firm, supportive, comfortable chairs with high backs allow rising from a sitting position with minimal assistance. Wide armrests, either wooden or metal, allow identification by touch when eyesight is poor or trunk rotation is limited. An aged individual should always be instructed to feel the chair seat with the back of his or her legs before attempting to sit down.

Environmental Design

Environmental designs for aged patients have been studied, and several factors are consistently identified as environmental hazards, including: poor illumination; inadequate color differentiation; cluttered furnishings; confusing room layout (such as a table in a dimly lit hallway); bland, nondistinct textiles; and complex architectural features (such as split level rooms).[69] Behavioral approaches (ie, using environmental cues like color coding, distinct color contrasting, or object labeling) have advantages over drugs in the treatment of cognitive impairments. Encouragement of independence, self-sufficiency, and social interaction is critical to prolonging cognitive functions.[70]

Visual limitations lead to a decreased ability to adapt to changes in lighting conditions requiring increased illumination to see and an increased sensitivity to glare. The older eye needs approximately 3 times the amount of light to function adequately. Depth perception and color differentiation can interfere with ambulation (ie, poor judgment in distance), ADL, and driving an automobile. Color vision deficiencies in the aged have been described by Andreasen.[71] Aged individuals have difficulty distinguishing between shades of blue-green, blue, and violet and are unable to distinguish between 2 shades of a similar color (aged individuals maintain the ability to differentiate between brighter colors, such as orange and red as long as they do not have any eye pathology [see Chapter 4] which may interfere with accurate color discrimination). Large pattern designs or solid bright colors in upholstery and textiles help to enhance visibility, interest, and appeal (reducing the likelihood of bumping into or falling over furniture). Small patterns can produce blurring of vision, eye fatigue, and dizziness.[72] Independence can be facilitated by bright and sharply contrasting colors. Contrasting colors or better lighting can provide safety in that room. Color coding of walls and corridors using bright colors can aid aged persons' finding of their own rooms, bathrooms, sitting rooms, and so on.

Different colors have differing effects on an individual's emotional state.[73] The colors red, yellow, and orange have been associated with excitement, stimulation, and aggression. Red increases muscular tension and increases blood pressure. It could be used as a visual stimulant with the elderly to alert them of environmental changes or hazards, such as stairs or level changes. It must be noted, however, that individuals with cataracts lose the shorter frequencies in the spectrum (which includes red, orange, and, in extreme cases, yellow). Although elderly persons often need to be stimulated, the aged individual with dementia requires soothing and warm colors, such as light oranges and blues, in their living quarters to enhance relaxation and comfort.

Conclusion

What do these age-related changes in body systems mean overall? First, with advancing age, we become less like each other biologically, so health care needs to be more individualized. Rehabilitation of the aged patient is one of the most challenging tasks for health care professionals. It is often difficult to separate the physiological aspect of aging and disability from cognitive changes when designing a rehabilitation treatment program. With increased knowledge, the natural history of normal aging may eventually be altered. Until then, rehabilitation of aged individuals needs to focus on obtaining the

maximal functional capacity within the care environment by simplifying that environment and providing activity to ensure that disabilities do not result from disuse. To maintain the highest level of functional ability for the longest amount of time, decline in all sensory integration and physical functioning capabilities must be considered when providing rehabilitative care. One of the most salient aspects of geriatric rehabilitation is the simultaneous management of multiple conditions and the concept of frailty. For the rehabilitation team, these multiple diagnoses translate into multiple—and often multidimensional—impairments that complicate the management of ADL and hinder maximal functional capabilities.

The primary goal of rehabilitation is to promote independent living. When working with aged people, rehabilitation teams need to be aware of the number of factors that make caring for them more complex, more challenging, and more fulfilling. The PTA is important in the provision of this care.

Pearls

- Geriatrics is the branch of medicine that focuses on the specialized care of aging populations, healthy living, and the prevention and treatment of disease and disability in later life.

- An interdisciplinary team approach is required because of the complexity of interventions needed in dealing with the aged.

- PTAs play an integral part on the geriatric team. Under the supervision of a PT, duties include: (1) assisting the PT in implementing treatment plans according to the plan of care; (2) training patients in exercises and ADL; (3) conducting treatments using specialized equipment, administering modalities and other treatment procedures; and (4) reporting to the PT regarding the patient's progress.

- The aging process varies from one individual to another and is determined by genetics, nutrition, lifestyle behaviors, exercise, sleep, and environmental factors.

- Maximal achievable lifespan is a measure of the maximum amount of time members of a group are observed to survive between birth and death.

- Medical complexity is common in older patients and primary diagnoses are complicated by co-existing diseases, impairments, and/or disabilities and frailty.

- Functional assessment is the cornerstone of geriatric rehabilitation.

- Chronological age is not a reliable indicator of functional ability. There is a great deal of variability from one older adult to another.

- Bed rest should be avoided at all costs.

- The goal of geriatric rehabilitation is to obtain optimum well-being and maximal functional capabilities through rehabilitation interventions.

- The PTA needs to pay close attention to the elderly patient's response to movement and allow frequent rest periods, progressing the patient only as tolerated.

REFERENCES

1. US Census Bureau. *65 in the United States: 2005.* Commissioned Report of the National Institute on Aging (ongoing and continually updated). Available at: http://www.census.gov. Accessed June 24, 2009; Re-accessed March 21, 2010.
2. Harman D. Aging: Overview. *Ann N Y Acad Sci.* 2001;928:1-21.
3. American Physical Therapy Association. *Guide to Practice.* 2nd ed. American Physical Therapy Association. *Phys Ther.* 2001;81:9-746.
4. National Bureau of Economics. How the aging process changed during the 20th century. *Natl Bur Econ Res Bull Aging Health.* 2003;1:1-2.
5. Yin D, Chen K. The essential mechanisms of aging: irreparable damage accumulation of biochemical side-reactions. *Exp Gerontol.* 2005;40:455-465.
6. Speakman JR. Correlations between physiology and lifespan–two widely ignored problems with comparative studies. *Aging Cell.* 2005;4:167-175.
7. Perls TT, Kunkel L, Pura A. The genetics of aging. *Curr Opin Genet Dev.* 2002;12:362-369.
8. US Census Bureau. *65 in the United States: 2005.* Commissioned report of the National Institute on Aging (ongoing and continually updated). Available at: http://www.census.gov. Accessed June 24, 2009.
9. US Census Bureau. *July 1, 2006 Population estimates by state.* Census 2000 Summary. http://www.census.gov. Re-accessed March 21, 2010.
10. Rauser CL, Mueller LD, Rose MR. The evolution of late life. *Ageing Res Rev.* 2006;5:14-32.
11. Topp R, Fahman M, Boardly D. Healthy aging: health promotion and disease prevention. The importance of function. *Nurs Clin North Am.* 2004;39:411-22.
12. Perls TT. The different paths to age one hundred. *Ann N Y Acad Sci.* 2005;1055:13-25.
13. Bryant LL, Corbertt KK, Kutner JS. In their own words: a model of healthy aging. *Soc Sci Med.* 2001;53:927-941.
14. National Center for Health Statistics. *Health, United States, 2005, with Health and Aging Chartbook.* Hyattsville, MD: National Center for Health Statistics, 2006;36-37.
15. Grossman T. Latest advances in anti-aging medicine. *Keio J Med.* 2005;54:85-94.
16. Lundin-Olsson L, Nyberg L, Gustafson Y. Attention, frailty, and falls: the effect of a manual task on basic mobility. *J Am Geriatr Soc.* 1998;46:758-761.
17. Fiatarone MA, O'Neill EF, Ryan ND, et al. Exercise training and nutritional supplementation for physical frailty in very elderly people. *N Engl J Med.* 1994;330:1769-1775.
18. Federal Council on the Aging. *The Need for Long-Term Care. A Chartbook of the Federal Council on Aging.* Washington, DC: US Government Printing Office; 2005. US Department of Health and Human Services publication No. (OHDS) 81-20704,29.
19. Rusk H. *Rehabilitation Medicine.* St Louis, MO: Mosby; 1958.
20. Lawton MP, Brody EM. Assessment of older people: self-maintaining and instrumental activities of daily living. *Gerontologist.* 1969;9:179-186.
21. Nagamautsu T, Oida Y, Kitabatake Y, Kohno H, Egawa K, Nezu N, Arao T. A 6-year cohort study on relationship between functional fitness and impairment of ADL in community-dwelling elderly. *J Epidemiol.* 2003;13:142-148.
22. Demura S, Sato S, Kasuga K. The interdisciplinary achievement patterns of activities of daily living for institutionalized dependent elderly. *J Physiol Anthropol Appl Human Sci.* 2002;21:167-175.
23. National Center for Health Statistics. *Health, United States, 2005, with Health and Aging Chartbook.* Hyattsville, MD: National Center for Health Statistics, 2006;64-65,71-73.
24. Branch LG, Jette A. The Framingham Disability Study: social disability among the aging. *Am J Public Health.* 1981;71:1202.
25. Wells JL, Seabrook JA, Stolee P, Borrie MJ, Knoefel F. State of the art in geriatric rehabilitation. Part I: review of frailty and comprehensive geriatric rehabilitation. *Arch Phys Med Rehabil.* 2003;84:890-897.
26. Woollacott MJ. Changes in posture and voluntary control in the elderly: research findings and rehabilitation. *Top Geriatr Rehabil.* 1990;5:1-11.
27. Woollacott MJ. Response preparation and posture control: neuromuscular changes in the older adult. *Ann N Y Acad Sci.* 1988;515:42-53.
28. Haegerstrom-Portnoy G. Vision in elders–summary of findings of the SKI study. *Optom Vis Sci.* 2005;82:87-93.
29. Kasper RL. Eye problems of the aged. In: Reichel W, ed. *Clinical Aspects of Aging.* Baltimore, MD: Williams and Wilkins; 1988.
30. Vandervoort AA. Aging of the human neuromuscular system. *Muscle Nerve.* 2002;25:17-25.
31. Wells JL, Seabrook JA, Stolee P, Borrie MJ, Knoefel F. State of the art in geriatric rehabilitation. Part II: clinical challenges *Arch Phys Med Rehabil.* 2003;84:898-903.
32. Schaie KW. Historical time and cohort effects. In: McCuskey KA, Reese HW, eds. *Lifespan Developmental Psychology: Historical and Generational Effects.* 3rd ed. New York: Academic Press; 2004.
33. Ferrara CM, Goldberg AP, Ortmeyer HK, Ryan AS. Effects of aerobic and resistive exercise training on glucose disposal and skeletal muscle metabolism in older people. *J Gerontol A Biol Sci Med Sci.* 2006;61:480-487.
34. Schneider El, Reed JD. Modulations of aging processes. In: Finch CE, Schneider EL, eds. *Handbook of the Biology of Aging.* New York: Academic Press; 1985.
35. Taylor HL, Henschel JB, Keys A. Effects of bed rest on cardiovascular function and work performance. *J Am Physiol.* 1949;2:223.
36. Yamada M, Tohno Y, Tohno S, et al. Age-related changes of elements and relationships among elements in human tendons and ligaments. *Biol Trace Elem Res.* 2004;98:129-142.

37. Miller PB, Johnson RL, Lamb LE. Effects of four weeks of absolute bed rest on circulatory functions in man. *Aerospace Med.* 1964;35:1194.

38. Koehn M. Embracing the aging process. *J Christ Nurs.* 2005;22:20-24.

39. Fries JF. Aging, natural death, and the compression of morbidity. *Bull World Health Organ.* 2002;80:245-250.

40. Eccleston NA, Jones J. International curriculum guidelines for preparing physical activity of older adults, in collaboration with aging and life course, World Health Organization. *J Aging Phys Act.* 2004;12:467-479.

41. Himann JE. Age-related changes in speed of walking. *Med Sci Sports Exerc.* 1998;44:161-165.

42. Siegler IC, Costa PT, Jr. Health behavior relationships. In: Birren JE, Schaie KW, eds. *Handbook of the Psychology of Aging.* 2nd ed. New York: Van Nostrand Reinhold; 1985.

43. Kaplan E. Psychological factors and ischemic heart disease mortality: a focal role for perceived health. Paper presented at the annual meeting of the American Psychological Association. Washington, DC; 1999.

44. Rosillo RA, Fagel ML. Correlation of psychologic variables and progress in physical therapy: I. degree of disability and denial of illness. *Arch Phys Med Rehabil.* 1970;51:227-228.

45. Stoedefalke KG. Motivating and sustaining the older adult in an exercise program. *Top Geriatr Rehabil.* 1985;1:78.

46. Van Maanen HM. Being old does not always mean being sick: perspectives on conditions of health as perceived by British and American Elderly. *J Adv Nurs.* 2006;53:54-61; discussion 61-64.

47. O'Connor BP, Rousseau FL, Maki SA. Physical exercise and experienced bodily changes: the emergence of benefits and limits on benefits. *Int J Aging Hum Dev.* 2004;59:177-203.

48. Wolfson L. Gait and balance dysfunction: a model of interaction of age and disease. *Neuroscientist.* 2001;7:178-83.

49. Knott M, Voss DE. *Proprioceptive Neuromuscular Facilitation: Patterns of Techniques.* 2nd ed. New York: Harper and Row; 1968.

50. Tremblay KL, Piskosz M, Sousa P. Effect of age and age-related hearing loss on the neural representation of speech cues. *Clin Neurophysiol.* 2003;114:1332-1343.

51. Goodpasters BH, Carlson CL, Visser M, et al. Attenuation of skeletal muscle and strength in the elderly: the health ABC study. *J Appl Physiol.* 2001;90:2157-2165.

52. Sinaki M. Nonpharmacologic interventions. Exercise, fall prevention, and role of physical medicine. *Clin Geriatr Med.* 2003;19:337-359.

53. Meyers J. Applications of cardiopulmonary exercise testing in the management of cardiovascular and pulmonary disease. *Int J Sports Med.* 2005;26(suppl 1):S49-S55.

54. Pautex S, Gold G. Assessing pain intensity in older adults. *Geriatrics Aging.* 2006;9:399-402.

55. Homers JP, Huizing AR. Why do we use physical restraints in the elderly? *Z Gerontol Geriatr.* 2005;38:19-25.

56. Center of Medicare and Medicaid Services. *State Operations Manual, Part II: Guidance to Surveyors for Long Term Care Facilities, Interpretive Guidelines.* 483.13a, 2000. http://www.cms.gov.

57. Omert L, Zakhary S, Wilson R, Diminno C, Rodriques A. Falling down and falling out: management and outcome analysis. *J Trauma.* 2004;56:58-63.

58. Stalenhoef PA, Diederiks JP, Knottnerus JA, Kester AD, Grebolder HF. A risk model for the prediction of recurrent falls in community-dwelling elderly: a prospective cohort study. *J Clin Epidemiol.* 2002;55:1088-1094.

59. Podsiadlo D, Richardson S. The timed up and go: a test of basic functional mobility for frail elderly persons. *J Am Geriatr Soc.* 1991; 39:142-148.

60. Kron M, Loy S, Sturm E, Nikolaus T, Becker C. Risk indicators for falls in institutionalized frail elderly. *Am J Epidemiol.* 2003;158:645-653.

61. Tideiksaar R. Fall prevention in the home. *Top Geriatr Rehabil.* 1987;3:57-64.

62. Kannus P, Sievanen H, Paluanen M, Jarvinen, Parkkeri J. Prevention of falls and consequent injuries in elderly people. *Lancet.* 2005;366:1885-1893.

63. Shumway-Cook A, Horak FB. Assessing the influence of sensory interaction on balance. *Phys Ther.* 1986;66:1548.

64. Bottomley JM. The use of T'ai Chi as a movement modality in orthopaedics. *Ortho Phys Ther Clinics North Am.* 2000;9:361-373.

65. Wolf SL, Coogler C, Xu T. Exploring the basis for T'ai Chi Chaun as a therapeutic exercise approach. *Arch Phys Med Rehabil.* 1997;79:886-892.

66. Bottomley JM. Gait in later life. *Ortho Phys Ther Clinics North Am.* 2001;10:131-149.

67. Alexander NB, Ulbrich J, Raheja A, Channer D. Rising from the floor in older adults. *J Am Geriatr Soc.* 1997;45:564-569.

68. Tinetti ME, Richman D, Powell L. Falls efficacy as a measure of fear of falling. *J Gerontol.* 1993;45:P239-P243.

69. Nelson A, Powell-Cope G, Gavin-Dreschnack D, Quigby P, Bulat T, Baptiste AS, Applegarth S, Friedman Y. Technology to promote safe mobility in the elderly. *Nurs Clin North Am.* 2004;39:649-671.

70. *Alzheimer's disease: Report of the Secretaries Task Force on Alzheimer's Disease.* Washington, DC; US Government Printing Office; 1999. Rockville, MD; US Dept of Health and Human Services, Public Health Service, Alcohol, Drug Abuse, and Mental Health Administration. DHHS pub. no. (ADM) 84-1323.

71. Andreasen MK. Making a safe environment by design. *J Gerontol Nurs.* 1985;11:18-22.

72. Zeisel J, Silverstein NM, Hyde J, Leukoff S, Lawton MP, Holmes W. Environmental correlates to behavioral health outcomes in Alzheimer's special care units. *Gerontologist.* 2003;43:697-711.

73. Sharpe DT. *The Psychology of Color and Design.* Chicago: Nelson-Hall; 1974.

2

Theories of Aging

The attempt to describe the circumstance called "old age" has interested many scientists for decades and inspired them to theorize and experiment with possible explanations for the aging process. Several theories of aging have been proposed and the most prominent theories will be reviewed and compared in this chapter, providing a basic framework for understanding normal and pathological aging (as discussed throughout the following chapters) and critically evaluating clinical observations and strategies for managing the care of elderly individuals.

HISTORICAL PERSPECTIVE

The study of aging has a long history. Much of the research in the biology of aging has focused on prolongevity studies (eg, extending length of cellular life) rather than on the actual mechanisms of aging. Freeman[1] presents a comprehensive monograph of research on aging over the last 2,500 years.

Research on aging began around the turn of the 20th century. According to Freeman in *Aging, Its History and Literature*, Metchnikoff introduced the concept that aging was caused by the continuous absorption of toxins from intestinal bacteria and, in 1908, received the Nobel Prize for his contributions to biology and the study of aging. Systematic studies that described the aging phenomena in terms of cell morphology, physiology, and biochemistry began in about 1950,[2] leading to improvements in experimental designs and the evolution of 2 major groups of aging theories.

The first group of studies conducted on aging presented *fundamentalist* or *developmental-genetic* theories. These theories are based on the premise of "wear and tear,"[3] such that aging is attributed to pathological changes that are tissue specific (eg, connective, nervous, vascular, endocrine tissue, etc).

The second group of aging theories, termed *nongenetic* or *stochastic* (random) theories of aging, view aging as an epiphenomenon in which environmental insults such as gravity, toxins, and cosmic rays result in the aging process.[4] Many additional theories not contained in these 2 theoretical groups view aging as a continuum, with development and tissue evolution and growth,[5] while others relate aging to a cessation of somatic cell growth[6] and energy depletion.[7]

Current modified versions of these theories have been introduced that involve the immune system, the neuroendocrine system, failures in deoxyribonucleic acid (DNA) repair, random mutation in somatic cells, errors in protein synthesis, and random damage from free radicals. These theories, although often presented as separate from each other, are not mutually exclusive. Clearly, there has not been just one theory that fully identifies all of the causes, mechanisms, or bases of aging. The processes regulating the rate of aging may be different in different cell types and tissues. The combined effects of environmental damage and intrinsic pathologies may further blur a simple explanation of a basic mechanism for aging.[8]

The evolutionary theories of aging are basically drawn from Darwin's theories of survival of the fittest. The evolutionary theories of aging are: (1) the theory of programmed death, (2) the mutation accumulation theory of aging, and (3) the antagonistic pleiotropy (control or determination of characteristics or function by a single gene) theory of aging.[9] All of these theories are contained in the classic evolutionary theory of aging that explains why mortality rises with age: as

Bottomley J. *Geriatric Rehabilitation: A Textbook for the Physical Therapist Assistant* (pp 29-42).
© 2010 SLACK Incorporated

individuals grow older, less lifetime fertility remains, so continued survival contributes less to reproductive fitness. Successful reproduction often involves intergenerational transfers as well as fertility. In the formal theory, age-specific selective pressure on mortality depends on the remaining fertility of a population (the classic effect) and the remaining intergenerational transfers to be made to others.[10] These theories of aging are useful because they open new opportunities for further research by suggesting testable predictions, but they have also been harmful in the past when they were used to impose limitations on aging studies. Currently, the evolutionary theories of aging are not seen as completed theories, but rather as a set of ideas that require further elaboration and validation.

From an historical perspective, the concept of aging as a cell-based phenomenon vs organismic (whole body) aging is comparatively new. Weissman[6] was the first to emphasize the distinction between body (somatic) cells which age, and germ cells which do not age. He suggested that the inability of somatic cells to replicate indefinitely was the reason for limited lifespan in the human compared with germ cells.

A landmark study by 2 then unknown cell biologists, Hayflick and Moorehead,[11] turned the study of the aging of cultured cells in a new direction. Conclusions from these in vitro studies on fetal cells were that, in culture, human cells have a limited lifespan. Hayflick and Moorehead reported that there was a period of rapid and vigorous cellular division followed by a decline in reproductive activity and characteristic aging of the cells. They proposed that aging was a cellular as well as an organismic phenomenon.

The loss in functional capacity of the aging person reflects the summation of the loss of critical functional capabilities within individual cells. For instance, the loss of fast-twitch (type II) fibers in the muscle that occurs with aging results in atrophy and a decrease in muscle force, strength, and stability, thereby decreasing functional capacity.

FUNDAMENTAL CONSIDERATIONS

A discussion of the theories of aging must include a review of the observations and correlations associated with the aging process. There is not a great deal known about the nature of the mechanisms involved in aging and the study of aging is intrinsically difficult. It is even difficult to define aging. Aging is characterized by an increasing vulnerability to physiological and environmental changes. Increasing chronological age brings with it an increasing incidence of disability and increasing probability of death. System-wide function and structural changes caused by the aging process are often identifiable by biomarkers of aging.[12]

The following fundamental considerations are an important basis on which to build further knowledge in the studying of aging.

Aging is developmental. This concept is very simple: we do not suddenly age. We evolve into mature adults and grow older developmentally, not chronologically. Aging is unique among all developmental stages. A 70-year-old person in chronological age may have the physiologic age of a 50-year-old; yet a 50-year-old person with chronic diseases and a sedentary lifestyle may parallel the physiologic decline of a 90-year-old.

Old age is a gift of 20th-century technology and scientific advancement. The gerontologist James Birren[12] has penned the notion that the extended life expectancy that we now have is really a gift of modern medicine and technology. Some biologists argue that the "survivorship kinetics" of biological aging may be an artifact of civilization and domestication. In nature, populations of species (including humans) only recently began to live long enough to show the characteristic kinetics of biological aging. Since the discovery of insulin, vaccination for diseases, improved sanitation, a decline in infant mortality, the development of modern surgical techniques, and the advanced treatment modes for formerly fatal diseases, humans now experience longer lives. We stayed older longer, not younger longer, in the 20th century and this is expected to expand further into the 21st century. The whole phenomenon of aging is new.

The effects of normal aging vs pathologic aging must be differentiated if possible. A confounding problem in understanding aging is the fact that there is a vast spectrum of aging changes. The process of aging is probably multifactorial in its regulation; however, it is virtually impossible to tell which changes are primary to an age-regulated event and which are secondary. Often we assume that a functional decline is due to aging. However, disease may often cause functional decline that is not part of a normal aging process, although it increases the speed at which a person ages because of his or her inactivity. For example, adult-onset diabetes (type II) increases one's probability of cardiovascular disease as a result of the effect of the diabetes. It is not normal to get diabetes; it is a function of lifestyle and heredity. Confusion exists between aging, disease, and dying. Aging characteristically brings a loss in homeostasis and with it increased vulnerability to diseases, some of which result in death. Death has been used as the endpoint measurement of aging. However, death can occur from many causes, some of which are related to the aging process only secondarily, and in some cases totally unrelated (ie, accidents).

There is no universally accepted theory of aging. Aging does not occur in all species or in all organisms of the same species in exactly the same way. While one tissue may be losing functional capacity rapidly, others may be comparatively quite "young" functionally (see Chapter 3 for a more comprehensive discussion on normal aging). Although aging is a universal phenomenon, no one really knows what causes it or why people age at different rates. Chronological age is a much less useful and definitive measure of functional capacity than scientists would like.

Amid all these confusing assumptions of aging there has been a set of aging characteristics that have been identified to be consistent:

- There is an increased mortality with age.[13]
- Consistent changes in the biochemical composition of the body with age have been well documented.[14] These changes include a decrease in lean body mass and an increase in fat; there are also characteristic increases in waste product deposition (lipofuscin) in certain tissues, and an increased cross-linking in molecules such as collagen and elastin, which impedes nutrition and hydration of the cells and results in tissue binding.[15]
- A broad spectrum of progressive deteriorative changes have been demonstrated in relation to inactivity.[16]
- There is a reduced ability to adapt or respond to environmental change, particularly when the cell is so deconditioned that it cannot reach a level of homeostasis (perhaps the hallmark of aging).[17] This can be demonstrated at all levels from individual molecule to the complete organism.[18] Thus, the changes of age are not so much the resting pulse rate or the fasting serum glucose, but the ability to return these parameters to normal after a physiological stress.

- There is an increased vulnerability to many diseases with age.[19] The age-associated increase in vulnerability to diseases occurs at the cellular level. Aging is a process that is distinct from disease. The fundamental changes of aging provide the substratum in which the age-associated diseases can flourish.

Aging theories are divided into 2 major categories: genetic (*fundamentalist*) and nongenetic (*environmental*). Genetic theories focus on the mechanisms for aging located in the nucleus of the cell. Nongenetic theories focus on areas located elsewhere, such as in organs, tissues, or systems within the body or extrinsic environmental causes. In order to understand both of the theories of aging, a basic understanding of 3 somatic cell types is necessary (see Table 2-1).

Somatic cells are the cells of the body. Not all somatic cells age at the same rate, nor do they have similar aging characteristics. Somatic cells are divided into 3 categories: *mitotic cells, reverting postmitotic cells,* and *fixed postmitotic cells.*[20]

Continuously proliferating mitotic cells never cease to replicate themselves, and injury done to these cells is healed through continuous cell division and regeneration. Such cells can be found as superficial skin cells, red blood cells, cells of the lining of the intestine, and bone marrow cells. Reverting postmitotic cells have a slower rate of division than the continuously proliferating cells, but when there is injury, the rate of division speeds up and regeneration is

Table 2-1

SOMATIC CELL TYPES

SOMATIC CELL TYPE	CHARACTERISTICS	TISSUE TYPE	
Mitotic cells	Replicate; continuous cell division and regeneration; continually replaced	Skin cells Red blood cells	Bone marrow Intestine lining
Reverting postmitotic cells*	Slower rate of proliferation; nucleus intact; division and regeneration will increase with injury	Kidney cells Liver cells	
Fixed postmitotic cells	Never replicate once maturity is reached; no new vital cells produced	Muscle cells Nerve cells	

*Postmitotic cells replicate and repair themselves only if the nucleus is intact.

possible. Kidney and liver cells are examples of reverting postmitotic cells. The final type of somatic cells, fixed postmitotic cells, never replicate once the cells reach maturity[21]; primary examples include muscle cells and nerve cells. In adult life, therefore, nerve and muscle cells replicate and repair themselves only if the nucleus is intact. Because the postmitotic cell will not replicate itself, no new vital cells are produced. For instance, the aging athlete who tears an Achilles tendon will replace the healing tissue with a fibrotic scar rather than muscle fibers. These tissues do not have contractile properties and often create fixed adhesions, and therefore, the need for residual fixed somatic cells to remain vital is crucial to the well-being and life expectancy of the individual.

THEORIES OF AGING

Historically, one of the major problems in gerontology is the ease and frequency with which new theories have appeared. There is currently no one theory that fully explains the process of aging. Researchers have viewed aging as "an event" that happens rather than as a period in the life of organisms that begins at maturity (or conception) and lasts for the rest of the lifespan. It seems that aging should be considered a developmental process. Numerous primary and secondary changes occur during development and aging. Some changes are genetically programmed and directed within the body, while some changes are caused by the environment.

THE DEVELOPMENTAL-GENETIC THEORIES

The developmental-genetic theorists consider the process of aging to be part of a continuum with development genetically controlled and programmed. Gerontologists agree that the maximum lifespan and the rate of aging are regulated intrinsically. The primary evidence of this is the species-specific maximum lifespan. Variation in lifespan is far greater among species than within species. For instance, the lifespan of a human averages about 76 years, while a sparrow might expect an average of 3 years. Certain breeds of turtles have lifespans recorded in the hundreds, whereas a house fly might only live for 3 days. Because maximum lifespan is a species characteristic, it would seem evident that this is genetically determined.[22]

Of interest are studies that compare the longevity of identical, fraternal, and non-twin siblings. It has been shown that there is a remarkable similarity in longevity between human fibroblast cell cultures in monozygotic twins that is not demonstrated in the other 2 groups.[23,24] A greater similarity of cell behavior and replicative lifespan is observed in these twins when compared to non-twin, age-matched controls.[25] One could argue that genetics governs susceptibility to certain diseases but not to aging per se. Alternatively, a certain "vigor" could be inherited that protects against the developmental susceptibility to a wide variety of diseases. It clearly is difficult to distinguish between the 2 mechanisms. Nonetheless, there is circumstantial evidence for genetically controlled mechanisms of aging that potentially operate in a similar way to developmental processes.

Hayflick Limit Theory

Hayflick and Moorehead, and subsequent researchers, have been able to show that a deterioration in cells (ie, mitotic and mitochondrial activity) is not dependent on environmental influences, but rather that cell aging is intrinsic to the cells.[26] It has been determined that there is a limited number of cell divisions ranging from 40 to 60 replications per life cycle of each cell. The developmental aging process of cultured cells includes 3 phases. Phase I is the beginning stage of cell life, phase II involves a rapid cell proliferation, and the final cessation of cell division occurs in phase III. The generality of the Hayflick phenomenon is that, in the absence of pathology in the cells, aging always occurs and ultimately results in the death of the cell. This finite ability to reproduce cells appears to be genetically based[27] (see Box 2-1).

Hayflick and Moorehead made one of the greatest contributions to the history of cellular biology by demonstrating the senescence of cultured human cells. Hayflick theorized that the aging process was controlled by a biological clock contained within each living cell. The 1961 study cited above concluded that human fibroblast cells (lung, skin, muscle, heart) have a limited lifespan.[27] The cells divided approximately

---

Box 2-1: Hayflick Limit Theory

- Cell deterioration is not dependent on environmental influences alone.
- Cell aging is intrinsic to cells.
- The aging process of cultured cells has 3 phases:
  - beginning stage of cell life
  - rapid cell proliferation
  - cessation of cell division
- Aging always occurs and ultimately results in the death of a cell.

50 times over a period of years and then suddenly stopped. Nutrition seemed to have an effect on the rate of cell division: Overfed cells made up to 50 divisions in a year; underfed cells took up to 3 times as long as normal cells to make divisions. Alterations and degenerations occurred within some cells before they reached their growth limit. The most evident changes took place in the cell organelles, membranes, and genetic material. This improper functioning of cells and loss of cells in organs and tissues may be responsible for the effects of aging.

Waste Accumulation Theory

In the course of their lifespans, cells produce more waste than they can properly eliminate. This waste can include various toxins that, when accumulated to a certain level, can interfere with normal cell function, ultimately killing the cell.

Evidence supporting this theory is found in the presence of a waste product called lipofuscin leading to age pigment. The cells most commonly found to contain lipofuscin are nerve and heart muscle cells, both of which are critical to life. Lipofuscin is formed by a complex reaction that binds fat in the cells to proteins, and accumulates in the cells in the form of small granules, which increase in size as a person ages. Because lipofuscin builds up over time, it has been described as "the ashes of our dwindling metabolic fires."[28]

Limited Number of Cell Divisions Theory

The number of cell divisions is directly affected by the accumulations of the cell's waste products. The more waste that is accumulated over time, the faster cells degenerate. Although an ordinary chicken does not live anywhere near 20 years, French surgeon Dr. Alexis Carrel was able to keep pieces of a chicken heart alive in a saline solution that contained minerals in the same proportion as chicken blood for 28 years. He believed that he had achieved this by disposing of the waste products daily. Although Carrel's theory was eventually overturned by Hayflick when it was found that fresh cells had been inadvertently added to the cultures making the chicken cells seem "immortal," the experiment helped explain why cells from older people with more waste divided fewer times than cells from embryos, which divided the most.[29]

"Wear and Tear" Theory

August Weismann, a German biologist, first introduced the "wear and tear" theory in 1882. He believed that the body and its cells were damaged by overuse and abuse. The organs, liver, stomach, kidneys, skin, and so on are worn down by toxins in our diet and in the environment; by the excessive consumption of fat, sugar, caffeine, alcohol, and nicotine; by the ultraviolet rays of the sun; and by the many other physical and emotional stresses to which we subject our bodies. Wear and tear is not confined to our organs, however, it takes place on the cellular level as well[30] (see Box 2-2).

Of course, even if you have never touched a cigarette or had a glass of wine, you have stayed out of the sun and eaten only natural foods, by simply using the organs that nature provided to you, your organs are going to wear out; abuse will only wear them out more quickly. Likewise, as the body ages, our very cells feel the effect, no matter how healthy our lifestyle.

When we are young, the body's own maintenance and repair systems keep compensating for the effects of both normal and excessive wear and tear. With age, the body loses its ability to repair damage caused by diet, environmental toxins, bacteria, or virus. Thus, many elderly people die of diseases that they could have resisted when they were younger. By the same token, nutrition, exercise, and other positive health behaviors can help reverse the aging process by stimulating the body's own ability to repair and maintain its organs and cells.

Box 2-2: Wear and Tear Theory

- Wear and tear occurs in every cell of the body due to exposure to the environment, overuse, and abuse throughout life.
- Parts wear out quicker if cells are poorly nourished and/or hydrated.
- Moderate exercise, good nutrition, and positive health behaviors can delay or reverse the aging process.

Neuroendocrine and Hormonal Theories

Neuroendocrine and hormonal theories regard functional decrements in neurons and their associated hormones as central to the aging process. Given the major interactive role of the neuroendocrine system in physiology, this is an attractive approach. Denckla, an endocrinologist turned gerontologist, believes that the center that controls aging is located in the brain.[31] He based his theory on past studies of hypothyroidism, a disease that mimics mature aging (eg, a depressed immune system, wrinkling of the skin, gray hair, and a slowed metabolic rate) (see Box 2-3).

The neuroendocrine theory developed by Dilman elaborates on the wear and tear theory by focusing on the neuroendocrine system, the complicated network of biochemicals that governs the release of our hormones and other vital bodily elements. When we are young, our hormones work together to regulate many bodily functions, including our responses to heat and cold, our life experiences, and our sexual activity. Different organs release various hormones all under the governance of the hypothalamus, a walnut-sized gland located within the brain.

The hypothalamus sets off various chain reactions whereby an organ releases a hormone that, in turn, stimulates the release of another hormone, that, in turn, stimulates yet another bodily response. The hypothalamus responds to the body's hormone levels as its guide to regulating hormonal activity.

When we are young, hormone levels tend to be high, accounting for, among other things, menstruation in women and high libido in both sexes. As we age, the body produces lower levels of hormones, which can have disastrous effects on our functioning. The growth hormones that help us form muscle mass, human growth hormone, testosterone, and thyroid, for example, drop dramatically as we age so that even if an elderly person has not gained weight, he or she has undoubtedly increased the ratio of fat to muscle.

Hormones are vital for repairing and regulating our bodily functions, and when aging causes a drop in hormone production, it causes a decline in our body's ability to repair and regulate itself as well. Moreover, hormone production is highly interactive. The drop in production of any one hormone is likely to have a feedback effect on the whole mechanism, signaling other organs to release lower levels of other hormones, which will cause other body parts to release lower levels of yet other hormones.

Hormone replacement therapy, a frequent component of any anti-aging treatment, helps to reset the body's hormonal clock and reverse or delay the effects of aging. If our hormones are being produced at youthful levels, in a very real sense, the cells of our bodies are stimulated to be metabolically active and, thus, we stay young.

Another aspect of the neuroendocrine basis of aging depends on the role of the pituitary hormones.[32] The anterior pituitary gland controls the thyroid gland by the thyroid stimulating hormone (TSH), and thus the secretion of thyroxine. Thyroxine is the master rate-controlling hormone within the body for metabolism and protein synthesis.[33] The focus of this theory is the proposed ability of the anterior pituitary to release a blocking hormone called the decreasing oxygen consumption hormone (DECO), which blocks the cell membrane from taking up thyroxine

as a check-balance in the human system. Unlike other cells, brain cells or neurons do not replicate. When DECO is released by the pituitary glands of rats, their immune system is revitalized, the rate of cross-linking in cells is reduced, and cardiovascular function is restored to levels of youth when tested in the laboratory setting. Denckla speculated that as we age the pituitary begins to release DECO, which inhibits the ability of cells to use thyroxine, thus, the rate at which cells convert food to energy. The increased metabolic rate brings on and accelerates the process of aging.

An important version of Denckla's theory proposes that the hypothalamic, pituitary, and adrenal axis is the master timekeeper for the organism and the primary regulator of the aging process. The neuroendocrine system regulates early development, growth, puberty, the control of the reproductive system, metabolism, and, in part, the activities of all the major organ systems.[34]

Satisfactory evidence to relate endocrine function to aging is not present to substantiate a significant contribution of endocrine gland function to the process of aging. In response to stress and trophic hormones, the adrenal cortex and thyroid gland remain intact. For women, menopause is a hormone-mediated event that chronicles but does not regulate aging.[35] The ovary is the sole endocrine gland whose functional capacity predictably declines with normal aging. On the other hand, androgen production by the testis is not as predictable because there are individual differences.

The importance of neuroendocrine research cannot be overemphasized. Critics of these theories, however, point out that the master timekeeper of aging, the neuroendocrine system, lacks universality. Many organisms that age (eg, higher vertebrates) have no complex neuroendocrine system. It can also be argued that the changes that occur in the

Box 2-3: Neuroendocrine & Hormonal Theory

- This theory states that the center controlling aging is located in the brain.

- It is proposed that the hypothalamic, pituitary, and adrenal axis is the master timekeeper and primary regulator of the aging process.

- Hypothyroidism mimics aging.

- There is an overall decrease in the available neuroendocrines in both males and females with aging.

- Glandular function decreases with age, leading to declines in both functional capacity and the maintenance of homeostasis.

neuroendocrine system are fundamental changes and occur in all tissues. Aging of the brain, however, produces additional secondary effects that, although not fundamental to aging, contribute to the development of the overall aging process.[36] What the neuroendocrine system contributes to the aging process is evidenced by the lack of estrogen with respect to its effects on bone density and vascularity. Its contribution to other aging processes remains to be determined.

Immunological Theory

The immunological theory of aging is another theory categorized as a developmental-genetic theory. This theory was proposed by Walford[37] and has two major observations on which it is based: (1) the functional capacity of the immune system declines with age as a result of reduced T-cell function[38] and a reduced resistance to infectious diseases, and (2) the efficiency and resiliency of the immune system declines with age as evidenced by the striking age-associated increase in autoimmune diseases (see Box 2-4).

As with the neuroendocrine theory, the immunological theory is attractive. The immune system has a primary integrative role and is of major importance in health maintenance.[39] Conversely, lifespan differences could simply be due to the prevention of diseases.

The thymus is the master gland of the immune systems. The size of this gland reduces from 250 to 200 grams at birth and then shrinks to around 3 grams by age 60. Scientists are investigating whether the disappearance of the thymus contributes to the aging process by weakening the body's immune system.

Studies have shown that thymic factors are helpful in restoring the immune systems of children born without them as well as rejuvenating the poorly functioning immune systems of the elderly. Thymic hormones may also play a role in stimulating and controlling the production of neurotransmitters and brain and endocrine system hormones, meaning that they may be the "pacemakers" of aging itself, as well as key regulators responsible for immunity.

Box 2-4: Immunological Theory

- Functional capacity of the immune system decreases with age as a result of reduced T-cell function and reduced resistance to infectious diseases.

- The immune system decreases in efficiency with age as evidenced by the age-associated increase in autoimmune disease.

Free Radical Theory

Another example of developmental-genetic theory has to do with free radicals.[40] *Free radical* is a term used to describe any molecule that differs from conventional molecules in that it possesses a free electron, a property that makes it react with other molecules in highly volatile and destructive ways.

In a conventional molecule, the electrical charge is balanced. Electrons and protons come in pairs so that their electrical energies cancel each other out. Atoms that are missing electrons combine with atoms that have extra electrons, creating a stable molecule with evenly paired electrons and a neutral electrical charge.

The free radical on the other hand has an extra negative charge. This unbalanced electrical energy tends to make the free radical attach itself to other molecules as it tries to steal a matching electron to attain electrical equilibrium. Some scientist speak of these free radicals as "promiscuous," breaking up the happy marriages of paired electrons in neighboring molecules in order to steal an electron "partner" for themselves. In doing so, they create free radicals that result in extensive damage at a cellular level.

Free radical activity within the body is not only, or even primarily, negative. Without free radical activity, which creates biochemical electricity, we would not be able to produce energy, maintain immunity, transmit nerve impulses, synthesize hormones, or even contract our muscles. The body's electricity enables us to perform these functions; that electricity comes from the unbalanced electron activity of free radicals.

But free radicals also attack the structure of our cell membranes, creating metabolic waste products, including lipofuscins. An excess of lipofuscins in the body is shown as a darkening of the skin in certain areas, the so-called "aging spots." Lipofuscins, in turn, interfere with the cells' ability to repair and reproduce themselves. They disturb DNA and ribonucleic acid (RNA) synthesis, interfere with synthesis of protein, lower energy levels, prevent the body from building muscle mass, and destroy cellular enzymes needed for vital chemical processes.

This type of free radical damage begins at birth and continues until we die. In our youth, its effects are relatively minor since the body has extensive repair and replacement mechanisms that, in healthy young people, function to keep cells and organs in working order. With age, however, the accumulated effects of free radical damage begin to take their toll. Free radical disruption of cell metabolism is part of what ages our cells; it may also create mutant cells leading ultimately to cancer and death.

Free radicals attack collagen and elastin, the substances that keep our skin moist, smooth, flexible, and elastic. These vital tissues fray and break under the assaults of free radicals, a process particularly noticeable in the face, where folds of skin and deep-cut wrinkles are testaments to the long-term effect of free radical damage.

Another way of looking at free radical changes is to think of it as oxidation, the process of adding oxygen to a substance. Another word for oxidation is rust and, in a sense, our aging process is analogous to the rusting away of a once intact piece of metal. Because forms of oxygen itself are free radicals, our very breathing and our otherwise healthy aerobic exercise generate free radicals that help along the aging process.

Substances that prevent the harmful effects of oxidation are known as antioxidants. Natural antioxidants include vitamin C, vitamin E, and beta carotene, the substance that our body uses to produce vitamin A. Specialists in anti-aging medicine prescribe a host of natural and manufactured antioxidants to help combat the effects of aging.

Another substance that combats free radical damage is known as a free radical scavenger. Free radical scavengers actually seek out free radicals and harmlessly bind them before they can attach themselves to other molecules and/or cause cross-linking. Many vitamins and minerals and other substances fight aging by acting as free radical scavengers.

Age pigments (lipofuscin) are seen at microscopic levels in self-selected tissues of the body, such as nerve and muscle tissue. Lipofuscin is the oxidation product of free radical action on polyunsaturated fatty acids. The rate of accumulation of age pigments is a good index of chronologic age and perhaps one of the few aging phenomena universally demonstrated in mammals. Age pigments as an entity are examples of degenerative change. When accumulated in tissue, they cut off oxygen and nutrient supplies to surrounding areas, causing further degeneration and eventual death of tissue.[41]

There is much support for free radical reactions and their implications in the aging process as well as their probable pathologic effects as a hypothesized cancer-causing and atherosclerosis-causing agent. This is an appealing theory because it provides a mechanism for aging that does not depend on tissue-specific action but is fundamental to all aerobic tissues (see Box 2-5).

Metabolic rate is related directly to free radical generation and inversely to lifespan.[42] It is reasonable to hypothesize that the rate of free radical production is in some way related to lifespan determination or to aging. Proponents of this theory suggest that caloric restriction can increase the mean and maximal lifespan of a species. The notion is that caloric restriction lowers the metabolic rate and therefore decreases the free radical production.

Box 2-5: Free Radical Theory

- Free radicals are highly charged ions whose outer orbits contain an unpaired electron.
- Rate of accumulation of age pigments is a good index of physiologic age. (Aging spots on the skin are examples of free radical degenerative changes.)
- Age pigment accumulation in tissue cuts off the supply of oxygen and nutrients.
- A slower metabolic rate is directly related to free radical generation.

Mitochondrial Theory

The free radical theory is supported by directed experimental observations of mitochondrial aging. Mitochondria are the energy-producing organelles in the cells that are responsible for producing adenosine triphosphate (ATP), our primary source of energy. They produce cell energy by a process that leads to the formation of potentially damaging free radicals. Mitochondria are also one of the easiest targets of free radical injury because they lack most of the defenses found in other parts of the cell. Evidence points to various kinds of accumulated DNA damage over time to be a contributing factor to disease, and new research in mitochondrial repair could play an important part in the fight against aging.[43]

Rate of Living Theory

German physiologist Max Rubner established the relationship among metabolic rate, body size, and longevity in the rate of living theory proposed in 1908. It simply states that we are each born with a limited amount of energy. If we use this energy slowly then our rate of aging is slowed. If the energy is consumed quickly, aging is hastened. Other rate of living theories focus on limiting factors such as the amount of oxygen inhaled or number of heartbeats spent.[44]

Order to Disorder Theory

From the time of conception to sexual maturation, our bodies are undergoing a system of orderliness. We are, as Hayflick states, "[d]irecting most of our energies to fulfilling a genetically determined plan for the orderly production and arrangement of an enormous number and variety of molecules."[27] According to the order to disorder theory, after sexual maturation, these same energies start to diminish in efficiency. Disorder occurs in molecules, causing other molecules to produce errors and so on. These chaotic changes in our cells, tissues, and organs cause aging. Disorderliness varies by individual and this may be the reason why our tissues and organs deteriorate at different rates.[45] In essence, this perspective combines several of the previously presented theories, including the limited number of cell divisions, Hayflick, cross-linkage, and neuroendocrine theories.

Caloric Restriction Theory

Calorie restriction, or energy restriction, is a theory proposed by respected gerontologist Roy Walford. After years of animal experiments and research on longevity, Walford developed a high-nutrient/low-calorie diet demonstrating that "under nutrition with malnutrition" can dramatically retard the functional, if not the chronological, aging process. An individual on this program would lose weight gradually until a point of metabolic efficiency was reached for maximum health and lifespan. Walford stressed the importance of not only the high-low diet but also moderate vitamin and mineral supplements coupled with regular exercise.[46] Walford himself serves as living evidence of the in vivo experiment—that a lifestyle committed to the high-nutrient/low-calorie diet, moderate vitamin and mineral supplementation, and a regular exercise regimen are beneficial. Caloric restriction and its effects on lifespan extension is perhaps one of the most promising probes of the mechanisms of aging. Caloric restriction may exert its effectiveness through the neuroendocrine system. Everitt has shown a striking similarity between dietary restriction and surgical removal of the pituitary gland.[47]

This high-nutrient/low-calorie diet is a result of years of animal in vivo experimentation, exploring longevity and maximum lifespan potential. Walford's caloric restriction program prescribes that an individual gradually lose weight over several years until a point of maximum metabolic efficiency is reached for maximum health and lifespan.[48] Despite more recent reports associating being a little overweight as "healthier" than being underweight, most recent results from the National Institutes of Health Nutrition Committee and the Centers for Disease Control have concluded that weights below those of the population have the greatest longevity, as long as such weights are not associated with diseases. The result of the high-quality but low-caloric diet serves to retard aging in the sense that one would be chronologically old but functionally younger.[48]

The calorie restricted diet influences both aging rate and disease susceptibility. It has been said that the immune system is the pacemaker of aging. Caloric restriction has been shown to affect the immune system. For example, it slows down the immune system's decline and inhibits the increased autoimmune reaction. Furthermore, pilot studies in mice provide supportive evidence that caloric restriction may also slow the decline in DNA repair capacity,[49] as well as affect the generation or persistence of free radicals[50] (see Box 2-6).

Box 2-6: Caloric Restriction Theory

- Caloric restriction can increase the maximal lifespan of a species.
- Caloric restriction lowers metabolic rate and decreases free radical production.
- High-nutrient/low-calorie diet serves to retard aging so one could be chronologically old, but physiologically and functionally younger.
- Caloric restriction influences both the aging process and disease susceptibility by slowing the immune system decline and inhibiting an autoimmune reaction.

Genetic Control Theory

This planned-obsolescence theory focuses on the genetic programming encoded within our DNA. We are born with a unique genetic code, a predetermined tendency to certain types of physical and mental functioning, and that genetic inheritance has a great deal to say about how quickly we age and how long we live. To use a macabre analogy, it's as though each of us comes into the world as a machine that is preprogrammed to self-destruct. Each of us has a biological clock ticking away, set to go off at a particular time, give or take a few years. When that clock goes off, it signals our bodies first to age and then to die.

However, as with all aspects of our genetic inheritance, the timing on this genetic clock is subject to enormous variation, depending on what happens to us as we grow up and on how we actually live (the old "nature vs nurture" debate).

STOCHASTIC THEORIES OF AGING

The second category of theories is described as stochastic theories. *Stochastic* is defined as random occurrences. These theories purport that aging is caused by an accumulation of insults from the environment. The result of these insults is that the organism eventually reaches a level incompatible with life.

Error and Repair Theory

Leslie Orgel suggested that because the "machinery for making protein in cells is so essential, an error in that machinery could be catastrophic."[51] The production of proteins and the reproduction of DNA sometimes is not carried out with accuracy. The body's DNA is so vital that natural repair processes kick in when an "error" is made. The system is incapable of making perfect repairs on these molecules every time; therefore, the accumulation of these flawed molecules can cause diseases and other age changes to occur. If DNA repair processes did not exist, scientists estimate that enough damage would accumulate in cells in 1 year to make them nonfunctional.

The error theory, also known as the error catastrophe theory, was first presented by Orgel in 1963.[51] This theory states that random errors in protein synthesis may occur and the error-containing protein molecule will be turned over. If the error-containing protein is one involved in the synthesis of the genetic material (such as DNA or RNA) or in the protein-synthesizing machinery, then this molecule could cause further replication errors. If this is the case, the number of error-containing proteins expands to result in an "error crisis," which would be incompatible with proper function and life. The theory specifies that "any accident or error in either the machinery or the process of making proteins would cascade into multiple effects"[52] (see Box 2-7).

This continued error in replication of the proteins can be compared to a photocopier, where reproduction of a single page continues through the life of the copier without ever changing the toner or cleaning the glass. Ultimately, the copies get fuzzier and less distinct, until the copies are unreadable.

Box 2-7: **Error Theory**

- Random errors in protein synthesis may occur and the error-containing protein molecule will be replicated.
- Any error or accident in the machinery or the process of making proteins would cascade and accelerate aging.

Redundant DNA Theory

Like the errors and repairs theory, the redundant DNA theory blames errors accumulating in genes for age changes. But as these errors accumulate, this theory also blames reserve genetic sequences of identical DNA that take over until the system is worn out. Different species' lifespans may be a function of the degree of these repeated gene sequences.[53]

Somatic or Gene Mutation Theory

One of the most prominent theories in the stochastic theories category is the somatic mutation theory of aging.[54] This theory emerged following World War II as a result of increased research in the area of radiation biology. The theory hypothesizes that mutations or genetic damage of the cells result from radiation and that radiomimetic agents accumulate and eventually create functional failure and ultimately death of the organism. The somatic mutation theory is based on the scientific observation that exposure to ionizing radiation shortens the lifespan[55] (see Box 2-8).

In the 1940s, scientists investigated the role of mutations with radiation exposure and aging. It was hypothesized that mutations would occur in the genes and disrupt the processes fundamental to life. Evidence supporting this idea came from experiments with radiation. It was observed that radiation not only increased animals' gene mutation but it also accelerated their aging process as well. However, later studies showed that radiation-induced changes were only mimicking age-related changes. This hypothesis further diminished in validity when experiments with moderate amounts of radiation actually increased the lifespan of rats.[56]

Box 2-8: **Somatic Mutation Theory**

- Mutations, or genetic damage of the cells, result from radiation.
- Accumulation of radioactive agents eventually creates functional failure and the death of an organism.
- Exposure to ionizing radiation shortens lifespan.

Cross-Linkage Theory

Developmental aging and cross-linking were first proposed in 1942 by Johan Bjorksten. He applied this theory to aging diseases such as sclerosis, a declining immune system, and the most obvious example of cross-linking, loss of elasticity in the skin. Collagen is one of the most common proteins found in the skin, tendons, ligaments, bone, and cartilage. Collagen protein can be compared to the legs of a ladder with very few rungs. Each protein is connected to its neighbors by other rungs forming a cross-link. In young people there are few cross-links and the ladders are free to move up and down. The collagen stays soft and pliable. With age, however, the number of cross-links increases, making the skin less soft and pliable. It is thought that as these cross-links increase, the skin becomes denser and begins to obstruct the passage of nutrients and waste between cells. This poor exchange decreases the health of the skin and increases its vulnerability to injury (see Box 2-9).

This theory is based on the observation of cross-linking in macromolecules such as protein molecules found in collagen and elastin fibers. Rather than maintaining a parallel alignment of collagen or elastin fibers, the fibers start to cross-hatch much like a Chinese finger puzzle. This increases the fibers' density restricting nutrition and hydration, and results in a decreased flexibility of the tissues. Although cross-linking is not restricted to proteins, most experimental research has been on collagen and elastin because these molecules are accessible, do not readily turn over, and show increased cross-linking with age. Bjorksten[57] looked at large reactive protein molecules within the body (such as collagen, elastin, and DNA molecules), and surmised that their cross-linkage was responsible for secondary and tertiary causes of aging because it restricted the absorption of nutrients and water, impeded the removal of waste products, and ultimately restricted activity of the entire organism. Bjorksten implies that cross-linking is the primary cause of sclerosis, failure of the immune system, and loss of elasticity in all the tissues of the body. Aging of the skin is perhaps the most obvious example of cross-linking and exposure to solar radiation promotes cross-linkage. Loss of flexibility of the aging body was thought to be due to the cross-linking of tendon, ligament, and muscle tissue fibers. We now see active aging individuals remain more flexible despite constant exposure to cross-linking agents (eg, unsaturated fats, polyvalent metal ions, aluminum, magnesium, zinc, radiation) and few if any researchers view collagen cross-linking as the primary underlying cause of aging as long as an individual remains active.[58]

Cross-linking also appears to occur when older immune systems are incapable of cleaning out excess glucose molecules in the blood. These sugar molecules react with proteins causing cross-links and the formation of destructive free radicals. Scientists once thought inflexibility of the body with age was due to cross-linking of tendon, bone, and muscle tissue. However, people who lead a more active lifestyle and follow a good diet seem to inhibit or delay the cross-linking process.

Box 2-9: Cross-Linkage Theory

- Cross-linking in protein molecules found in collagen and elastin fibers decreases flexibility of tissues.

- Increased fiber density restricts nutrients and hydration at the cellular level.

A Newer Theory—The Telomerase Theory of Aging

A new theory of aging that holds many promising possibilities for the field of anti-aging medicine is the *telomerase* theory of aging. This theory was born from the surge of technological breakthroughs in genetics and genetic engineering. First discovered by a group of scientists in Menlo Park, California, *telomeres* are sequences of nucleic acids extending from the ends of chromosomes. Telomeres act to maintain the integrity of our chromosomes. Every time our cells divide, telomeres are shortened, leading to cellular damage and cellular death associated with aging.

Scientists discovered that the key element in rebuilding our disappearing telomeres is the "immortalizing" enzyme telomerase, an enzyme found only in germ cells and cancer cells. Telomerase appears to repair and replace telomeres, manipulating the "clocking" mechanism that controls the lifespan of dividing cells. Future development of telomerase inhibitors may be able to stop cancer cells from dividing and presumably may convert them back into normal cells.

CONCLUSION

Despite the monumental progress in aging research, there has yet to be a unanimous vote on one specific theory of aging. Most of these theories have been disputed by scientists over and over again and many of them, as Hans Kugler, editor of the *Journal of Longevity Research*, said, "...are dying of old age." Table 2-2 provides a summary of the theories presented in this chapter. Age-related changes do not occur uniformly in individuals; rather, they are controlled jointly by genetic and environmental factors, which further heightens the difficulty of finding a universal theory. What is universal is that we are all involved in a global aging phenomenon. Through theoretical gerontology and anti-aging medicine, we may eventually discover there is no limit to human lifespan.

Table 2-2

SUMMARY OF THEORIES ON AGING

AGING THEORY	DESCRIPTION
Developmental-Genetic	
Hayflick Limit Theory	Limited number of cellular divisions; genetically determined based on cell type
Waste Accumulation Theory	Lipofuscin accumulates; binds fat in cells to protein; decreases metabolism
Limited Number of Cell Divisions Theory	Genetic predisposition to the number of times a cell can divide; similar to Hayflick Limit; adds environmental influence and wear and tear
Wear and Tear Theory	Poor hydration and lubrication; cells and tissues wear out
Programmed Senescence	Aging is the result of the sequential switching on and off of certain genes
Neuroendocrine Theory	Biological clocks act through hormones to control the pace of aging
Immunological Theory	A programmed decline in immune system functions leads to an increased vulnerability to infectious disease and thus aging and death
Free Radical Theory	Accumulated damage caused by oxygen radicals causes cells, and eventually organs, to stop functioning
Mitochondrial Theory	Free radical injury; DNA damage; decreased energy production
Rate of Living Theory	The greater an organism's rate of oxygen basal metabolism, the shorter its lifespan
Order to Disorder Theory	Disorder of production and arrangement of cells over time
Caloric Restriction Theory	Decreased weight associated with greatest longevity; nutrient rich/low caloric diet retards aging process
Genetic Control Theory	Genetic programming encoded in our DNA; unique genetic code/fingerprint
Telomerase Theory	Shortening of telomeres leads to cellular damage and eventual death
Nongenetic (Stochastic)	
Error and Repair Theory	Environmental damage to DNA over time results in faulty replication of cells
Error Catastrophe Theory	Associated with illness or injury; damage to mechanisms that synthesize proteins results in faulty proteins that accumulate to a level that causes catastrophic damage to cells, tissues, and organs
Redundant DNA Theory	Errors accumulating in genes; passed on from generation to generation (survival of the fittest)
Somatic or Gene Mutation Theory	Genetic mutations occur and accumulate with increasing age, causing cells to deteriorate and malfunction; damage of cells from radioactive and radiomimetic agents
Cross-Linkage Theory	An accumulation of cross-linked proteins damage cells and tissues, slowing down bodily processes; increasing inelasticity leads to poor nutrition and waste removal

Two major categories of scientific theories on aging exist: the genetic-based and the nongenetic-based (stochastic) theories. Gerontology has evolved into a sophisticated scientific realm enabling us to distinguish between logical, plausible explanations and idealistic searches for the fountain of eternal youth. But, the question still remains: what causes us to age?

PEARLS

- Aging research began in the early 1900s, and the 2 major groups of aging theories that have evolved are the developmental-genetic theories and the environmental-stochastic theories.

- Hayflick and Moorehead conducted a landmark study that showed that, in culture, human fibroblasts have a limited lifespan.

- Theoretical gerontology uses these fundamental considerations: (1) aging is developmental; (2) old age is a gift of modern technology; (3) we must differentiate normal vs pathological aging; and (4) there is not an universally accepted theory of aging.

- Neuroendocrine and hormonal theory regards functional decrements in neurons and their associated hormones as central to the aging process.

- Immunological theory states that the immune system declines with age.

- According to free radical theory, free radicals accumulate with age and cause destruction to important biological structures.

- Caloric restriction theory prescribes that an individual gradually loses weight until a point of maximum metabolic efficiency is reached for maximum health and lifespan.

- The error theory specifies that any error in the process of making proteins will cascade into multiple effects.

- Somatic mutation theory hypothesizes that genetic damage will result from radiation, and that radiometric agents accumulate and create functional failure and death of the organism.

- In the cross-linkage theory, cross-linkage of proteins in collagen and elastin fibers is responsible for tissue aging.

REFERENCES

1. Freeman JT. *Aging, Its History and Literature.* New York: Human Science Press; 1979.

2. Comfort A. *The Biology of Senescence.* 3rd ed. New York: Elsevier; 1979.

3. Pearl R. *The Rate of Living.* New York: Vropfu; 1928.

4. Yin D, Chen K. The essential mechanisms of aging: irreparable damage accumulation of biochemical side-reactions. *Exp Gerontol.* 2005;40:455-465.

5. Warthin AS. *Old Age, the Major Revolution: The Philosophy and Pathology of the Aging Process.* New York: Hoeber; 1929.

6. Weissman A. *Uber die dauer des lebens.* Jena, Germany: 1882.

7. Rubner M. *Das problem der lebensdaver und seine beziebungen zum wachstum und ernabrung.* Munich: Oldenbourg; 1908.

8. Barzilai N, Rossetti L, Lipton RB. Einstein's Institute for Aging Research: collaborative and programmatic approaches in the search for successful aging. *Exp Gerontol.* 2004;39:151-157.

9. Gavrilov LA, Gavrilov NS. Evolutionalry theories of aging and longevity. *Scientific World Journal.* 2002;2:339-356.

10. Lee RD. Rethinking the evolutionary theory of aging: transfers, not births, shape senescence in social species. *Proc Natl Acad Sci USA.* 2003;100:9637-9642.

11. Hayflick L, Moorehead PS. The serial cultivation of human diploid all strains. *Exp Cell Res.* 1961;25:585-593.

12. Kriete A. Biomarkers of aging: combinatorial or system model? *Sci Aging Knowledge Environ.* 2006;2006:pe1.

13. Strehler BL. *Time, Cells and Aging.* 2nd ed. New York: Academic; 1977.

14. Cristofalo VJ. Overview of biological mechanism of aging. *Ann Review Gerontol Geriatr* 1991;6:1-22.

15. Sun XJ, Lu QC, Cai Y. Effect of cholecystokinin on experimental neuronal aging. *World J Gastroenterol.* 2005;11:551-556.

16. Shock NW. Longitudinal studies of aging in human. In: Finch CE, Schneider EL, eds. *Handbook of the Biology of Aging.* New York: Van Nostrand Reinhold; 1985:721-739.

17. Miller RA. Accelerated aging: a primrose path to insight? *Aging Cell.* 2004;3:47-51.

18. Adelman RC. Hormone interaction during aging. In: Schimke RT, ed. *Biological Mechanisms in Aging.* Washington, DC: US Dept of Health and Human Services; 1980:31-47.

19. Rauser CL, Mueller LD, Rose MR. The evolution of late life. *Ageing Res Rev.* 2006;5:14-32.

20. Fries I, Crapo L. *Vitality and Aging.* San Francisco: WH Freeman; 1981.

21. Hayflick L. *Senescence and cultured cells.* In: Shock N, ed. *Perspectives in Experimental Gerontology.* Springfield, IL: Charles C Thomas; 1966.

22. Hamet P, Tremblay J. Genes of aging. *Metabolism.* 2003;52(suppl 2):5-9.

23. Martin GM, Turker M. Genetics of human disease, longevity and aging. In: Hazzard EG, ed. *Textbook of Genetic Medicine.* New York: McGraw-Hill; 1990.

24. Kallman JF, Jarvik LF. Twin data on genetic variations in resistance to tuberculosis. In: Gedda L, ed. *Genetica della tuberculosi e dei tumori.* Rome: Gregorio Mendel; 1957:15-41.

25. Jarvik LF. Survival trends in a senescent twin population. *Am J Hum Genet.* 1960;12:170-181.

26. Effros RB. From Hayflick to Walford: the role of T cell replicative senescence in human aging. *Exp Gerontol.* 2004;39:885-890.

27. Hayflick L, Moorehead PS. The serial cultivation of human diploid all strains. *Exp Cell Res.* 1961;25:585-593.

28. Gray DA, Woulfe J. Lipofusion and aging: a matter of toxic waste. *Sci Aging Knowledge Environ.* 2005:re1.

29. Wright WE, Shay JW. Historical claims and current interpretations of replicative aging. *Nat Biotechnol.* 2002;20:682-688.

30. Goldsmith TC. Aging as an evolved characteristic–Weismann's Theory reconsidered. *Med Hypotheses*. 2004;62:304-308.

31. Walford RL, Weindruch RH, Gottesman SRS, Tam CF. *Immunopathology of aging*. In: Eisdorfer C, ed. *Annu Rev Gerontol & Geriatr*. vol. 2. New York: Springer; 1981.

32. Brody H, Jayashankar N. Anatomical changes in the nervous system. In: Finch CE, Hayflick L, eds. *Handbook of the Biology of Aging*. New York: Van Nostrand Reinhold; 1977:17-29.

33. Everitt AV. The hypothalamic pituitary control of aging and age-related pathology. *Exp Gerontol*. 1973;8:265-269.

34. Kelly KM, Nadon NL, Morrison JH, Thibault O, Barnes CA, Blalock EM. The neurobiology of aging. *Epilepsy Res*. 2006;68(suppl 1):S5-S20.

35. Rosenfeld A. Are we programmed to die? *Sat Rev*. 1976; 10:10.

36. Zarchin N, Meilin S, Rifkind J, Mayevsky A. Effect of aging on brain energy-metabolism. *Comp Biochem Physiol A Mol Integr Physiol*. 2002;132:117-120.

37. Walford RL. Immunopathology of aging. In: Eisdorfer C, ed. *Annu Rev Gerontol & Geriatr*. vol. 2. New York Springer; 1981.

38. Walford RL. *The Immunologic Theory of Aging*. Copenhagen: Munksgaard. 1969.

39. Hawley LC, Cacioppo JT. Stress and the aging immune system. *Brain Behav Immun*. 2004;18:114-119.

40. Harmon D. Aging: a theory based on free radical and radiation chemistry. *J Gerontol*. 1956;11:298-311.

41. Harmon D. Prolongation of life: roles of free radical reactions in aging. *J Am Geriatr Soc*. 1969;17:721-723.

42. Harmon D. The aging process. *Proc Nat Acad Sci USA*. 1981;78:7124-7141.

43. Wei YH, Ma YS, Lee LC, Lee CF, Lu CY. Mitochondrial theory of aging matures–roles of mtDNA mutation and oxidative stress in human aging. *Zhonghua Yi Xue Za Zhi* (English translation). 2001;64:259-270.

44. Noveoseltseua VN, Noveoseltseua J, YaShin AL. A homeostatic model of oxidative damage explains paradoxes in earlier aging experiments. *Biogerontology*. 2001;2:127-138.

45. Gavrilov LA, Gavrilov NS. The reliability of theories of aging and longevity. *J Theor Biol*. 2001;213:527-545.

46. Walford RL, Harris S, and Weindruch R. Dietary restriction and aging: historical phases, mechanisms and current directions. *J Nutr*. 1987;117:1650-1654.

47. Everitt AV. The effects of hypophysectomy and continuous food restriction, begun at ages 70 and 400 days, on collagen aging, proteinuria, incidence of pathology and longevity in the male rat. *Mech Aging Dev*. 1980;12:161-169.

48. Walford RL. *The 120-Year Diet*. New York: Pocket Books; 1986.

49. Weindruch R, Chia D, Barnett EV, and Walford RL. Dietary restriction in mice beginning at 1 year of age: effects in serum immune complex levels. *Age*. 1982;5:111-112.

50. Harmon D. Free radical theory of aging: role of free radicals in the origination and evaluation of life, aging, and disease processes. In: Johnson JE, Walford RL, Harmon D, Miguel, eds. *Free Radicals, Aging, and Degenerative Diseases*. New York: Liss; 1986:3-50.

51. Orgel LE. The maintenance of the accuracy of protein synthesis and its relevance to aging. *Proc Nat Acad Sci USA*. 1963;49:517-531.

52. Sonneborn T: The origin, evolution, nature and causes of aging. In: Behnke J, Fince C, Moment G, eds. *The Biology of Aging*. New York: Plenum Press; 1979:341.

53. Zhang Y, McEwen AE, Crothers DM, Levene SD. Statistical-mechanical theory of DNA looping. *Biophys J*. 2006;90:1903-1912.

54. Failla G. The aging process and carcinogenesis. *Ann NY Acad Sci*. 1958;71:1124-1130.

55. Szilard L. On the nature of the aging process. *Proc Nat Acad Sci USA*. 1959;45:30-51.

56. Koehn M. Embracing the aging process. *J Christ Nurs*. 2005;22:20-24.

57. Bjorksten J. Crosslinkage and the aging process. In: Rockstein M, ed. *Theoretical Aspects of Aging*. New York: Academic; 1974:43-56.

58. Bjorksten J. The crosslinkage theory of aging: clinical implications. *Compr Ther*. 1976;2:65.

Age-Related Changes in Anatomy, Physiology, and Function

Aging is a progressive and cumulative process involving a number of biological, anatomical, physiological, and functional changes that occur over time. Some of these changes that were once thought to be "normal" aging have turned out to be the result of disease. The longer we live, the greater the chances of acquiring some disease that will impact normal functioning. Recent research clearly shows that activity, proper nutrition and hydration, a positive attitude, and reduction of stress result in a longer and healthier life.[1]

Most of the changes that occur with aging have no impact on normal functioning, although they become apparent when the body is placed under stress, such as an acute illness or physical exertion. For example, the maximum heart rate achievable by older adults is lower than that of younger adults; the resting pulse, however, would not show this change.[2]

It is important to be able to recognize the changes of normal aging vs the effects of disease or inactivity. Untreated disease can result in excess disability and reduce the quality of life of individuals. In this chapter, the changes in the body that occur with aging will be identified and described. Healthy aging is an issue of increasing importance as the size of the older population continues to grow. Poor health in later life is not inevitable.[3] Much of the illness and disability associated with aging is related to inactivity and other modifiable lifestyle factors that are present throughout life.

Although we have more wrinkles, more gray hair, and stiffer arteries, the normal changes of aging are unlikely to kill us. No one dies only of old age per se; infections or other diseases, most of which might not be life threatening in youth, are the usual cause of death in old age. This chapter covers changes in anatomy, physiology, and function that occur with aging. It reviews each body system and discusses the consequences of what is considered *normal aging*, the wearing and slowing of systems with the passage of time.

AGING: FUNCTIONAL RESULTS

While the process of aging is very complex, this survey of the body's systems will be based on the functional changes that the physical therapist assistant (PTA) is likely to see in the clinic. Some changes in function go hand in hand with anatomical or structural changes. Skeletal muscle is one such example; while muscle mass decreases as muscle fibers are lost, the remaining muscle mass is capable of maintaining and actually increasing muscle strength and stability. In some aging processes there are no anatomic losses, but rather a reduction in physiological efficiency. For example, although the structural integrity of the nerves is maintained, there is a reduced conduction velocity in aging nerve fibers that results in slower reactions when balance is lost.

Homeostasis and Aging

Normal changes of aging reduce the capacity to regain *homeostasis*, a concept describing the body's

Bottomley J. *Geriatric Rehabilitation: A Textbook for the Physical Therapist Assistant* (pp 43-64).
© 2010 SLACK Incorporated

ability to maintain balance.[4] This ability to maintain an internal balance enables humans to survive in many environments and to withstand many biological and physiological challenges. Perhaps the single most important age-related change is the diminishing ability of the body to respond to physical and emotional stress and return to the pre-stress level, especially when the individual is deconditioned due to a sedentary lifestyle.[5] Contracting the flu, for example, may be experienced more intensely by an elder, frequently resulting in dehydration, electrolyte imbalances, and a loss in the ability to resume activities of daily living (ADL).

Different Rates of Aging

It is important to keep in mind that individuals will age at different rates. Everyone ages differently compared to others (eg, comparing twins) and the rate of aging can vary markedly within individuals. Age-related changes in one organ system are not predictive of changes in other systems in the same person. For example, an individual may have cataracts that severely restrict vision and yet have excellent heart function. There is a tremendous diversity among individuals of similar chronological age. A physically fit 70 year old can have the functional capacity of a 40 year old, while a 50 year old who has poor nutritional status or a sedentary lifestyle may function as if he or she was several decades older than 70.

THE BASICS

Cellular Function

General changes in the basic unit—each cell—of the body have been found to occur with the aging process. This is related to lower levels of activity, poorer nutrition, and dehydration, which result in a decrease in physiological efficiency at the cellular level. Aging causes functional changes in cells. For example, the rate at which cells multiply tends to slow down as we age. Certain cells that are important for our immune system to work properly (called T-cell lymphocytes) also decrease with age. As a result, these changes diminish the efficiency of our responses to environmental stresses. For example, exposure to sunlight, extreme heat and toxins, inadequate oxygen, and poor nutrition may result in illness with a significantly lower capacity to regain a healthy state again.[6]

Cells can be classified in many different ways. For our purposes, cells will be classified as *mitotic*, which are cells capable of reproductive division (eg, skin cells, blood cells) and as *postmitotic* (eg, nerve cells, muscle cells), which are not capable of division (refer to Table 2-1). This is an important distinction as we review each system of the body.

Age interferes with an important process called *apoptosis*, which programs cells to self-destruct or die after multiplying a genetically determined number of times (postmitotic) or die under certain conditions (both mitotic and postmitotic). This process is necessary for tissues to remain healthy, and it is especially important in slowing down immune responses once an infection has been cleared.[7]

Different diseases (discussed further in Chapter 4) can affect this process in different ways. For example, cancer results in a loss of apoptosis; the cancer cells continue to multiply and invade or take over surrounding tissue, instead of dying as originally programmed. Other diseases may cause cells to die too early. In Alzheimer's disease for instance, a substance called amyloid (a hard protein deposit) builds up and causes the early death of brain cells through tissue degeneration. This deposit blocks connections (synapses) between one area of the brain and another, resulting in a progressive loss of memory and other vital brain functions.

Body Composition

The most notable of aging changes occurs with the body's fat and water content. Extracellular water remains constant while intracellular water decreases. Dehydration is a common consequence of activity, medications, or ambient room temperature and leads to poor homeostasis.

In general, there is a decrease in lean muscle mass and an increase and redistribution of fat. The proportion of the body that is made up of fat doubles between the age of 25 and 65. Increases in body fat occur until middle age, stabilizes until later life, then decreases. In men, body weight generally increases until their mid-50s, stabilizes, and then decreases, with a loss of weight at a faster pace in their late 60s and 70s. In women, body weight increases until their late 60s, stabilizes, and then decreases at a rate significantly slower than that of men; the distribution of fat also shifts. Fat moves from just beneath the skin to surrounding deeper parts of the body. Women are more likely to store it in the lower body (eg, hips and thighs). Men tend to increase fat concentration in the abdominal area.[8]

Clinically, it is important to note that people who live in less technologically developed societies do not show this pattern of weight change. Observation of these populations indicates that they do not slow down as they age; they stay engaged in functional activities (both basic and instrumental ADL) and tend to maintain higher activity levels right up until the very end of their lives. They also tend to eat low-fat, high-nutrient diets, many maintaining their own gardens.[9] This suggests that reduced physical activity and changes in eating habits may be causes of the change in body weight in the inactive elderly—rather than the aging process.

Exercise programs may prevent or reverse much of the proportional decrease in muscle mass and increase in total body fat. Attention to nutritional planning and level of activity requires closer attention. The change in body composition also has an important effect on how the body handles various drugs. For example, when our body fat increases, drugs that are dissolved in fatty tissues remain in the body much longer than when our body was younger and more muscular.

Connective Tissue Changes

Connective tissue changes with age significantly impact functional abilities. Collagen and elastin are a part of every body structure and system. In younger individuals, collagen fibers are strong and flexible, and elastin fibers are elastic and very agile. Collagen and elastin fibers are arranged in organized bundles that form structure in the body. With age and inactivity, the collagen and elastin structures become more stiff and dense from accumulated waste products and dehydration. The cell wall becomes thicker and less porous. This increased density impairs molecular movement of nutrients and wastes at the cellular level. Dehydration and inadequate lubrication cause stiffening and inelasticity, which results in wear and tear of tissues.[10]

Collagen is the building block of fibrous connective tissue including bone, tendon, ligament, and cartilage. Generally, the flexibility of connective tissue in older persons is less than that of younger individuals. It becomes cross-linked due to inactivity and poor nutrition. The clinical significance is increased cross-linking as seen in contractures. Older people get "stuck" in the physical positions they maintain the most. Because collagen stiffens, elders are simply unable to move their bodies as much, or in as many ways, as they did when they were younger.[11] For instance, if older individuals spend a great deal of time in the seated position, they often get hip and knee flexion contractures and the extensor muscles at those joints lose strength. These bonds are strong and cannot often be broken by mechanical stretching.

Elastin molecules join together in an end-to-end and branching manner to form a lattice-like network, which gives elastin its ability to return to its original length after being stretched. There is a reduction in the amount of elastin in the skin, walls of the arteries, and the bronchial tree (branching of the respiratory system into the lobes of each lung) with age.[12] The result is inelasticity of these tissues. If the elastin fibers are overstretched to the point of tearing, scarring occurs, which further decreases the elasticity of the tissues.

The presence of *glycoproteins* outside the cell produces osmotic force. *Osmosis* is the diffusion of fluid through a semi-permeable membrane, such as a living cell wall. Osmosis is important in attracting nutrients and fluid into the tissues. Glycoproteins are produced at rest (ie, during nonweight-bearing activity).[13] The higher metabolic rate produced by exercise and activity results in higher glycoprotein levels and healthier tissues. The production and release of glycoproteins is reduced with prolonged inactivity (bed rest) and with age. As a result, it becomes increasingly difficult for the tissues to maintain a normal nutritional and fluid balance. Poorly nourished tissues and dehydration are commonly found in the tissues of sedentary elderly individuals.

Hyaluronic acid helps to regulate the viscosity of tissues by lubricating structures of the cell[14] (eg, like oil in a machine or an engine). This substance helps to decrease the friction between cellular components during movement. Hyaluronic acid is produced during weight-bearing and activity. There is a reduction in the amount of hyaluronic acid associated with inactivity and age, reducing the ease of movement of the connective tissues.[15] With poor lubrication, tissue degradation occurs due to wear and tear. Exercise becomes particularly important for maintaining the lubrication of tissues. Inactivity will affect the production of hyaluronic acid-producing tissue restrictions,[16] resulting in decreased functional mobility and pliability of the tissues in the muscles and joints.

Contractile proteins provide waste removal within the tissues. This substance provides removal of waste products or debris and enhances mobility within the tissue spaces. Contractile proteins are not needed as much in individuals with high levels of exercise and activity,[17] as circulation and muscle contractions are enough to remove the trash without them. Production of contractile proteins is increased in those who are inactive and/or immobile. For instance, more contractile proteins are found in the tissues surrounding the shoulder with shoulder-hand syndrome or in tissues affected by chronic pathologies that prohibit normal movement, such as stroke or Parkinson's disease. Inactivity results in soft tissue restrictions and contractures.

The importance of activity for the elderly cannot be overstressed. Anything above rest is enough to prevent the accumulation of contractile proteins.

Cartilage Changes

Hyaline cartilage is found in the joints as well as the nose and the rings of the respiratory passages. *Elastic cartilage* is found in parts of the larynx and the outer ear. *Articular cartilage* is found between each articular joint surface of the skeletal system. Cartilage tends to dehydrate, become stiff, and thin out in weight-bearing areas. These changes occur more rapidly in an individual who is poorly hydrated and poorly nourished. Inadequate exercise or not maintaining a balance between rest and activity will also speed up the breakdown of cartilage.[18]

Cartilage has no direct blood supply. Adjacent bones and synovial fluid provide nutrients to the cartilage. Glycoprotein produces an osmotic force providing nutrients necessary for normal metabolism within the cartilage.

In synovial joints, the articular surfaces are covered by hyaline cartilage. Lubrication at the interface of the hyaline cartilage is provided by the secretion of hyaluronic acid during weight bearing.[16] This "oils" the joints by forming a viscous layer covering over the cartilage.[19] Nutrients enter the cartilage at rest, and fluid and nutrient substances are squeezed out with weight bearing, which is why a balance between rest and exercise is needed for joint health. The movement of nutritional and waste substances in and out of the cartilage could enhance the health of the cartilage.[20] Degenerative changes of the cartilage are not reversible and rehabilitation efforts need to be directed toward regular compression and release of compression in the aging joint. Normal weight-bearing exercises are recommended to maintain cartilaginous health. If an elder is unable to ambulate, providing weight-bearing forces through approximation, or for example, the use of a tilt table, can be very helpful in preserving the viability of the joints. While tilt tables are often put into storage in elder care facilities, they can play a remarkably important role in the conservative treatment of older individuals.

Since connective tissue exists everywhere in the body, the effects of aging of these tissues can be widespread. Increased rigidity of tissues results in a greater amount of energy expenditure during movement. As connective tissues progressively tighten, there is a point of no return when the force needed to produce a stretch in a tissue could result in fraying and tearing. Skin becomes less elastic and more wrinkled. Lungs lose elasticity, arteries become more rigid, and the heart becomes less distensible. Joints become stiff while decreased nourishment and hydration in the intervertebral discs and extremity joints results in reduced height. With less activity, cellular repair, nutrition, and waste removal are impaired. Other effects of connective tissue changes will be discussed further below as various systems are reviewed.

Muscle Changes

Quantitatively, all muscle measures—strength, endurance, flexibility, and speed of contraction—decline with age. With aging there is a decrease in the number of active functional units (ie, motor units or muscle fibers) and a loss in concentration of specific enzymes or fiber types. A decrease in conduction velocity and synaptic transmission impacts the speed and strength of muscle contraction. Central nervous system (CNS) changes (discussed later in this chapter) will affect muscle tone and sensory input to the periphery and alter the production of neuroendocrines. All of these factors will affect muscle function.

Normal aging in humans is associated with a progressive decrease in skeletal muscle mass and strength, referred to as *sarcopenia*, which contributes to frailty and falls. Muscle mass declines with aging, especially in the absence of exercise.[21] As we age, our muscles generally decrease in strength, endurance, speed of contraction, size, and weight. Typically, we lose about 23% of our muscle mass by age 80, as both the number and size of muscle fibers decrease. The greatest loss is in the fast type II fiber (phasic fiber). As these are the muscle fibers that contract quickly in response to balance perturbation, the decrease in type II fibers has a significant impact on function and safety. Type I fibers (core stabilizers) are relatively stable, but proportionally increase when compared to the type II fibers. Type II fibers also provide the "bulk" in a muscle, so as they are lost, an older person tends to look like he or she is atrophying.[22]

Several factors may be occurring simultaneously during this process. Loss of strength, seen as a decrease in muscle hypertrophy and changes in muscle function, is a result of a complex interaction of factors. For instance, there is a reduced ability of the cardiovascular system to deliver oxygen and nutrients to working muscles.[23] It is estimated that 20% to 40% of maximal strength is lost by the age of 65 in nonexercising adults. Clinically, it is apparent that aging affects certain muscles more than others. For example, flexor muscles of lower extremities show age-related changes relatively early compared to other muscle groups.[24] Proximal muscles of the lower extremity and trunk, for example, iliopsoas and gluteus medius, tend to be affected prior to distal musculature. These changes are the result of less time spent walking and moving around for functional activities and more time spent sitting. Balance, posture, and functional abilities, for tasks such as getting up from a seated position or standing erectly, are affected.

These muscle changes may be more the result of inactivity, poor nutrition, and chronic illness or disease than the result of aging per se.[25] Sedentary lifestyles exacerbate the aging of the musculoskeletal system. Movement dysfunction due to pathological conditions can also speed this loss. These changes can often been worsened or exacerbated by changes in vision, peripheral and central synaptic nerve abilities, motivation, musculoskeletal disorders (such as osteoarthritis), or structural imbalances caused by tonal changes (such as in stroke or other neurological syndromes and nutritional deficits).

Skeletal Changes

Bone loss appears to be a normal aging process and has been characterized by a decreased bone mineral composition, an enlarged medullary cavity, a normal mineral composition, and biochemical abnormalities in plasma and urine. Because structural changes occur in ligaments, joints, and bones, it is important to keep in mind that the age of onset and rate of bone loss depends on nutrition, exercise, gender, and type of bone. Nearly 90% of adult skeletal mass is formed by the end of the teenage years.[26] The rate of bone loss is about 1% per year for women starting between ages 30 and 35 and for men between ages 50 and 55.

Although bone loss occurs normally as we age, osteoporosis is not an inevitable consequence of aging. Osteoporosis has been described as a "pediatric disease with geriatric consequences due to the fact that osteoporosis begins early, often due to poor nutrition, and exacerbates as one ages."[27] Prevention must begin early to give the individual a strong foundation of bone mass. Once peak bone mass is reached, exercise and nutrition will assist in maintaining this mass. If bone mass is lost, it is much more difficult to regain. The decrease in muscle bulk and strength increase the rate of loss of bone mass. The tugging of muscle on bone enhances bone build-up. Regular exercise helps to slow the process of bone loss and muscle mass, thus enhancing the overall health of the musculoskeletal system.[27] The skeletal system functions to support, protect, and shape the body. Additionally, bone has the metabolic functions of blood cell production, the storage of calcium, and a role in acid-base balance (see Box 3-1).

The appearance of an older person typically changes as we age. We lose height due to:

- Loss of bone mass
- Changes in the shape of vertebrae (the bones of the spine) and posture
- A forward bending of the spine
- Compression of the discs between the vertebrae
- Increased flexion of the hips and knees
- Decreased joint space in the extremities and spine
- Flattening of the arches in the feet.

The most commonly known age-related change involving bone is calcium availability and absorption leading to loss of mass and density. Bone density is lost from within by a process termed *reabsorption*. As we grow older, an imbalance occurs between *osteoblast* activity (bone buildup) and *osteoclast* activity (bone breakdown). Osteoclast activity proves to be stronger. A decline in circulating levels of activated vitamin D_3 occurs with age.[28] This causes less calcium to be absorbed from the gut and more calcium to be absorbed from the bones to meet the other body needs (ie, heart contraction, muscle contraction, nerve impulse, etc).

Box 3-1: Musculoskeletal Changes with Aging

- Muscle mass and strength decreases at a rate of about 30% between the ages of 60 and 90.
- Change occurs in muscle fiber type, both type I and type II. Type II fibers decrease by about 50%.
- There is a change in the clear differentiation of fiber type.
- There is a decrease in recruitment of motor units.
- There is a decrease in the speed of muscle contraction and movement.
- There is a decrease in tensile strength of bone (eg, greater than 30% of women over age 65 have osteoporosis).
- Females lose about 30% of bone mass by age 70; males lose about 15% by age 70.
- Joint flexibility is reduced by 25% to 30% in individuals over the age of 70.
- There is a decrease in enzymatic activity, cell count, and metabolic substrates in cartilage (ie, collagen fibers increase their cross-linking and result in an increase in soft tissue density).

CARDIOVASCULAR CHANGES WITH AGE

Cellular Changes

The cardiovascular system includes the heart, which pumps the blood throughout the body and the network of vessels through which the blood is transported. The changes that normally occur in the cardiovascular system with aging do not significantly limit the normal work capacity of the heart. Most of the changes that cause clinically significant declines in cardiovascular function are the result of disease.

As we age, the heart muscle becomes stiffer and may increase slightly in size. Despite this increase in heart size, the amount of blood that the chamber can hold may actually decrease because of the heart wall's thickness. The heart shows a slight increase in the thickness of the left ventricular wall with age. The elastic tissue, fat, and collagen content of the myocardium (the middle and thickest layer of the heart wall) shows only a slight increase in end-stage aging and small areas of fibrosis in the myocardium show an age-related increase. There is a thickening of the endocardium (innermost layer of tissue that lines the chambers of the heart) and valves due to an increase in the density (cross-linking) of the tissue. As a result of mechanical stresses induced by repeated contact, nodular thickenings are often noted to form along the line of closure in the atrioventricular valves.[29] Stiffening of the arterial tree alters afterload and left ventricular shape and, although resting left ventricular systolic function is maintained, left ventricular diastolic function changes substantially.[30]

The maximum heart rate obtainable (the highest rate at which your heart can pump) decreases even among the most fit older athlete. Heart rate response is usually not affected at submaximal exercise levels. Resting cardiac rate and cardiac output (amount of blood pumped over a period of time) do not change, although peripheral resistance (blood pressure) is increased. In response to stress or exertion, older adults compensate for their lower maximum heart rate by increasing their stroke volume (ie, amount of blood pumped with each contraction of the heart) to maintain cardiac output.

The baroreceptors, which monitor the blood pressure and adjust the blood pressure when the position is changed, become less sensitive with aging. This can cause orthostatic hypotension (a condition where the blood pressure falls when going from a lying to a sitting position and from a sitting to a standing position) and will cause dizziness for an older patient when he or she changes positions. In addition, the heart rate response has been shown to decrease in response to various physiological stimuli such as coughing, postural changes, or during the Valsalva maneuver (ie, forcible exhalation).

The rate with which the heart rate peaks also becomes prolonged with increasing age.[31] At rest, in sitting, the cardiac output does not show a change with age; however, in supine and in standing, there is often an age-related decrease in cardiac output. There is also a similar position-associated change in stroke volume. This can result in orthostatic hypotension, which may cause an individual to become dizzy or even to pass out with positional changes.[32] Following a moderately sized meal, the elderly tend to show a decrease in systemic blood pressure. The blood is shunted to the intestinal area to assist in digestion. Therefore, the PTA should be aware that an individual who has just eaten a meal may experience orthostatic hypotension with positional changes.

Heart rate may be slightly slower as we grow older due to a loss in the number of pacemaker cells. A marked decline in the total number of pacemaker cells at the sinoatrial (S-A) node occurs and decreases the ability of the heart to respond rapidly to increasing levels of activity. It has also been found that, as we age, heart tissue becomes less elastic and therefore less efficient as a pump. The electrical pathway may develop tissue and fat deposits that can make dysrhythmias more common. Shifts in the circulation of blood to various organs can also change—the blood flow to the kidneys may decrease by 50% and to the brain by 15%. Finally, heart murmurs are more common with old age because heart valves become less flexible and calcium deposits build up.

With aging there is a decrease in cardiac output at rest, a decline in the cardiovascular system's response to stress, an increase in the systolic blood pressure, and a progressive increase in the peripheral vascular resistance to blood flow. The effect of these changes on the cardiovascular system is seen in changes in cardiac output, stroke volume, and blood pressure at rest and in response to stress. Resting blood pressures, both diastolic and systolic, tend to show an increase with age. It is not clear whether this increase in blood pressure is a reflection of normal aging or the result of heredity and/or environmental factors. It is clear, however, that these changes are not as pronounced in an active older population. Systolic pressure is increased with age. These changes are due to arteriosclerosis and fibrotic changes in the vessel walls. The arterial walls become hard. The amount of elastin in the vessel walls is also less, resulting in an increase in peripheral vascular resistance. The tendency for there to be an increase in blood pressure combined with a decrease in heart rate results in a decrease in stroke volume. The overall effect of this is to decrease cardiac output (heart rate/min × stroke volume = cardiac output).[33] Among older adults, it takes longer for the heart rate and blood pressure to return to normal resting levels following stress.

Cardiovascular function in older people can be significantly improved by exercise training. Regular physical activity positively affects cardiac condition and attenuates the effects of aging.[34] In the absence of pathology, the cardiovascular response to higher activity levels consistently seen with increasing age and the effects of exercise on the cardiovascular system are positive.[35]

Age-related changes in structure and function of the heart lower the threshold at which cardiac diseases become apparent. The convergence of normal alterations and distinct cardiovascular conditions, such as disorders of rhythm, disorders of the heart itself, and vascular disease compound the challenge of clinical management. Pathologic conditions of the heart will be discussed in greater detail in Chapter 4.

Blood Vessels

Our blood vessels, including the aorta and other arteries, also become stiffer and less responsive to hormones that relax the blood vessel walls. The stiffening of blood vessels contributes to the increasing systolic blood pressure with aging as previously discussed. Vascular changes with age include a thickening of the supporting membranes of the vessels including capillaries; an elongation of the arteries, which become twisted and calcify; and an increase in deposits of excess starch-like material in the vessels (see Box 3-2). The aging process affects each area of the vascular tree differently. Changes appear first in the proximal vessels progressing to involve the distal vasculature. It is also noted that the distal vessels undergo the most pronounced changes. Changes in the coronary arteries appear first in the left branches and do not appear in the right and posterior descending coronary arteries until well into the fifth decade of life.[36]

PULMONARY CHANGES WITH AGE

The respiratory system reflects changes that occur in many other body systems. Respiratory function is one of the best predictors of mortality. Most of the normal respiratory changes with age are of little functional significance in healthy older adults; however, they do reduce reserve capacity and increase vulnerability to respiratory disease.

Box 3-2: Cardiovascular Changes With Aging

- There is a decrease in maximum heart rate.
- It takes longer for an older adult's heart rate and blood pressure to return to normal resting levels after exertion.
- The aorta and other arteries become thicker and stiffer and may result in an increase in systolic blood pressure.
- The valves between the chambers of the heart thicken and become stiffer.
- Heart murmurs are fairly common among older adults.
- The pacemaker of the heart loses cells and develops fibrous tissue and fat deposits.
- Irregular heart rhythms and extra heartbeats become more common with age.
- The baroreceptors, which monitor blood pressure, become less sensitive. Quick changes in position can cause orthostatic hypotension.
- There is a decrease in cardiac output (CO) by about 0.7% per year after 20 years of age (5 L/min CO at age 20 vs 3.5 L/min by age 75).
- There is a decrease of cardiac reserve, as well as a decrease in physical and psychological responses to stress.
- The efficiency of heart muscle and lipid catabolism are decreased, causing an increased risk of atherosclerosis.
- Work capacity declines about 30% between the ages of 40 to 70.
- Healthy lifestyles reduce the risk of having cardiac pathology.

As we age, the lungs become stiffer, respiratory muscle strength and endurance diminishes, and the chest wall becomes more rigid. The supporting membranes between the alveoli and the capillaries thicken, total lung capacity declines, residual volume (the amount of air remaining in the lungs after maximum expiration) increases, vital capacity (the volume of air that can be forcibly exhaled) is reduced, and there is a decrease in the resiliency of the lungs. Mechanical properties that are altered in the pulmonary system with age include decreases in chest wall compliance and lung elastic recoil tendency. Increased calcification of the ribs, a decline in intercostal muscle strength, and changes in the spinal curvature all result in a lower compliance and increased work of breathing.[37]

In the normal aging lung, alveolar surface area decreases, reducing the maximal oxygen uptake (the volume of air that can be moved in and out by forced voluntary breathing) by as much as 55% by age 85. Fibrotic changes of the lungs combined with postural changes, a decrease in rib cage compliance, and an increase in rigidity of the respiratory tract result in a decrease in breathing capacity, although respiratory rates remain unchanged at 12 to 14 breaths per minute. These changes increase the work of breathing compared to younger individuals. Thus, over time, our exercise capacity declines because we have less reserve. In addition, the alveoli of older adults tend to collapse sooner on expiration than in younger people. This tendency is exacerbated by reduced mobility, illness, and hypoventilation, and increases the risk for respiratory diseases such as atelectasis (the collapse of part or all of a lung). The ability to provide oxygen to working tissues is more difficult, although in spite of these changes, the respiratory system remains capable of maintaining adequate gas exchange at rest and during exertion throughout the entire lifespan. In the absence of pathology, the heart and lungs can generally meet the body's needs; however, reserve capacities are diminished. With any challenge, the body's demand for oxygen and perfusion may exceed available supply.[38] Clinically, the patient may present with shortness of breath and diminished oxygenation within the arterial blood (PaO_2). The PTA will frequently use a finger pulse oximeter to monitor this while an elderly patient is exercising and ambulating. Additionally, many elderly patients receive oxygen through a nasal cannula or a face mask in order to enhance pulmonary efficiency.

The number of cilia decline in number as we grow older. Cilia protect against infection by clearing irritants and obstruction. At the same time, the number of mucus-producing cells may increase resulting in mucus clogging the airways. These changes make older adults more vulnerable to respiratory infections, and less efficient in monitoring and controlling breathing. For example, they are less sensitive to hypoxia and less able to recognize acute bronchoconstriction. Although the causes are not well understood, the implications are clear: older adults may be at greater risk for mortality from acute respiratory problems if they are less aware of respiratory symptoms and seek medical care later rather than sooner (see Box 3-3).

It is difficult to completely separate pulmonary changes resulting with age from those associated with the pathology of emphysema or chronic bronchitis. Throughout a lifetime, exposure to occupational and environmental inhalants, as well as cigarette smoke, may result in chronic pulmonary changes and lung pathologies. These disease states closely parallel those of the aging process and also increase in incidence with advancing age. Normal pulmonary aging that parallels disease states include a loss of elastic tissue leading to expiratory collapse of the larger airways, difficulty with expiration, and dilatation of the terminal air passages.[39]

In a clinical setting, exercise monitoring by the PTA is important. The recovery period following effort is prolonged in the elderly. Among other factors, this reflects a greater relative work rate, an increased proportion of anaerobic metabolism, slower heat elimination, and a lower level of physical fitness. The cool-down phase of exercise needs to be lengthened to allow for a more gradual return to the baseline vital signs. Abrupt cessation of exercise without considering an adequate recovery period could have negative effects for a person of any age, but is particularly important in the elderly.

Box 3-3: **Pulmonary Changes With Aging**

- Lungs become stiffer, muscle strength and endurance diminish, and the chest wall becomes more rigid.

- Lung function decreases. Between age 25 to 85 there can be as much as a 50% decrease in maximal voluntary ventilation due to an increase in air resistance and a 40% decrease in vital capacity.

- Respiratory gas exchange surface decreases at a rate of about 0.27 square meters per year. (The maximum oxygen consumption for sedentary individuals of any age is 0.6 to 0.7 mL/min.)

- There is a decrease in elastin in the lungs and chest wall soft tissues, which results in a decrease in chest wall compliance.

- Total lung capacity remains constant while vital capacity decreases and residual volume doubles.

- Changes in posture and muscle strength result in decreased lung capacity and efficiency.

- The alveolar surface decreases by about 20% and tends to collapse sooner on expiration.

- There is an increase in mucus production and a decrease in the activity and number of cilia.

- Life-long exposure to pollutants, damage from disease, and habits such as smoking decrease the efficiency of the lungs.

- The effects of changes in the respiratory system, including shortness of breath and fatigue, may lead to decreased activity for older adults.

NEUROMUSCULAR CHANGES WITH AGE

The aging of the CNS is often portrayed as an irreversible loss of functions and decline in abilities. In the past, it was thought that millions of neurons were lost every day. Fortunately, that's not correct. The brain retains a remarkable plasticity in its ability to compensate functionally for those losses that do occur. Further, cognitive abilities are stable or may actually increase with age. Older people are an amazing resource to our society. They have the potential of providing a remarkable source of wisdom and life experience.

The nervous system is the communication system of the body, relaying information to and from the brain from all parts of the body. The transmission of messages can be affected with aging. Slower reflexes, decreased speed, poorer balance, and a slower response time are factors in how an individual reacts to and with the environment. Moving and reacting at a slower pace can affect driving skills or lead to falls. (See Box 3-4 for neuromuscular changes with aging.)

The weight of the brain peaks around age 20. After peaking in the early decades of life, brain mass (or weight) slowly decreases by as much as 6% to 7% by the time a person reaches 80. This modest decline is limited primarily to the loss of gray matter (outer surface of the brain). Although the brain stem appears to be minimally affected by cell loss, widely varied but significant losses occur in the cerebral cortex lobes and cerebellar area. Older nerve cells may have fewer dendrites (branches) and some may become demyelinated (lose their coating), which can slow the speed of transmission.[40] Most of these changes do not appear to affect ordinary ADL.

The loss of cells from the motor system that occurs during the normal aging process leads to a reduction in the complement of motor neurons and muscle fibers. The latter age-related decrease in muscle mass, termed *sarcopenia* (discussed earlier), is often combined with the detrimental effects of a sedentary lifestyle in older adults, leading to a significant reduction in reserve capacity of the neuromuscular system. Conduction velocity decreases with advancing age. A loss of the myelin sheath and a loss of large myelinated fibers decrease the axon's abilities to transmit impulses, especially in the posterior spinal column tracts. These tracts provide reflex-positive righting responses. Remembering that balance impairment partially results from cerebellar losses coupled with CNS delays, one can begin to see why an older person has a greater tendency to fall and less ability to quickly correct a center of balance before injury occurs.[41]

The Brain's Blood Supply

Another important consideration involves the morphological and functional changes in cerebral vasculature. Diminished brain function may occur over time as a result of ischemia due to fluctuation of blood flow.[42] Subclinical transient ischemic events may cause progressive changes in cerebral functioning due to lack of circulation to localized areas of the brain. Transient ischemic attacks (TIAs) are defined as transient neurologic deficits lasting no longer than 24 hours; longer-lasting deficits are considered to be indicative of a cerebral infarction ("brain attack"). Infarction from ischemia is typically confined to a vascular territory. Ischemia and nutritional deficits often result in cognitive changes that dramatically affect function.[43]

The PTA needs to consider these changes in the absence of a pathological condition when delivering care. For example, when working on weight-bearing exercises following orthopedic surgery, proper guarding techniques need to be utilized for safety.

Box 3-4: **Neuromuscular Changes With Aging**

- Myoneural junction decreases in transmission speed.
- Mitochondrial activity decreases.
- Nerve conduction velocity is decreased by about 0.4% per year after age 70.
- There is a decrease in reflexes, resulting from a decrease in nerve conduction.
- There is a decrease in reaction time (simple reflexes less than complex).
- There is increased postural sway during gait, increasing risk of falls.

COGNITIVE CHANGES WITH AGE

There is little change in intellectual ability if a person remains healthy, however, changes in cognitive function do increase as we age. Cognitive changes affect memory, reasoning, and abstract thinking. As we get older, more time is required to learn new things but the ability is retained. One of the things that compensates for the mild changes is experience and judgment gained over a lifetime. In general, the changes that occur in normal aging do not preclude people from doing things that are meaningful to them. It is important for older adults to "exercise" their mind as well as their body, as decline in intellectual function can result from lack of stimulation.

Long-term memory remains intact but there may be some changes in short-term memory. Under normal conditions, memory aids solve the problem. Remember that we all use memory aids, such as lists and notes, so this is not isolated to a particular age group.

The process of memory is difficult to separate from the total process of learning. After information is perceived, it is stored in either short-term or long-term areas of memory. The elderly typically have more difficulty recalling recently experienced, short-term recall information. In order to be properly perceived, information needs to be presented to an older person at a slower rate and with an increased number of repetitions. If the information is presented in a manner that compensates for age-related sensory changes (decreased vision and hearing) and if the information is made to have some personal relevance to the older person, recall of the information is greatly improved. This is particularly important with regard to patient education and establishing a home program (see Chapter 11).

"Intelligence" may be affected by pathology, but even in advanced years, it remains unaffected by the physiologic changes of normal aging. A significant decline in mental function may be an important clinical sign of illness and should always be investigated (see Box 3-5).

Box 3-5: Cognitive Changes With Aging

- There is little change in intellectual ability if a person remains healthy.

- Changes in cognitive function increase as we age, affecting the memory, reasoning, and abstract thinking.

- Experience and judgment gained over a lifetime can compensate for mild changes in cognition.

- It is important for older adults to "exercise" the mind as well as the body. Decline in intellectual function can result from a lack of stimulation, as well as other factors.

- Long-term memory remains intact, but there is some change in short-term memory. Memory aids can solve the problem.

- A significant decline in mental function may be an important clinical sign of illness or pathology.

PERIPHERAL NEUROLOGICAL CHANGES WITH AGE

Aging is often characterized by reduced sensibility, reduced coordination, reduced cognitive abilities, and reduced ability to react to changing environmental conditions. A general assumption is made that loss of nerve tissue (ie, reduced cell number) is a predominant feature of aging. In reality, although some loss of nerve cells does take place during the aging process, the extent to which this loss occurs is less than usually assumed. The reduced level of nervous system functioning in the elderly is better explained in terms of biochemical changes that take place in neurons during aging and senescence.[44]

As people age, peripheral nerves may conduct signals more slowly. Usually, this effect is so minimal that no change in function is noticeable. The peripheral nervous system's response to injury is also reduced. When the axon of a peripheral nerve is damaged in younger people, the nerve is able to repair itself as long as the cell body is undamaged. This self-reparation occurs more slowly and incompletely in older people than in younger people, making older people more vulnerable to injury and disease.

One source of falls in the elderly may be an inability to sufficiently adjust to transient postural perturbations or slips. Loss of sensation, proprioception, and kinesthetic sense are factors that affect the ability of an individual to detect movement, changes in the standing support surface, and resulting postural stability. Changes in peripheral nerve sensitivity and proprioception affect the older person's perception of acceleration and weight shifting/displacement during ambulation and create a risk for falls.[45,46]

SENSORY CHANGES WITH AGE

Sensory changes can have a tremendous impact on lifestyle, such as problems with communication, enjoyment of activities, and social interactions. Sensory changes can contribute to a sense of isolation. All of the senses receive information of some type from the environment (light, sound vibrations, etc). This is converted to a nerve impulse and carried to the brain where it is interpreted into a meaningful sensation. Everyone requires a certain minimum amount of stimulation before a sensation is perceived. This minimum level is called the threshold. Aging increases this threshold so that the amount of sensory input needed to be aware of the sensation becomes greater. Changes in the body part related to the sensation account for most of the other sensation changes. Hearing and vision changes are the most dramatic, but all senses can be affected by aging. Fortunately, many of the aging changes in the senses can be compensated for with equipment such as glasses and hearing aids or by minor changes in lifestyle[47] (see Box 3-6).

The primary change in senses as one grows older is a loss of acuity in the senses. By ages 65 to 70, 90% of adults have some visual loss and 30% have significant hearing loss. Losses in hearing and vision can cause inappropriate responses, confusion, anger, disorientation, or social isolation. Deficits must be properly addressed and corrective measures taken whenever possible. Losses in sensory function affect the ability to interact with the environment. In the body, information is gathered, interpreted, and transmitted through the integration of the neurosensory system. The neurosensory system includes the nervous system and each of the 5 senses (ie, touch, smell, taste, vision, hearing). Each of these systems is highly complex and structural changes are known to occur with aging. The sum of these changes results in a decline of neurosensory function.[48] Changes in the sensory system will impact the PT's approach to intervention and needs to be incorporated into the treatment approach. The alterations in communication and educational approaches to an individual with sensory losses will be discussed further in Chapter 11.

Box 3-6: **Sensory Changes With Aging**

- By age 90, there is a 10% to 20% decrease in brain weight.

- A decrease in mechanoreceptors alters an elder's proprioception and kinesthetic sense.

- Normal age-related changes in the skin can result in wrinkles, dryness, and thinning.

- Sensitivity to touch is decreased.

- There is a decrease in visual acuity and the ability to accommodate to lighting changes due to an increased density of lens.

- There is a decrease in hearing, smell, and taste capabilities.

- There is a loss, thinning, and graying of the hair.

- Nail growth slows and nails become thicker and more brittle.

- Sweat glands shrink and sweat production decreases.

Touch

In later life, the sense of touch and response to painful stimuli decreases. The actual number of touch receptors decreases, resulting in a higher threshold for touch. A concern for personal safety is certainly presented by a loss in overall sensitivity to touch and pain. For example, older adults do not sense heat as quickly so they tend to have worse burns.

Peripheral receptors are responsible for the sense of touch. As with the other senses, touch also declines with age. Specific receptors for touch, pressure, pain, and temperature are found within the dermis and epidermis of the skin. Receptors can be free-standing or arranged in small corpuscular masses.[49] *Meissner's corpuscles* (touch-texture receptors), *Pacinian corpuscles* (pressure-vibration receptors), and *Krause corpuscles* (temperature receptors), as well as peripheral nerve fibers, are noted to decline. Sensitivity to touch, temperature, and vibration frequently decline with age. Although quantitative studies have produced inconclusive results, since free nerve endings remain relatively unchanged, the ability to sense pain should remain intact. The elderly person must take special care to avoid injury from concentrated pressures or temperature on the skin (eg, pressures from shoes that are too tight, bath water that is too hot, etc).[50] The PTA can play a critical role in educating an elder about this tendency for diminishing sensation, and ways to modify the environment and perform self-inspection to prevent potential maladies.

One of the most common physical changes that people associate with aging is the wrinkling, pigment alteration, and thinning of the skin. It is now known that these changes reflect exposure to ultraviolet light more than aging; most of the aging of the skin is due to the effects of environment and disease. The most common changes in the skin include:

- Thinning of the area between the dermis and epidermis by about 20%

- Elastin and collagen decrease

- Reduction in cell size

- Inability of skin to retain moisture.

The skin is a very important element in touch. In general, skin wrinkles increase with advancing age. The dermis thins, loses elasticity, and has a diminished vascularity. Loss of tissue support for remaining capillaries results in fragility and easy bruising (senile purpura). Although tanning response diminishes, the appearance of flat pigmented age spots increases with exposure to the sun. The skin has a reduced resiliency and an increased susceptibility to hypothermia or hyperthermia (which involves more than just the skin, but depends on temperature sensitivity at the onset). As discussed earlier in this text, the decline in cellular division results in a slower rate and efficiency of tissue repair following any trauma. Normal age-related changes in the skin can result in wrinkles, dryness, and thinning, making it more susceptible to breaks and slower to heal.[51]

One factor in aging of the skin involves changes in 2 important proteins—elastin and collagen—which determine the elasticity and resiliency of the skin. The skin becomes less able to retain fluids and is more easily dried and cracked. As a result, both the thickness and elasticity of the skin decrease. Moisturizing creams play an important role in protecting the aging skin.[52]

In addition to changes in the skin itself, the subcutaneous layers of fatty deposits dwindle with age; this is what gives some very elderly people an emaciated appearance. Using a microscope, a dermatologist can estimate a person's age by examining changes in skin structure, usually to within 5 years of accuracy. This is because the dermis thins almost 20% with aging as the number of skin cells decrease.[53]

Protecting the skin throughout the life cycle can reduce some of these changes. Prevention of most, but not all, of the aging changes in the skin is done by avoiding sun exposure. Ultraviolet light causes the pathological effects that produce wrinkles, thin skin, pigmentation changes, and benign and malignant tumors. The use of sunscreen with a sun protective factor (SPF) of at least 30, wearing broad-brimmed hats to shade the face, sunglasses to protect the eyes, and light-colored long-sleeved clothing and pants are recommendations for life-long skin care.

Hair

Changes in the hair also occur with age. A reduction in hair follicles produces a reduction of hair. In contrast, after menopause, facial hair tends to increase in women.[54] The degree to which hair becomes gray is largely genetically determined. Hair grays because of a gradual decrease in the production of melanin, the pigment cells in the hair bulbs. The graying of hair is also influenced by heredity and hormones.[55] By age 50, the hair of more than half of all White Americans is 50% gray. By contrast, gray hair occurs less frequently in Black Americans and other nationalities living in America. Men tend to gray earlier and to have more "graying" than women.

As one ages, fewer hair follicles remain on the scalp and the growth rate of new hair decreases in the scalp, armpits, and pubic areas. However, hair growth actually accelerates and thickens in places like the nostrils, ears, and eyebrows, especially in men; older women often have an increase in facial hair as their estrogen levels decrease.[56] Men who are bald have either one or two genes for baldness, but women go bald only when they have both genes.

Nails

Nails grow more slowly and develop longitudinal ridges. They become thicker, more brittle, and

caution—especially for the feet—is very important to ensure safe nail care. Differences in the structure and quality of the nails at an advanced age are determined mainly by age-dependent variations in the lipid content of the nail plates.[57] The number and size of sweat glands is diminished resulting in a reduction of sweat production. This leads to a condition of hypohidrosis or anhidrosis, a reduced or absent ability to generate sweat for the purpose of evaporative heat dissipation. The result is an increased risk of hyperthermia in the elderly.[58] The PTA needs to consider this with regard to the therapy environment.

Vision

Visual impairment is the most common sensory problem of older adults. About 95% of individuals ages 65 and older report wearing glasses or needing glasses to improve their vision. However, the effectiveness of glasses decreases with age. Among those over age 85, only 45% report that their glasses correct all their visual problems and 12% are legally blind.

Humans are strongly visual creatures and the eye is vulnerable to many age-related changes. Externally, the eyelids show an increased wrinkling and *ptosis* (drooping eyelid) resulting from losses of elastic tissue, orbital fat, and muscle tone. Very often, the older person will develop an *entropian* (a turning inward of the eyelid), or an *ectropian* (an outward relaxation of the eyelid), which is particularly apparent with the lower lids. Aging results in diminished tear production, and ocular inflammation or infection may occur in some elderly as the lens of the eye becomes yellowed, stiffer, slightly cloudy, and the iris becomes more rigid over time.[59] Supplementary artificial tears can be provided to prevent or relieve the problem.

In addition to becoming smaller with age, the ocular pupil reacts more slowly to light and the ability to focus quickly from far to near distances declines. The pupil's response to darkness or bright lights is slower and acuity is poor. This loss of accommodation is termed *presbyopia*. The ability to focus is dependent on the ability of the ocular lens to change shape as needed. Presbyopia is partially caused by a decline in ciliary muscle efficiency. As a person ages, the ocular lens continues to grow while becoming more dense and inelastic. With increased stiffness comes decreased flexibility resulting in a decreased ability to change shapes and focus on desired objects. Far vision is more easily achieved because the ciliary muscles relax and allow the lens to thin. Near vision requires the ciliary muscles to contract to increase the thickness of the lens. This is why older people may require bifocals or reading glasses that offer a weaker lens for far vision and a thicker one for near vision. Along with reduced accommodation, older people experience a decreased ability to adapt comfortably and quickly to changes of light and dark (eg, many older people give up nighttime driving).

In the aging eye, the corneal surface flattens, admitting less light into the eye. This change reduces the transmitted light into the eye. The transparency of the lens diminishes with age, which weakens available light to receive colors with short wavelengths, such as violet and blue. When new lens fibers naturally multiply at the edge of the lens, older fibers move inwards to create a dense center. Over time, the lenses accumulate yellow substances that filter out the blue part of the color spectrum. Blue actually appears more green. Warm colors, like red and orange, seem stronger in comparison.

The most sensitive part of the retina gradually functions less well with age due to decreased blood supply and the cumulative effects of radiation damage from the sun. The result is decreased spatial discrimination, black and white contrast, and flicker sensitivity. The eye is less able to tolerate glare and has more trouble adapting to darkness or bright light.[60] This may be a reason for falls in the home and can be modified to improve safety.

A decline in visual acuity may ultimately be produced by many age-related changes. Even when errors of age refraction are corrected, a loss of visual receptors in the aging retina will result in a decrease of acuity. Fortunately, with modern technology, the majority of older people are able to maintain a high degree of visual function and independence.

Hearing

Hearing loss is very common with aging and is one of the most correctable yet often unrecognized problems, contributing significantly to social isolation. About 25% of people between 65 and 74 years of age, and 50% of people age 75 or older, report difficulty with hearing. Unfortunately, although 65% of those ages 85 and older report hearing difficulty, only 8% use a hearing aid or other assistive listening device. After age 60, there is approximately a 10 decibel reduction in hearing sensitivity with each successive decade. Older men are more likely to have hearing loss than older women, and people with Alzheimer's disease have a higher rate of hearing impairment than others.[61]

A number of age-related changes occur in the ear. Membranes in the middle ear (including the eardrum) become less flexible and the small bones in the middle ear (the ossicles) become stiffer. Both of these factors somewhat decrease hearing sensitivity but are not thought to cause significant impairment. Changes also occur in the inner ear but it is unclear whether it is aging or exposure to environmental noise that causes these problems that result in hearing loss.

Although a hearing loss may develop at any age, hearing losses occur more frequently in the older years. A sensorineural hearing loss, often called *presbycusis*, is most common in the elderly. Presbycusis results in a decreased ability to hear and discriminate speech, particularly at higher and lower frequency levels. Because normal speech contains a broad range of frequencies, the older person may realize that someone is speaking but may not understand all that is being said.[62] Because of the loss of high and low frequencies, the individual only hears the "soft" sounds of language, often missing the beginnings and endings of words (harder sounds). Difficulties increase when the speaker talks too quickly or when the hearing impaired individual is unable to observe the speaker's face.

Contrary to common belief, a sensorineural hearing loss does not always preclude the use of a hearing aid. Vision should be corrected so the skill of visual speech conception can be used as much as possible. When speaking with an elder with sensorineural loss, words should be spoken slowly in a medium-pitched voice and face-to-face communication should always be maintained.

Changes in the middle ear with advancing age also contribute to a weakening sense of balance. The vestibular system is responsible for our sense of balance. The vestibular apparatus begins to degenerate with age in a similar way to the hearing apparatus. Equilibrium becomes compromised and older individuals may complain of dizziness, finding it difficult to move quickly without losing their balance.

Proprioception/Kinesthesia

Proprioception or kinesthetic sense is provided by sensory nerves that give information concerning movements and position of the body. These receptors are located primarily in the muscles, tendons, and the labyrinth system. Although a greater degree of sensory-perceptual loss results from local system changes (ie, impaired vision from increased lens density), cerebral cortex cell loss may result in less cellular availability for sensory interpretation. This is very important from a clinical stance in that, as one ages, there may be an accompanying loss of position and movement sense. Coupled with losses in the other sensory systems (eg, vision) this could significantly impact an elderly individual's awareness of limb or body position, affecting safety during transfers and ambulation.[63]

Vestibular System

The vestibular system changes during the aging process in that there is degeneration in the sensory receptors in both the otoliths and semicircular canals. The function of the vestibular system is to monitor head position and to detect head movements. When an individual is deprived of visual and lower extremity somatosensory information, the vestibular system is left to provide sensation for control of balance. Healthy young adults are able to balance without meaningful visual or support surface information. Healthy elderly, on the other hand, lose their balance and might even fall when vestibular input is the only spatial orientation information available. All of the major sources of orienting information are compromised during the aging process. Diseases further compound this problem.[64]

Taste and Smell

The ability to smell and taste becomes less acute with age. This diminishes the gratification of eating and impedes good nutrition. As much as 80% of the taste buds may atrophy and perception of taste sensation (sweet, salty, bitter, acidic, etc) becomes less sharp. A reduction of saliva flow occurs as a person ages and may aggravate an already dulled sense of taste. The olfactory bulb demonstrates age-related cell losses that seem to be associated with decreased perceptions of various smells. It is proposed that these declines contribute to the appetite decline often observed in and experienced by the majority of elderly people.[65]

As we age, the number of functioning smell receptors decreases, which increases the threshold for smell. An odor must be more intense for it to be identified and differentiated from other odors. After the age of 50, the sense of smell decreases gradually. By age 80, the sense of smell is reduced as much as 50%.[66] The lack of ability to smell spoiled food can lead to indigestion and food poisoning. Even more seriously, studies have shown that older persons may not be able to detect high levels of mercaptan, an odorant added to natural gas so that individuals can detect gas leakage. Thus, older persons can miss detecting natural gas leakage at levels that could cause explosions.

Taste also diminishes with age, and older persons often complain that food doesn't taste as good as it used to. Some atrophy of the tongue occurs with age and this may diminish sensitivity to taste. Receptor cells for taste are found in the taste buds on the tongue and are replaced continuously. Another factor that contributes to changes in taste among seniors is dentures that fit poorly.[67]

NEUROENDOCRINE CHANGES AND INTERSYSTEM HOMEOSTASIS

The way the body regulates certain systems is often dictated by neuroendocrine changes, which affect intersystem homeostasis. Some examples include:

1. Progressive changes in the heart and blood vessels interfere with the body's ability to control blood pressure.

2. The body cannot regulate its temperature as it could during younger years, which can result in a dangerously low body temperature from prolonged exposure to cold or in heat stroke in warm environments.

3. There are aging-related changes in the body's ability to develop a fever in response to an infection due to a suppressed immune system response.

4. The regulation of the amount and makeup of body fluids is slowed down in healthy older persons.

Usually (resting) levels of the hormones that control the amount of body fluids are unchanged, but problems in fluid regulation commonly develop during illness or other stress. Also, elderly people tend to not feel as thirsty after water deprivation as they did when they were younger, often leading to dehydration.[68]

Thermal Regulation

There is an age-related decline in the body's ability to regulate temperature. The CNS control center for regulating the body's response to ambient, locally applied, and internal temperature gradients is less responsive. Many acute conditions in the elderly, such as an increase in body weight, increased serum cholesterol, or a decrease in glucose tolerance are due to faulty thermoregulation.[69]

The hypothalamic thermostat sensitivity and basal metabolic rate decreases. The overall reactivity of the autonomic nervous system declines with age, altering skin hydration and circulation. The vasomotor system is less responsive to warming and cooling, and the normal transient bursts of vasoconstrictor activity are reduced. It is unclear whether or not thermoreceptors in the skin are altered. Because cold receptors are dependent on a good oxygen supply, it may be reasoned that decreased circulatory supply may decrease perception of cold because of the vulnerability of cold receptors to hypoxia.

The changes in the thermal regulatory response in the elderly have great clinical significance. The aged individual's ability to maintain homeostasis with increasing exercise levels is poor. The cooling time following exercise is often prolonged. In addition, a decrease in the receptiveness of temperature gradients impacts the application of heat and cold modalities in treatment interventions. Consideration of these changes needs to be employed when treating the elderly patient.

ENDOCRINE CHANGES WITH AGE

The endocrine system is a complex network of glandular tissues that secrete hormones directly into the blood, which are then used by "target" organs. The endocrine system controls a variety of important functions such as energy metabolism, reproduction, and stress response.[70] The pituitary gland is often referred to as the master gland because it regulates the hormones used by the thyroid, adrenal cortex, ovaries, testes, and breasts. The pituitary gland is located in the brain below the hypothalamus. It peaks in size in middle age and then gradually shrinks[71] (see Box 3-7).

Proper functioning of the endocrine system is essential to maintain the majority of the body's regulatory processes. In some cases (reproductive hormones), age-related changes are well known; in other cases, specific information is nonexistent or unclear. Much available information remains highly controversial.

The pancreas secretes insulin, a hormone that is critical to the metabolism of glucose (blood sugar). Insulin continues to be produced in sufficient quantities in older adults but their muscle cells may become less sensitive to its effects. It is thought that this lack of sensitivity may be due to the loss of the number of insulin receptor sites in the cell wall that occurs with age. After age 50, the normal fasting glucose level rises 6 to 14 mg/dL every 10 years. Adult-onset diabetes, or type II diabetes, occurs when the body develops resistance to insulin. It is usually managed through diet, exercise, and oral hypoglycemic medications. Sometimes people stop producing insulin and then insulin injections are needed. A number of studies indicate that adult-onset diabetes is related to obesity and inactivity.[72]

Although age-related structural changes in the thyroid do occur, in the absence of pathology, its function tends to remain adequate for bodily needs. A decrease in the basal metabolic rate (BMR) is shown in elderly people but seems related to the reduction of lean body mass rather than neuroendocrine function. While the elderly are at risk for both hypothyroid and hyperthyroid problems, these problems are unrelated to changes that occur with normal aging.[73]

The adrenals are located just above the kidneys and secrete several hormones including glucocorticoid, aldosterone, and cortisol. Tests of adrenal function show plasma glucocorticoid levels to be similar in the young and old. The adrenal cortex response to adrenocorticotropic hormone (ACTH) remains intact as does the pituitary's release of ACTH in response to stress. Circulating levels of aldosterone decrease with aging. Aldosterone is important in regulating fluid and electrolyte balance. On average, aldosterone levels are 30% lower in an adult ages 70 to 80 years than in younger adults. Lower aldosterone levels may cause orthostatic hypotension (a drop in blood pressure with changes in position). Cortisol is a stress response hormone that has anti-inflammatory and anti-allergy effects. Secretion of cortisol diminishes by 25% with age, although the significance of this remains unclear. Dehydroepiandrosterone (DHEA) blood levels decline with age; however, the functional consequences of this decline are not well understood.[74]

The most dramatic age-related changes in the reproductive system occur with women at *menopause* when their estrogen production ceases and they lose their capacity to reproduce. Following menopause, estrogen and progesterone levels significantly decrease. Serum androgen levels remain relatively unchanged. Many men also experience declines in testosterone production but they maintain their reproductive ability in extreme old age. An age-related decrease in hormones, primarily blood levels of testosterone, results in *andropause*. Both sexes experience *somatopause*, or the decrease in glandular production of hormones and a physiologic slowing of all organ systems.[75]

Box 3-7: Age-Related Changes in the Endocrine System

- The endocrine system controls a variety of important functions such as stress response, energy metabolism, and reproduction, and becomes less efficient due to a loss of neuroendocrines with age.

- Proper functioning of the endocrine system is essential to maintain the majority of the body's regulatory processes.

- A decrease in the BMR is shown in elderly people and seems related to the reduction of lean body mass.

- Insulin resistance may prevent the efficient conversion of glucose into energy.

- A decrease in aldosterone and cortisol may affect immune and cardiovascular function.

Changes in Women

Menopause, in which the cycle of ovulation ceases, is one of the most widely studied age-related changes in biology. Menopause generally occurs in women between the ages of 45 and 52. The ovaries are the female reproductive glands that secrete estrogen and produce the reproductive cells (ova). At menopause, the production of estrogen decreases by about 95% and there is a rapid decline in oocytes. With menopause, the ovaries become fibrotic and atrophy; lower estrogen levels cause atrophic changes in the uterus and vagina, making the uterine lining thin and the vagina decrease in elasticity. Vaginal secretions are reduced. Most of the signs and symptoms of menopause are the result of a 95% decrease in the levels of circulating estrogen. Common symptoms include hot flashes, palpitations, irritability, headaches, depression, fatigue, weight gain, insomnia, night sweats, forgetfulness, and inability to concentrate. The vaginal walls become thinner and less elastic and there is a decrease in lubrication. Many of these symptoms can be avoided through Estrogen Replacement Therapy (ERT).[76]

In the years following menopause, the circulating follicle stimulating hormone (FSH) and luteinizing hormones (LH) are greatly increased. Over subsequent years, FSH and LH levels fall slowly before leveling off about 30 years after menopause. These hormonal changes cause a relaxation of ligaments and a loss of muscular tone that alter the contour of the breast. Women who are not on ERT face an increased risk for osteoporosis, heart attack, stroke, and possibly Alzheimer's disease[77] (see Box 3-8).

Box 3-8: Age-Related Changes in the Female Reproductive System

- Ovulation ceases and estrogen levels drop by 95%.
- Vaginal walls become thinner and lose elasticity.
- Most women experience a decrease in the production of vaginal lubrication.

Changes in Men

In men, the decline in reproductive ability is more gradual. The male reproductive glands are the testes, which are located in the scrotum. They secrete testosterone and produce spermatozoa. With aging, the rate of sperm production slows, but there are few changes in sperm number so this does not significantly affect fertility. However, there may be an increase in chromosomal abnormalities. By the age of 85, there is a 35% decrease in the level of testosterone and a reduction in the size of the testes. The amount of fluid ejaculated remains the same. Declining levels of testosterone may be partly responsible for losses in muscle strength.[78]

With aging, a decrease in sex drive may occur and sexual response may become slower and less intense. These changes may be related to testosterone levels as well as other factors such as disease, medications, or psychosocial aspects of aging. Erectile dysfunction (impotence) increases with age; about 15% of men age 65 cannot achieve or maintain an erection. All of these symptoms comprise male menopause, termed *andropause*[79] (see Box 3-9).

Box 3-9: Age-Related Changes in the Male Reproductive System

- In some men, testosterone levels drop by up to 35%.
- The size of the testes decreases.
- The rate of sperm production declines, although the extent varies among individuals.
- Erectile dysfunction (impotence), in which an erection cannot be achieved, is experienced by 15% of men by age 65 and increases to 50% by age 80.

HORMONAL BALANCE WITH AGE

Aging is marked by a deterioration in the functional efficiency of individual cells and organs, and by a failure of hormonal mechanisms for the coordination of function between various body parts. A weakening of both neural and hormonal controls reduces the ability to adjust to external and internal stresses and maintain homeostasis. Among other responsibilities, the body hormones contribute to (1) the regulation of circulating fluid volumes and cardiovascular performance; (2) the mobilization of fuels for exercise (eg, maintenance of blood glucose, liberation of fat, and breakdown of protein); and (3) the repair of body structures with the synthesis of new protein (anabolism).

All of the changes in these functions impact exercise tolerance and the healing process in the elderly. The aged are slower to reach homeostasis during exercise, and the return to a balanced homeostatic state following exercise is prolonged. In addition, the healing process is slower due to a diminished synthesis of new proteins.[80]

GASTROINTESTINAL CHANGES WITH AGE

The gastrointestinal (GI) system consists of the esophagus, the stomach, the small intestine, the large intestine or colon, the liver, the gallbladder, and the pancreas. Generally, the physiological changes of an aging digestive system are minor. With this in mind, it is important to recognize and actively treat most new GI problems in healthy older people, rather than ascribing symptoms to aging. The following changes are considered to be a part of normal aging; pathologies of the GI system will be dealt with in Chapter 4 (see Box 3-10).

Declines in salivation, taste, and smell have already been reviewed. It is a fallacy to believe that teeth must be lost with aging. Improved dental hygiene and nutrition can prevent common pathologies of tooth loss (dental caries and periodontal disease).

The esophagus in the aged demonstrates a reduction of motility and a hesitance of the lower esophageal sphincter to relax with swallowing. To define these changes, the term *presbyesophagus* was coined. When eating, the older person may experience an often uncomfortable substernal sense of fullness as food entry into the stomach is delayed. In contrast, the lower esophageal resting pressure declines with age. This weakening allows gastric contents to more easily reflux into the lower areas of the esophagus causing heartburn to occur. *Hiatal hernias* (the protrusion of the upper part of the stomach into the thorax through a tear or weakness in the diaphragm) frequently develop in the older person who has a reduced resting pressure of the lower esophageal sphincter.[81]

An age-related reduction in motility also affects the stomach, colon, and probably the small intestine. Gastric emptying time often is delayed. A reduced blood supply to the gut and a decrease in the number of absorbing cells can hinder nutrient absorption in the small intestine. Decreased motility in the colon causes the elderly to have a tendency to develop constipation. If the elderly person is particularly immobile or dehydrated, constipation can easily lead to more serious conditions such as fecal impaction and bowel obstruction.[82]

The liver plays an important role in processing the body's waste products of metabolism, as well as affecting the uptake of medications and serum cholesterol. The major functional changes with age include reduced blood flow, altered clearance of some drugs, and a diminished capacity to regenerate damaged liver cells. Among older adults, the half-life of many drugs may be doubled due to decreased metabolism.[83]

In general, aging does not affect the transport of food through the intestines. Our intestines do not change significantly in their ability to absorb foods and drugs, although there are a few exceptions. For example, changes in the metabolism and absorption of lactose, calcium, and iron can occur. As we age, the small intestines absorb less calcium, therefore, we need more calcium to prevent bone mineral loss and osteoporosis in later life. Some enzymes, such as lactase (which aids in the digestion of lactose, a sugar found in diary products), decline with age.[84]

The prevalence of diverticulosis increases with age. Almost all of us, if we live long enough, will have diverticula—small out-pouches in the colon. This condition is caused by increased pressure in the colon as a result of impaired intestinal muscle function and weakness in the intestinal wall. Diverticula can be uncomplicated or they can become inflamed (called *diverticulitis*) and result in great pain. Diverticulitis can be prevented by maintaining a high intake of fiber.[85]

Studies of motility in older adults show reduced peristalsis (intestinal muscle contractions) of the large intestine (colon). This slower rate of food transport can contribute to constipation. However, constipation is aggravated by a low intake of fiber and water, inactivity, medications, and overuse of laxatives.

Box 3-10: Gastrointestinal Changes With Aging

- Declines in salivation, taste, and smell occur with advancing age.

- Reduction in saliva production can lead to a dry mouth and cause chewing problems.

- The esophagus of an elderly person demonstrates a reduction of motility and a hesitance of the lower esophageal sphincter to relax with swallowing.

- Reduction in digestive enzymes can cause some problems with digestion.

- An age-related reduction in motility also affects the stomach, colon, and probably the small intestine.

- The liver is less efficient in metabolizing drugs and repairing damaged liver cells.

- Diverticuli in the colon may cause pain.

- Reduced peristalsis of the colon can increase risk for constipation (which is worsened by sedentary lifestyle).

- Changes in the mucosal lining of all parts of the digestive tract can affect absorption of nutrients.

URINARY SYSTEM CHANGES WITH AGE

The urinary system includes the kidneys, urethra, and bladder. It undergoes substantial changes in function as we grow older. In both men and women, urinary changes are often associated with changes in the reproductive system (see Box 3-11).

There are several important changes that occur in kidney function with age. The kidneys filter the blood and dispose of wastes and excess fluid as urine; they also play a vital role in the "acid-base" balance of the body. Beginning around the mid-40s, many people experience a decline in kidney function, although they continue to function more than adequately under ordinary circumstances.

Most of the clinically important changes in renal function with age are probably due to changes in the intrarenal vasculature. Blood flow to the kidneys decreases by as much as 10% per decade and can be decreased by nearly half that of younger people (600 mL/min) in those who are age 80 or older (300 mL/min). As we age, the kidneys lose one-quarter to one-third of their mass, as both the number and size of nephrons (filtering units) decreases. By age 80, the total number of glomeruli decreases by 30% to 40%, and another 30% may become sclerotic and nonfunctional. These changes reduce the rate at which the blood is filtered by the kidneys.[86]

In addition, the regulation of hormones that respond to dehydration (ie, vasopressin) and the ability to conserve salt may decline. These renal changes make older adults particularly vulnerable to dehydration. As a result of physiologic changes, the kidneys are less efficient in concentrating urine and eliminating solutes from the blood stream.

For the most part, kidney function is well preserved, although it may be slower. Most changes do not cause disease or disability, but they do leave the kidney vulnerable to illness or medications that can depress renal function and lead to acute or chronic renal failure. Medication dosages often need to be reduced in the elderly because the reduction in kidney function can affect clearance of some drugs and lead to adverse effects or toxicity.

The aging bladder is characterized by a decrease in capacity and urinary flow, and an increase in urgency and amount of residual urine. These changes contribute to an increase in *nocturia* (frequent urination at night) as well as a higher rate of urinary tract infections among the elderly.[87]

There is a strong relationship between incontinence and impaired mobility and/or cognitive functioning. Tissue changes with aging affect the bladder just as they do with the other systems discussed, becoming stiffer and losing extensibility. Additionally, situations such as childbirth and intra-abdominal pressures created during defecation (in conjunction with obesity, heavy lifting, hard coughing, sneezing, or laughing) may result in the leakage of urine if the outlet closure of the bladder is weakened. In postmenopausal women, the loss of adequate estrogen diminishes the strength and tone of the bladder. Inadequate hydration will also cause overconcentrated urine to irritate the walls of the bladder, creating a contraction at the wrong time.[88]

Box 3-11: Urinary System Changes With Aging

- Kidney mass decreases by 25% to 30%, and the number of glomeruli decrease by 30% to 40% with age.

- There is a reduction in the ability to filter and concentrate urine and to clear drugs.

- With aging, there is a reduced hormonal response (vasopressin) and an impaired ability to conserve salt, which may increase risk for dehydration.

- Bladder capacity decreases and there is an increase in urinary frequency and residual urine.

- Increased incidence of urinary infections, incontinence, and urinary obstruction may occur.

IMMUNE SYSTEM CHANGES WITH AGE

Age-related changes in the immune (lymphatic) system increase vulnerability to infections, tumors, and immune diseases. Factors that affect immune system function include hormonal changes, age, nutrition, and psychological factors (eg, stress). As we grow older, our bodies are less able to produce antibodies, which are important in fighting infections. As a result, older adults are at a greater risk for infections and the mortality rate from infection is much higher than in the young. Older adults are 3 times more likely to die of pneumonia or sepsis, 5 to 10 times more likely to die of urinary tract infections, and 15 to 20 times more likely to die of appendicitis.

The thymus gland produces hormones that are important for the development of white blood cells. White blood cells are the "phages" of the immune system—they attack and isolate foreign materials. The involution (shrinking) of the thymus gland begins after adolescence and the level of thymic hormones decreases by age 30. By the age of 60, thymic hormones frequently cannot be detected in the blood.[89]

As we age, the immune system also responds less vigorously to skin tests in which a foreign substance is injected below the skin surface, indicating a diminished response to antigens (see Box 3-12).

Box 3-12: **Immune System Changes With Aging**

- There is a decreased production of thymic hormones.
- There is a decrease in levels of antibody response.
- The system's response to antigens diminishes.

SLEEP CHANGES WITH AGE

The phenomenon of sleep is not yet totally understood, but it is known that quality sleep positively influences health and slows the aging process (see Box 3-13). Sleep is one of the most often altered functions in elderly people, with insomnia as one of the main complaints. Additionally, conditions such as *sleep apnea syndrome* and *restless legs syndrome* cause frequent waking. Four progressively deeper levels of sleep plus an intermediate level associated with rapid eye movements (REM) are known to exist. Once asleep, a younger person seldom awakens and the deeper sleep levels

---

Box 3-13: **The Stages of Sleep**

- Stage 1: Drowsiness—lasts about 5 to 10 minutes, eyes move slowly under eyelids, muscle activity slows, individual is easily awakened.
- Stage 2: Light Sleep—eye movements stop, heart rate slows, body temperature decreases.
- Stages 3 & 4: Deep Sleep—difficult to wake, groggy and disoriented if woken, allows the brain to rest, replenishes energy stores, immune functions increase, gets progressively deeper as you move from Stage 3 to Stage 4.
- Stages 5: REM Sleep/Dream Sleep—occurs about 30 minutes into sleep, about 3 to 5 REM episodes per night, processes emotions, retains memories, relieves stress, breathing becomes rapid and irregular, heart rate and blood pressure increase.

---

of 3 and 4 are maintained. In the elderly, consecutive sleep time is decreased, awakenings are more frequent, and less sleep time is spent in levels 3 and 4, although total sleep time is normally only slightly reduced. Because of side effects, such as drowsiness and confusion, the use of sedatives should be discouraged in the aged. In most cases, actual sleep loss is minimal. Other therapeutic supports such as increased daytime activity and decreased naps can be effective in relieving the elderly person's feelings of impaired nocturnal sleep.[90]

WHAT DO THESE AGE-RELATED CHANGES MEAN?

Currently, it is impossible to prevent normal aging. The challenge is to determine which changes are the results of factors that can be altered. With normal aging, people retain the capacity to do things that have meaning and remain physically and mentally active.

Looking at one example of an elderly patient with decreased lung efficiency, we know that lifestyle habits, such as smoking, cause damage to the body systems. Therefore, the PTA can work with the patient to maximize lung function and minimize the effects of normal aging by using exercise to increase lung efficiency. Although changes in lifestyle and environment cannot halt the aging process, they can improve the quality of life for the patient working through therapy and adjusting to life changes. Changes include both making the environment more accessible (both physically and sensory) and by reducing the risk of contracting diseases to which the aged may be more susceptible.

In a second example, we consider joint stiffness with aging. Suppose a man has some arthritis (thus, there is a disease coupled with the effects of normal aging) and leads a sedentary life. His inactivity will lead to more joint problems, increased loss of muscle, bone mass, and strength. His inactivity will also affect other systems; for example, his digestive system may become sluggish, leading to constipation. The man may take in too many calories and put on weight, putting further stress on the joints and creating challenges for other systems. If he is taking some medication for arthritis, this may cause more digestive problems. The reduced metabolic rate will also decrease the absorption of drugs and nutrients. Therefore, the question arises—what is caused by normal aging and what is caused by other factors?

In determining an "answer" to this question, it is important to keep in mind the following:

- Age-related changes are usually not noticed in a day-to-day routine.

- Changes become apparent when the system is stressed (running to catch the bus, recovering from injury or surgery, etc).

- In the absence of disease, people continue to function very well into old age.

- To fully understand aging, we need to look at more than biological change—nutrition, social situations, medications, and outlook will also play a role in how successfully a person ages.

CONCLUSION

Normal aging in the absence of disease is a remarkably benign process. In other words, the body can remain healthy as it ages. Although organs may gradually lose some function, these changes may not even be noticed except during periods of great exertion or stress. Conceptually, this seems clear enough, but when applied to specific cases, the boundaries become blurred. Some degree of decline is noted with age in all biological, anatomical, physiological, and functional components of the human body and it is not considered pathological. Aging has been excluded from the domain of disease because it is considered *normal*.

Aging and disease are related in subtle and complex ways. Aging is viewed as the result of the accumulation of unrepaired injuries resulting from mostly unavoidable changes. A variety of degenerative processes are repeatedly termed "normal aging" until they proceed far enough to cause clinically significant disability and become "disease." Several conditions that were once thought to be part of normal aging have now been shown to be due to disease processes that can be influenced by lifestyle. For example, heart and blood vessel diseases are more common in people with high fat diets. Similarly, cataract formation in the eye largely depends on the amount of exposure to direct sunlight.

In summary, there is a range of individual responses to aging. Biologic and chronologic ages are not the same. In addition, body systems do not age at the same rate within any individual. For example, one aged patient might have severe arthritis or loss of vision, while the functioning of the heart and kidneys is excellent. Even those aging changes that are considered "usual" or "normal" are not inevitable consequences of aging.

Healthy aging is an issue of increasing importance as the size of the older population continues to grow. Poor health in later years is not inevitable. Much of the illness and disability associated with aging is related to modifiable lifestyle factors that are present during earlier stages of the life cycle.

PEARLS

- Individuals age differently depending on activity levels, nutrition, and hydration of the body systems.

- The process of homeostasis helps to keep the internal environment balanced.

- Normal weight-bearing and a balance of rest are recommended to maintain the health of cartilaginous tissues.

- Many persons have a misconception that they cannot build strength in their muscles as they age. PTAs should educate their patients in how participation in a structured exercise program will benefit them.

- The decrease in muscle mass is associated with a decrease in protein and nitrogen and an increase in connective tissue and fat.

- Cardiovascular changes with age are numerous and include anatomical changes in the heart and vasculature, a decrease in maximal achievable heart rate, and a decrease in cardiac output.

- Due to the structural and physiologic changes expected in the absence of cardiovascular pathology, it is imperative for the PTA to pay careful attention to the elderly patient's response to movement, especially positional changes, and proceed accordingly.

- In the pulmonary system, age-related changes affect mechanical properties of respiration, blood flow, gas exchange, and a decrease in lung defenses.

- Due to the change in thermal regulatory response, the aged have a prolonged cooling time following increased activity, as well as a decrease in receptiveness to heat and cold.

- The immune system is suppressed with age and older adults are more vulnerable to infections that can result in disability and death.

- All 5 senses as well as proprioception/kinethesia show a decline associated with disuse and aging.

- Aging is a progressive and cumulative process of change occurring over time. Many normal changes of aging do not cause clinically significant declines in function.

- Age-related changes that affect function are noticed most often in vision, hearing, memory, and bladder (eg, nocturia, frequency).

- Encouraging any movement in the elderly is better than no movement at all. If the patient is not likely to adhere to a longer exercise program, incorporate increased activity throughout the day versus one long exercise session.

- Incorporate weight-bearing activities as well as nonweight-bearing activities for improving overall fitness.

- Include drinking water as a part of an older person's exercise program.

References

1. Koehn M. Embracing the aging process. *J Christ Nurs.* 2005;22:20-24.
2. Melo RC, Santos MD, Silva E, Quiterio RJ, Moreno MA, Reis MS, et al. Effects of age and physical activity on the autonomic control of heart rate in elderly men. *Braz J Med Biol Res.* 2005;38:1331-1338.
3. Harman D. Aging: overview. *Ann N Y Acad Sci.* 2001;928:1-21.
4. Speakman JR. Correlations between physiology and life–two widely ignored problems with comparative studies. *Aging Cell.* 2005;4:167-175.
5. Walston J, Hadley EC, Ferrucci L, et al. Research agenda for frailty in older adults. *J Am Geriatr Soc.* 2006;54:991-1001.
6. Yin D, Chen K. The essential mechanisms of aging: irreparable damage accumulation of biochemical side-reactions. *Exp Gerontol.* 2005;40:455-465.
7. Zheng J, Edelman SW, Tharmarajah G, Walker DW, Pletcher SD, Seroude L. Differential patterns of apoptosis in response to aging in Drosophila. *Proc Natl Acad Sci USA.* 2005;102:12083-12088.
8. Zamboni M, Zoico E, Scartezzini T, et al. Body composition changes in stable-weight elderly subjects: the effect of sex. *Aging Clin Exp Res.* 2003;15:321-327.
9. Mitchell D, Haan MN, Steinberg FM, Visser M. Body composition in the elderly: the influence of nutritional factors and physical activity. *J Nutr Health Aging.* 2003;7:130-139.
10. Labat-Robert J. Age-dependent remodeling of connective tissue: role of fibronectin and laminin. *Pathol Biol.* 2003;51:563-568.
11. An KN, Sun YL, Luo ZP. Flexibility of type I collagen and mechanical property of connective tissue. *Biorhelology.* 2004;41:239-246.
12. Umeda H, Takeuchi M, Suyama K. Two new elastin cross-links having pyridine skeleton. *J Biol Chem.* 2001;276:12579-12587.
13. Luchansky SJ, Argada S, Hayes BK, Bertozzi CR. Metabolic functionalization of recombinant glycoproteins. *Biochemistry.* 2004;43:12358-12366.
14. Wang CT, Lin J, Chang CJ, Lin YT, Hou SM. Therapeutic effects of hyaluronic acid on osteoarthritis of the knee. A meta-analysis of randomized controlled trials. *J Bone Joint Surg Am.* 2004;86-A:538-545.
15. Pavelka K, Forjtova S, Olejarova M, et al. Hyaluronic acid levels may have predictive value for the progression of knee osteoarthritis. *Osteoarthritis Cartilage.* 2004;12:277-283.
16. Kakehi K, Kinoshita M, Yasueda S. Hyaluronic acid: separation and biological implications. *J Chromatogr B Analyt Technol Biomed Life Sci.* 2003;797:347-355.
17. Wakayam J, Tamura T, Yagi N, Iwamoto H. Structural transients of contractile proteins upon sudden ATP liberation in skeletal muscle fibers. *Biophys J.* 2004;87:430-441.
18. Yoo HS, Lee EA, Yoon JJ, Park TG. Hyaluronic acid modified biodegradable scaffolds for cartilage tissue engineering. *Biomaterials.* 2005;26:1925-1933.
19. Loeser RF. Aging cartilage and osteoarthritis–what's the link? *Sci Aging Knowledge Envir.* 2004;:pe31.
20. Walker J. Connective tissue plasticity: issues in histological and light microscopy studies of exercise and aging in articular cartilage. *JOSPT.* 1991;14:189-197.
21. Brown M, Rose SJ. The effects of aging and exercise on skeletal muscle-clinical considerations. *Top Ger Rehabil.* 1985;1:20-30.
22. Nikoli M, Bajek S, Bobinac D, Vrani TS, Jerkovi R. Aging of human skeletal muscles. *Coll Antropol.* 2005;29:67-70.
23. Vandervoot AA, Symons TB. Functional and metabolic consequences of sarcopenia. *Can J Appl Physiol.* 2001;26:90-101.
24. Sowers MR, Crutchfield M, Richards K, et al. Sarcopenia is related to physical functioning and leg strength in middle-aged women. *J Gerontol A Biol Sci Med Sci.* 2005;60:486-490.
25. Bales CW, Ritchie CS. Sarcopenia, weight loss, and nutritional frailty in the elderly. *Annual Rev Nutr.* 2002;22:309-323.
26. Parsons LC. Osteoporosis: incidence, prevention, and treatment of the silent killer. *Nurs Clin North Am.* 2005;40:119-133.
27. Grahn Kronhed AC, Blamberg C, Karlsson N, Lofman O, Timpka T, Moller M. Impact of a community-based osteoporosis and fall prevention program on fracture incidence. *Osteoporos Int.* 2005;16:700-706.
28. Prentice A. Diet nutrition and prevention of osteoporosis. *Public Health Nutr.* 2004;7:227-243.
29. McLaughlin MA. The aging heart. State-of-the-art prevention and management of cardiac disease. *Geriatrics.* 2001;56:45-49.
30. Oxenham H, Sharpe N. Cardiovascular aging and heart failure. *Eur J Heart Fail.* 2003;5:427-434.
31. Pugh KG, Wei JY. Clinical implications of physiological changes in the aging heart. *Drug Aging.* 2001;18:263-276.
32. Schrezenmair C, Gehrking JA, Hines SM, Low PA, Benrund-Larson LM, Sandrani P. Evaluation of orthostatic hypotension: relationship of a new self-report instrument to laboratory-based measures. *Mayo Clin Proc.* 2005;80:330-334.
33. Sander GE. Hypertension in the elderly. *Curr Hypertens Rep.* 2004;6:469-476.
34. Melo RC, Santos MD, Silva E, et al. Effects of age and physical activity on the autonomic control of heart rate in healthy men. *Braz J Med Biol Res.* 2005;38:1331-1338.
35. Laung JE, Benson WF, Anderson LA. Aging and public health: partnership that can affect cardiovascular health programs. *Am J Prev Med.* 2005; 29(suppl 1):158-163.
36. Fioranelli M, Piccoli M, Mileto GM, et al. Modifications in cardiovascular functional parameters with aging. *Minerva Cardioangiol.* 2001;49:169-178.
37. Zeleznik J. Normative aging of the respiratory system. *Clin Geriatr Med.* 2003;19:1-18.
38. Dervelle F, Nourry C, Mucci P, et al. Incremental exercise tests in master athletes and untrained older adults. *J Aging Phys Act.* 2005;13:254-265.
39. Janssens JP. Aging of the respiratory system: impact on pulmonary function tests and adaptation to exertion. *Clin Chest Med.* 2005;26:469-484.
40. Zhang YT, Zhang CY, Zhang J, Li W. Age-related changes of normal adult brain structure: analyzed with diffusion tensor imaging. *Chin Med J (Engl).* 2005;118:1059-1065.
41. Vandervoort AA. Aging of the human neuromuscular system. *Muscle Nerve.* 2002;25:17-25.
42. Zarchin N, Meilin S, Rifkind J, Mayevsky A. Effect of aging on brain energy-metabolism. *Comp Biochem Physiol A Mol Integr Physiol.* 2002;132:117-120.
43. Fewel ME, Thompson BG, Hoff JT. Spontaneous intracerebral hemorrhage: assessment and management of stroke and transient ischemic accidents. *Neurosurg Focus.* 2003;15:1-8.

44. Kelly KM, Nadon ML, Morrison JH, Thibault O, Barnes CA, Blalock EM. The neurobiology of aging. *Epilepsy Res.* 2006;68(suppl 1):S5-S20.

45. Richerson SJ, Morstalt SG, Vanya RD, Hollister AM, Robinson CJ. Factors affecting reaction times to short anterior postural disturbances. *Meng Eng Phys.* 2004;26:581-586.

46. Brumagne S, Cordo P, Verschueren S. Proprioceptive weighting changes in persons with low back pain and elderly persons during upright standing. *Neurosci Lett.* 2004;366: 63-66.

47. Desaie M, Pratt LA, Lentzner H, Robinson KN. Trends in vision and hearing among older adults. *Aging Trends.* 2001;1:1-8.

48. Anstey KJ, Luszcz MA, Giles LC, Andrews GR. Demographic, health, cognitive, and sensory variables as predictors of mortality in very old adults. *Psychol Aging.* 2001;16:3-11.

49. Donat H, Ozcan A, Ozdirenc M, Aksako lu G, Aydino lu S. Age-related changes in pressure pain threshold, grip strength and touch pressure threshold in upper extremities of older adults. *Aging Clin Exp Res.* 2005;17:380-384.

50. Bee HL. *The Journey of Adulthood: Physical Changes.* 4th ed. Upper Saddle River, NJ: Prentice Hall; 2000.

51. Giacomoni PU, Rein G. A mechanistic model for the aging of human skin. *Micron.* 2004;35:179-184.

52. Hashizume H. Skin aging and dry skin. *J Dermatol.* 2004;31:603-609.

53. Guinot C, Malvy DJ, Ambroisine L, et al. Relative contribution of intrinsic and extrinsic factors to skin aging as determined by a validated skin age score. *Arch Dermatol.* 2002;138:1454-1460.

54. Van Neste D, Tobin DJ. Hair cycle and hair pigmentation: dynamic interactions and changes associated with aging. *Micron.* 2004;35:193-200.

55. Nishimura EK, Granter SR, Fisher DE. Mechanisms of hair graying: incomplete melanocyte stem cell maintenance in the niche. *Science.* 2005;307:720-724.

56. Mandt N, Blume-Peytavi U. Aging of hair and nails. *Hautarzt.* 2005;56:340-346.

57. Brosche T, Dressler S, Platt D. Age-associated changes in integral cholesterol and cholesterol sulfate concentrations in human scalp hair and finger nail clippings. *Aging (Milano).* 2001;13:131-138.

58. Cheshire WP, Freeman R. Sweating disorders in the elderly. *Semin Neurol.* 2003;23:399-406.

59. Spry PG, Johnson CA. Senscent changes of the normal visual field: an age-old problem. *Optom Vis Sci.* 2001;78(6):436-441.

60. Wang YZ. Effects of aging on shape discrimination. *Optom Vis Sci.* 2001;78:447-754.

61. Levy BR, Slade MD, Gill TM. Hearing decline predicted by elders' stereotypes. *J Gerontol B Psychol Sci Soc Sci.* 2006;61: P82-P87.

62. Scholtz AW, Kammen-Jolly K, Felder E, Hussl B, Rask-Anderson H, Schrott-Fischer A. Selective aspects of human pathology in high-tone hearing loss of the aging inner ear. *Hear Res.* 2001;157:77-86.

63. Teasdale N, Simoneau M. Attentional demands for postural control: the effects of aging and sensory integration. *Gait Posture.* 2001;14:203-210.

64. Alpini D, Cesarani A, Fraschini F, Kohen-Raz R, Capobianco S, Cornelio F. Aging and vestibular system: specific tests and role of melatonin in cognitive involvement. *Arch Gerontol Geriatr Suppl.* 2004;38:13-25.

65. Davenport RJ. The flavor of aging. *Sci Aging Knowledge Environ.* 2004;12:ns1. http://sageke.sciencemag.org/cgi/content/full/2004/12/ns1. Accessed March 24, 2009.

66. Tuorila H, Niskanen N, Maunuksela E. Perception and pleasantness of a food with varying odor and flavor among the elderly and young. *J Nutr Health Aging.* 2001;5:266-268.

67. Mathey MF, Siebelink E, de Graaf C, Van Staveren WA. Flavor enhancement of foods improves dietary intake and nutritional status of elderly nursing home residents. *J Gerontol A Biol Sci Med Sci.* 2001;56:M200-205.

68. Walston J, Hadley EC, Ferrucci L, et al. Research agenda for frailty in older adults. *J Am Geriatr Soc.* 2006;54:991-1001.

69. Kenney WL, Munce TA. Invited review: aging and human temperature regulation. *J Appl Physiol.* 2003;95:2598-2603.

70. Mobbs CV. Not wisely but too well: aging as a cost of neuroendocrine activity. *Sci Aging Knowledge Environ.* 2004;2004:pe33.

71. Chen H. Gene expression by the anterior pituitary gland: effects of age and caloric restriction. *Mol Cell Endocrinol.* 2004;222:21-31.

72. Leslie M. Tuning up the pancreas. *Sci Aging Knowledge Environ.* 2005;34:nf67. http://sageke.sciencemag.org/cgi/content/full/2005/34/nf67.

73. Habra M, Sarlis NJ. Thyroid and aging. *Rev Endocr Metab Disord.* 2005;6:145-154.

74. Nawata H, Yanase T, Goto K, et al. Andrenopause. *Horm Res.* 2004;62(suppl 3):110-114.

75. Harman SM. What do hormones have to do with aging? What does aging have to do with hormones? *Ann N Y Acad Sci.* 2004;1019:299-308.

76. Landgren BM, Collins A, Csemicsky G, Burger HG, Baksheev L, Robertson DM. Menopause transition: annual changes in serum hormonal patterns over the menstrual cycle in women during a nine-year period prior to menopause. *J Clin Endocrinol Metab.* 2004;89:2763-2769.

77. Ossewaarde ME, Bots ML, Verbeek AL, et al. Age at menopause, cause-specific mortality and total life expectancy. *Epidemiology.* 2005;16:556-562.

78. Tan RS. Novel treatment options for overlapping yet distinct erectile dysfunction and andropause syndromes. *Curr Opin Investig Drugs.* 2003;4:435-438.

79. Hochreiter WW, Ackermann DK, Brutsch HP. Andropause. *Ther Umsch.* 2005;62:821-826.

80. Sator PG, Schmidt JB, Rage T, Zouboulis CC. Skin aging and sex hormones – clinical perspectives for intervention by hormone replacement therapy. *Exp Dermatol.* 2004;13(suppl 4):36-40.

81. Pilotto A. Aging and upper gastrointestinal disorders. *Best Pract Res Clin Gastroenterol.* 2004;18(suppl):73-81.

82. Bitar KN, Patil SB. Aging and gastrointestinal smooth muscle. *Mech Ageing Dev.* 2004;125:907-910.

83. Schmucker DL. Liver function and phase I drug metabolism in the elderly: a paradox. *Drugs Aging.* 2001;18:837-851.

84. Watson R. Assessing the gastrointestinal (GI) tract in older people: 2. the lower GI tract. *Nurs Older People.* 2001;13:27-28.

85. Chapman JR, Dozois EJ, Wolff BG, Gullerud RE, Larson DR. Diverticulitis: a progressive disease? Do multiple recurrences predict less favorable outcomes? *Ann Surg.* 2006; 243:876-830.

86. Hoang K, Tan JC, Derby G, et al. Determinants of glomerular hypofiltration in aging humans. *Kidney Int.* 2003;64:1417-1424.

87. Van der Horst C, Junemann KP. The aging bladder: anatomy and physiology. *Urologe A.* 2004;43:521-526.

88. Staskin DR. Overactive bladder in the elderly: a guide to pharmacological management. *Drugs Aging.* 2005;22:1013-1028.

89. Prelog M. Aging of the immune system: a risk factor for autoimmunity? *Autoimmun Rev.* 2006;5:136-139.

90. Lemoine P, Nicolas A, Faivre T. Sleep and aging. *Presse Med.* 2001;30:417-424.

Common Pathological Conditions in the Elderly: Impact on Function and Treatment Approaches

Aging is considered a normal physiological process because of its universality. As much as the aging process may influence the predisposition to disease, aging in and of itself is not considered to be pathological.

This distinction seems conceptually clear, however, the fine line between aging and disease is often blurred when applied to specific cases. Some degree of decreasing biological, physiological, anatomical, and functional capabilities occurs as one ages (as discussed in Chapter 3). Some degree of atrophy and altered physiology and function is evident in all tissues of the body. A variety of degenerative processes are called "normal aging" until they proceed far enough to cause clinically significant disability.

The incidence of many diseases and the resulting death rate is influenced markedly as age advances (see Figure 4-1). The death rates for atherosclerosis, myocardial degeneration, cerebrovascular disease (stroke), hypertension, and cancer all increase more steeply than the overall death rate, arousing the suspicion that aging predisposes an individual either to the development of the condition or to a fatal outcome. With some conditions, such as respiratory infections, the incidence is not increased in the elderly, but the likelihood of fatality from the insult is greater than in younger persons.[1] The good news is that with better health care and changes in lifestyle over the past decade, the death rate from cardiac diseases and stroke has actually seen a downward trend. In a child or young adult, death is most commonly caused by some form of accident. However, in the elderly, the main problems are coronary heart disease, cerebrovascular accidents, respiratory diseases, diabetes, peripheral vascular diseases, and neoplasms[2,3] (see Figure 4-2).

The 15 leading causes of death in the elderly in 2004 according to the Centers for Disease Control[4] were:

- Diseases of heart
- Malignant neoplasms (cancer)
- Cerebrovascular diseases (stroke)
- Chronic lower respiratory diseases
- Accidents (unintentional injuries)
- Diabetes mellitus (diabetes)
- Alzheimer's disease
- Influenza and pneumonia
- Nephritis, nephrotic syndrome, and nephrosis (kidney disease)
- Septicemia
- Intentional self-harm (suicide)
- Chronic liver disease and cirrhosis

Bottomley J. *Geriatric Rehabilitation: A Textbook for the Physical Therapist Assistant* (pp 65-94).

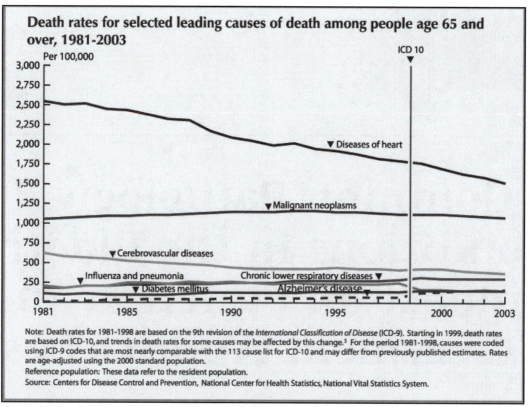

Figure 4-1. Death rates among people ages 65 and older. Reprinted from the Centers for Disease Control and Prevention. National Center for Health Statistics. National Vital Statistics System. 2003.[3]

- Essential (primary) hypertension and hypertensive renal disease (hypertension)
- Parkinson's disease
- Pneumonitis due to solids and liquids.

This chapter will review the pathologies that are common manifestations in the aged population. It will not attempt a detailed consideration of all pathology seen in a geriatric population; rather, it will examine some of the more common conditions that afflict the elderly and affect functional activities of daily living (ADL). Etiology of pathologies, signs and symptoms, medical interventions, and the impact on function will be covered in this chapter. Chapter 10 will deal specifically with the physical therapy interventions that a PTA would employ in the treatment of elderly patients.

AGING AS DISEASE

There is the assumed implication that aging, like growth and development, is a normal physiological process lying outside the domain of disease. Although aging may not be considered a disease process, the time-dependent loss of structure and function in all organ systems leads to pathological end states. There is a general decline in structure, function, and the number of many kinds of cells with age. Cellular aging is accompanied by changes of protein structures. The collagen and elastin of the skin become irreversibly frayed and rigid. The hyaline cartilage on articular surfaces of joints becomes pitted and fragmented, and the beautifully ordered structure of the lens of the eye becomes brittle and chaotic as lens protein is gradually lost.

The aging process proceeds slowly over the life course, resulting in a loss of structure and function within every organ or tissue. This process is exacerbated by inactivity, poor hydration, and poor nutrition. Countless micro-traumas occur and accumulate in small increments as imperceptible injuries. Over a lifetime, the skin elastin is exposed to micro-insults from the ultraviolet rays of the sun, repetitive mechanical stresses cause degeneration of articular cartilage, and the opacity of the lens of the eye diminishes due to reactions with metabolites. These are just a few examples of the changes that occur. The most important aging changes occur at the molecular level, as reviewed in Chapter 2. Small injuries occurring within the cell result in the loss of genetic memory and progressive cross-linking of collagen, the chief structural protein in the body.

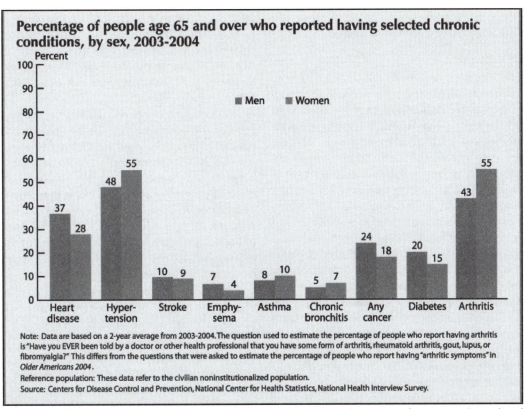

Figure 4-2. Chronic health conditions in the elderly. Reprinted from the Centers for Disease Control and Prevention. National Center for Health Statistics. National Vital Statistics System. 2003.[3]

Disease is often described as the reaction to injury. If aging is a gradual accumulation of incompletely repaired injuries due to micro-trauma through the life course, it may not be normal, despite its universality. Perhaps the pathological process resulting from the tissues reactions to imperceptible injuries could have been avoided. Nonetheless, the longer we live, the more likely we are to experience the cumulative effects of lifelong micro-trauma and pathology.

A FOCUS ON FUNCTION

Clinicians involved in rehabilitation therapies should play a major role in preventing disabilities. Preventive strengthening and conditioning exercises, positioning, joint and tissue mobilization, stretching, endurance exercises, and working to improve all functional capabilities could play a major role in healthy aging, in all age groups. Preventing disabilities that can result from pathological processes greatly improves the level of function and the quality of life.

COMMON CAUSES OF DISABILITY IN THE ELDERLY

Musculoskeletal Manifestations of Aging

The musculoskeletal system is comprised of muscles and tendons, the fascia, the bony skeleton, and joints (including ligaments and cartilage). The individual experiences gradually decreasing strength, control, and mobility as the components of this system age.

Muscle Changes With Aging

The composition of muscles changes over time with replacement of myofibrils by fat, collagen, and scar tissue. Individual muscle fibers also change in their permeability to water, sodium, and chloride, which increases with age. Blood flow to muscles decreases with age, thereby reducing the amount of nutrients and energy available to the muscle; strength declines. This process begins early in life and accelerates rapidly after the fifth decade, especially when overshadowed by inactivity. By age 60, the total loss in lean muscle mass represents 10% to 20% of the maximum muscle power attained at age 30.[5]

Myopathy and Myositis

Sarcopenia, the loss of muscle mass, is a hallmark of aging commonly attributed to a decreased capacity to maintain muscle tissue in old age (as discussed in detail in Chapter 3). Over time, this leads to other muscle pathologies, such as *myopathy* (any disease of a muscle) and *myositis* (inflammation of a muscle). Muscle dysfunction in the aged is usually the result of toxic or metabolic factors acting on muscle, rather than due to any intrinsic disease of the muscle.[6] Symptoms suggesting myopathy include weakness in the hip girdle muscles with difficulty rising from a chair and the development of a waddling gait or shoulder girdle weakness manifested by inability to lift objects above shoulder level. Muscle soreness is not a usual finding with any myopathy, and is more common with myositis in which there is infiltration of muscles by inflammation. *Polymyositis* (myositis affecting more than one muscle) can be idiopathic or related to the presence of underlying carcinoma. Myositis usually responds to steroids or other anti-inflammatory agents.[7]

Muscle weakness can result from several correctable causes including conditions such as hyperthyroidism, alcoholism, adrenocortical steroid excess (Cushing's disease or administration of steroids), and hypocalcemia (from diarrhea or diuretic use). Correction of the underlying cause usually results in resolution of the weakness.

Skeletal Manifestations of Aging

Aging brings many complex changes in bone structure. Both women and men show a progressive decline in bone mass after the age of 50, with women losing about 25% and men approximately 12%. Although bone growth continues into old age, reabsorption of the interior of the long and flat bones (trabecular bone) increases until reabsorption occurs at a greater rate than the formation of new bone. As a result, bone strength and stability decline. This is particularly true of trabecular bone, which is found in the highest proportions in vertebral bodies, wrists, and hips. This correlates with the clinical observation of the increased incidence of fractures at these sites with age.[8]

Osteoporosis

Osteoporosis is a heterogeneous condition characterized by an absolute decrease in the amount of normal bone, that is, loss of bone. Osteoporosis results when the production of new bone mass is exceeded by the reabsorption of old bone; in other words, osteoporosis is the failure of bone formation to keep pace with bone resorption, or *coupling*. The result is that bone becomes structurally weakened. Age-related trabecular bone loss starts at age 35, and cortical bone loss from about age 40. The loss proceeds at about 0.5% per year; but, at female menopause, the rate is accelerated to 2.0% to 8.0% due directly or indirectly to lowered estrogen production. The greater the bone mass attained at the time resorption exceeds the creation of new bone, the more time is needed before significant structural changes result. This in part accounts for the higher incidence of clinically significant osteoporosis in women than men because men have greater bone mass. However, the reasons for the differential rates of demineralization of bone between men and women are not understood, although there are several factors that appear to have a role in the process.[9]

Estrogen deficiency occurring with menopause, and testosterone deficiency occurring with andropause, lead to accelerated bone loss in women and men, respectively, and is partially reversed by replacing estrogen or testosterone.[10]

Other factors contributing to skeletal weakness include malabsorption of calcium leading to poor bone mineralization (osteomalacia), which affects both sexes. Negative calcium balance can result from many factors including calcium deficiency in the diet, malabsorption, and accelerated loss. Impaired absorption of calcium from the intestine can be due to insufficient vitamin D because of diet, or renal or hepatic disease. Calcium absorption can be affected as part of intestinal malabsorption syndromes such as irritable bowel syndrome or diverticulosis. Endocrine disorders affecting calcium balance include hyperthyroidism, excess corticosteroids as in Cushing's disease or steroid administration, hyperparathyroidism leading to excess bone resorption, as well as hypoparathyroidism resulting in poor calcium absorption. Immobility for any reason and at any age can lead to marked negative calcium balance. When a limb is immobilized, localized osteoporosis occurs. Thus, for the elderly, decreased mobility for any reason adds to the already abundant factors present for the development of osteoporosis. The presence of osteoporosis requires a thorough review of potentially treatable causes. Treatment is a judicious balance of exercise, medication, and dietary manipulation.[11]

Calcium supplementation is often recommended to prevent postmenopausal bone loss in women undergoing menopause or who have undergone menopause within 5 years before. In women who have been postmenopausal for 6 or more years, calcium citrate malate can significantly reduce bone loss at a dosage of 800 mg/day. Studies that have looked at the same supplementation regime effects in men are limited and inconclusive.[12]

Although the entire skeleton loses mass with aging, the distribution of bone loss is not uniform. Those areas of the skeleton with the highest content of trabecular bone (such as vertebral bodies and bones of the wrist and hip) will lose the greatest amount of their mass. Exercise has been found to be very effective in maintaining bone mass. Specific exercise protocols for osteoporosis prevention and bone mass maintenance will be presented in Chapter 10.

Joint Changes With Aging

Aging joints can have a tremendous impact on the functionality of elderly people with and without disabilities. Degenerative changes in joints begin as early as the second or third decade, and after age 40 progress more rapidly. These changes occur mainly in the weight-bearing joints such as the ankles, knees, hips, and lumbar spine. Cartilage forms the weight-bearing surfaces of these joints, and by age 30 begins to crack, shred, and fray. Over time, deep vertical fissures appear and the cartilage-producing cells die or become less effective. Ultimately, the cartilage layers are eroded exposing the bone beneath to direct contact with the opposing bone. This contact causes pain and produces the physical sign of crepitus or grinding when the joint is moved. New bone formation is stimulated, but the bone growth is irregular and often interferes with joint mobility as the resulting osteophytes enlarge. Synovial membranes, which surround and protect joints, also exhibit changes due to age. The synovial lining thickens and the synovial fluid becomes more viscous with age. Other changes include the shrinkage of the intervertebral discs in the lumbar spine due to loss of water content in the discs. Coupled with vertebral body collapse, disc shrinkage can produce a significant loss of height.[13] The aging changes associated with bone, cartilage, and synovial membranes are covered in Chapter 3.

Osteoarthritis

Osteoarthritis (OA) is the wear and tear of joint surfaces due to inflammation, resulting in joint corrosion. Age-related changes in the musculoskeletal system increase the risk of developing OA if other risk factors are also present. The joint is a functioning biomechanical unit of the neuromuscular system. Factors that contribute to the development of joint pain and loss of joint function include those associated with aging, those associated with underuse or misuse, and those associated directly with the development of OA. Complex interactions exist among many of these factors including strength, balance, and proprioception, which are affected by aging, underuse, and OA. Many older adults who have joint pain and loss of function do not exhibit the structural changes of OA that can

be detected by standard radiography. When structural damage is present, its contribution to pain and disability is not always clear. In the absence of pharmacologic agents that can prevent the progression of structural damage in OA, management of older adults who have joint pain and loss of function should focus on improving neuromuscular function and preventing further decline.[14] Physical therapy is a crucial component in the care of the OA patient.

Degenerative arthritis is an inflammation within the joint space that causes pain, loss of mobility, and deformity of the joint. There are several different types of arthritis, but all lead to a common final pathway known as *degenerative joint disease* (DJD) or OA. Recurrent joint trauma leads to intra-articular damage, which results in the release of proteolytic enzymes that often cause bleeding. A cycle is set up with increased cartilage damage, bleeding, and the release of potentially destructive enzymes. Over time, cartilage is eroded, new bone growth stimulated, and the joint gradually loses its ability to respond to trauma, thereby making it even more susceptible to additional trauma and damage. Because of irritation of the periosteum (joint capsule) and fibrotic changes of the muscles surrounding the joint, pain and decreased motion are the ultimate outcome. Over time, the joint can become fibrotic as a result of this primary degenerative process. The joints most often affected by DJD are the hands, knees, hips, lumbar, and cervical spine. It is manifested clinically by stiffness and pain, which increase with use. Impaired mobility makes it difficult to accomplish routine ADL.[15]

Functional movements require concerted actions of the joint's muscle agonists and antagonists. Understanding age-related changes in muscle function and their effects on performance requires an understanding of the contributions of different muscles to joint movements. It has been found that the decreased strength of muscle around the joint actually results in less joint movement. Muscle weakness also changes how the joint is held. Typically the muscle weakness results in a joint, such as the knee, being held in a slightly flexed position. This will affect performance and destabilize the joint. It also results in an inappropriate positioning of the joint, leading to undue stresses and wear.[16]

The development of effective anti-inflammatory medications and improvement of surgical interventions in joint disease has changed the current management of endstage DJD. Joint replacement can be very effective in restoring function and limiting pain. Joint fusion and anti-inflammatory medications are often effective in pain control.

Exercise is important in OA management. Benefits appear to be additive when exercise is delivered with other interventions such as weight loss. Supervised exercise sessions appear to be superior to home exercises for pain reduction. That result may be caused by improved compliance as opposed to the type of exercise (ie, those patients may not be doing home exercises). Regardless, research is clear that patients with OA benefit from strengthening, stretching, and functionally-based exercises.[17]

Rheumatoid Arthritis

Rheumatoid Arthritis (RA) can occur at any age and is characterized by the abrupt onset of symmetrical joint swelling, redness, and pain. Inflammation of the synovial membrane results in the release of proteolytic enzymes, which perpetuate inflammation and joint damage. Morning stiffness is more pronounced and has a longer duration than in DJD. The involved joints tend to be the small joints of the hands and feet, the wrists, shoulders, elbows, hips, knees, and ankles. Essentially every joint is involved in this autoimmune systemic condition. Eventually deformities occur, affecting mobility and basic ADL. RA is a systemic disease; therefore, other signs and symptoms are often present. These include fever, fatigue, malaise, poor appetite, weight loss, nutritional deficiencies, weakness, anemia, enlarged spleen, and lymphadenopathy (disease of the lymph nodes).[18]

Response to therapy is usually quite good. Given the ease with which the elderly develop muscle atrophy with disuse, aggressive physical therapy is essential to maintain strength and joint mobility during phases of remission. During exacerbation, physical therapy should be directed toward pain management through decreasing swelling in the joint (ice, electrical stimulation), maintaining joint mobility and decreasing discomfort (oscillation joint mobility techniques, active motion), and encouraging participation in functional ADL.[19] Keep in mind that fatigue is a common complaint among patients with RA and is regarded as an extra-articular symptom of the disease. Unlike normal tiredness, fatigue is chronic, typically not related to overexertion, and poorly relieved by rest. RA-related fatigue appears to be strongly associated to psychosocial factors.[20] Whatever the cause, short exercise sessions work much better in RA patients than longer exercise programs. In other words, several brief exercise periods per day are more beneficial than one long one.

Cardiovascular Manifestations of Aging

In the United States, cardiovascular disease (eg, atherosclerosis and hypertension, which lead to heart failure and stroke) is the leading cause of mortality. Age is a major risk factor for cardiovascular disease, which accounts for more than 40% of deaths in those ages 65 years and above. There are no clinically significant effects on heart function that can be solely ascribed to aging. Cardiovascular dysfunction attributed to the aging process closely mimics the decline in cardiac function seen with inactivity.[21]

Aging is associated with complex and diversified changes of cardiovascular structure and function. The heart becomes slightly hypertrophic and hyporesponsive to sympathetic (but not parasympathetic) stimuli, so that exercise-induced increases in heart rate and myocardial contractility are blunted in older hearts.[22] It is important for the PTA to pay close attention to the older adult's report of perceived exertion, as vital signs may not change consistently with the increasing level of activity.

Clinical manifestations and prognosis of cardiovascular diseases are altered in persons of advanced age because interactions occur between age-associated cardiovascular changes in health and specific pathophysiologic mechanisms that underlie a disease. A fundamental understanding of age-associated changes in structure and function of the cardiovascular systems ranging in scope from the impact of lifestyle, lifelong exercise and activity patterns, and nutrition to environmental and genetic influences is important when considering cardiac and vascular diseases (see Chapter 3). The following is a review of common pathologic manifestations in the cardiovascular system seen in an aged population.

Atherosclerosis

Atherosclerosis is the major cause of mortality in the Western world. It is a functional and vascular change leading to angina, myocardial infarct, transient ischemic cerebrovascular attacks, stroke, ischemic attacks in peripheral circulation (claudication), and thrombo/embolic complications. In fact, *arteriosclerosis* is a generally used term to describe any form of vascular degeneration associated with a thickening and loss of resilience in the arterial wall. Aging, lipids (primarily low-density lipoproteins, or LDL), infective agents, inflammation, increased glucose levels, hypertension, smoking, increased homocysteine levels, and oxidized stress (ie, free radical reaction—see Chapter 2) are recognized as factors that lead to atherosclerosis. It is associated with an accumulation of fat in the lining of the vessels, and an increase of connective tissue in the underlying vessel wall. Almost all animal species show some degree of atherosclerosis, and it has, for this reason, been considered an inevitable accompaniment of aging.[23]

The pathological consequences of atherosclerosis depend on the site. Weakness in the aorta can cause an aneurysm. Ischemic heart disease can result from atherosclerotic changes in the coronary arteries. A cerebrovascular accident (stroke) can result from involvement of the cerebral vessels.

Signs and symptoms of atherosclerosis may vary depending on the extent of vessel blockage. The arteries may not be entirely blocked, although the deposit of fat plaques can be great enough to produce symptoms during exercise when there is a need to increase the flow of oxygenated blood to the heart. With insufficient oxygen, the heart will ache—a symptom termed *angina* (eg, chest pain). Due to the changes in pressure sensation (see Pacinian corpuscles discussed in Chapter 3), chest pain may not occur in an older patient. Instead, the patient will become short of breath as he or she fights to increase the oxygen supply to the blood. As a result, the respiratory rate will increase, though the patient may not report angina at all. The older individual, besides being short of breath with poor exercise tolerance, may also report burning indigestion, nausea, or the need to belch. He or she may also become confused and disoriented and be unable to continue with therapy after what seems to be little effort. It is important that the PTA frequently ask how the individual is tolerating exercise or activity levels.

Currently, the most popular interventions of atherosclerosis are statin drugs (lipid-lowering therapy)[24] and attempts to reduce cholesterol through exercise and dietary modifications. In addition to modifying body mass through exercise and diet, estrogen replacement in women has gained much popularity in recent years. Estrogen has been found to be beneficial in preventing the progression of atherosclerosis in postmenopausal women not receiving lipid-lowering therapy, regardless of their initial body mass index (BMI).[25]

Ischemic Heart Disease

Ischemic heart disease, commonly called *coronary artery disease* (CAD), results from blockage of blood flow to cardiac muscle. Some 40% of those ages 65 to 74 years and 50% of those ages 75 years and older have evidence of heart disease. When there is a reversible lack of oxygen in the cardiac muscle in response to an increased activity level or emotional stress, chest pain results from atherosclerotic changes in the coronary arteries. The effect of ischemia can be reversed and the muscle cells will gradually regain their ability to contract as circulation is restored. A rapid loss of blood flow lasting 30 to 60 minutes can cause death of the myocardial cells. Irreversible damage to a part of the heart muscle from vascular narrowing can result from plaque formation that totally blocks the coronary vessel, an embolus, or a thrombosis, the consequence of which is a heart attack or myocardial infarction. Myocardial degeneration can progress with repeated minor episodes of irreversible oxygen depletion in the cardiac muscle. As degeneration progresses, the heart muscle functions poorly and can result in congestive heart failure. A muscle deprived of its blood supply becomes prone to chaotic and unregulated contractions, which can result in life-threatening arrhythmias.[26]

Oxygen extraction in the coronary circulation is relatively complete even at rest. When the work demands on the heart are increased, additional oxygen is required to meet the energy needs of the cardiac muscle cells. This occurs by dilatation of the coronary vessels. With rigid atherosclerotic vessels, vascular resistance is increased due to the inelastic quality of the vessels as well as resistance to blood flow by plaque obstruction; dilatation does not readily occur. Gross obstruction of the major coronary vessels results in chest pain typically brought on by vigorous exercise. In the elderly, however, angina pain is not a consistent symptomatic indicator of ischemia of the cardiac tissue. The elderly more commonly report dyspnea (shortness of breath). Clinically, shortness of breath is a much more reliable indicator of ischemia than angina in the elderly individual.[27] Respiratory frequency (eg, the breaths per minute) is an important objective measurement for the PTA to monitor and document when working with an elderly person. In addition to information regarding patient safety, information regarding respiratory response to increasing levels of activity provides input to the PT in determining the need to change the plan of care.

Early intervention in ischemic heart disease takes several forms. The most important is to reduce the "risk factors" that predispose individuals to the development of CAD such as cigarette smoking, high blood pressure, and serum cholesterol. Secondary prevention of heart attacks once CAD is established require attention to reduce risk factors, aspirin to prevent platelet aggregation (which may initiate obstruction of a coronary artery), and beta blockers (which appear to limit the extent of muscle injury). Management of symptomatic CAD is similar in all age groups and consists of medical and surgical interventions.[28]

Since the pathophysiology of CAD is the imbalance between the metabolic demands of the heart muscle and the ability of the coronary arteries to supply blood, interventions are directed at decreasing the metabolic needs of the heart muscle or increasing the ability of the coronary arteries to carry blood. Calcium channel-blocking agents and beta blockers reduce the metabolic demands on the heart muscle, and nitroglycerine reduces the pressure against which the heart has to pump by causing dilatation of the coronary vessels. Beta blockers and calcium channel blockers often improve function by reducing myocardial contractility. It is still debated how far the effectiveness and toxicity of these drugs is modified by aging, although it is felt that drug interventions greatly improve the quality of life by reducing symptoms.[29]

There are a number of reasons why exercise is helpful to the patient with angina. Development of an enhanced "collateral" flow has not been established; however, the cardiac oxygen demand is decreased by a drop in both heart rate and blood pressure at a given work load. The lengthening of the diastolic phase facilitates coronary perfusion. Although progress is slow in the elderly, dramatic gains of maximum oxygen intake can be achieved if the exercise periods are of sufficient lengths. Many ADL can be brought below threshold of angina by exercise training. Strengthening of the skeletal muscles may help to reduce blood pressure, and therefore reduce the likelihood of developing angina symptoms during functional ADL.

Surgical intervention is directed at increasing the capacity of the coronary arteries to provide blood to the heart muscle. Obstructions can be circumvented by grafts or removed by angioplasty if the narrowing occurs in larger branches of the coronary arteries. The results of coronary artery bypass graft (CABG) surgery and angioplasty are determined more by the preoperative function of the patient's heart than by the patient's age. In the absence of other severe coexisting diseases, the elderly are good candidates for cardiac surgery.[30]

Cardiomyopathy/Congestive Heart Failure

Cardiomyopathies are conditions in which the heart muscle hypertrophies and cardiac function is impaired leading to *congestive heart failure*. It is often associated with endocardial, and sometimes pericardial involvement, but not with atherosclerosis.[31] The muscle of the heart weakens because of poor nutrition, toxins, infections, or genetic factors. The weakening results in dilatation of the heart and can lead to congestive heart failure because the heart cannot contract strongly enough to empty a sufficient amount of blood into the peripheral vasculature to meet the body's needs. Hypertrophy of cardiac muscle tissue can be the end result of hypertension, outflow obstruction, or genetic factors. The cardiovascular changes resulting from cardiomyopathy impairs

function through several pathological mechanisms. The hypertrophied heart is stiff and does not easily fill with blood. As a result, the heart contracts vigorously but there is little forward circulation to show for the effort, and the body's energy and oxygen needs are not met. In hypertrophic cardiomyopathy, the muscle abnormally contracts, actually creating an obstruction to the outflow of blood from the heart. The stronger the heart contraction, the greater the obstruction.[32]

The general decline of cardiac performance with age and with inactivity affects elderly individuals' abilities to function at their maximum.[33] While a young person readily accepts a sustained increase of cardiac work rate, in old age, an equivalent relative stress may give rise to cardiac failure, particularly if there are other circulatory problems such as a high systemic blood pressure, a minor disorder of the heart valves, or an excessive intake of fluids. Complaints of shortness of breath in the elderly frequently reflect problems with getting enough oxygen to the working muscle through a failing circulatory system.

Exercise is often problematic and exercise tolerance may be limited in the patient with severe cardiomyopathy. Nonetheless, exercise training has been found to improve exercise tolerance in these patients, if initiated at very low levels and gradually increased in intensity. The extent to which there is a reversal in congestive heart failure or any other cardiomyopathy, however, remains to be seen. There is certainty, however, that exercise does improve the strength and the efficiency of the heart as a pump.[34] Medical treatment is directed at correcting or ameliorating the pathophysiology of the underlying cause of the heart failure. Rehabilitative efforts need to be directed toward maintaining the maximal functional capabilities of the elderly individual and preventing the debilitating effects of immobility.[35]

Individuals with a seriously reduced cardiac reserve report a marked need for rest even after mild physical activity. In addition to persistent and undue fatigue, an inadequate cardiac response to exercise usually causes acute shortness of breath, while a restriction of blood flow to the heart itself may produce angina pain. Inadequate blood flow to the peripheral tissues may give the skin a bluish hue (peripheral cyanosis). The pulse rate typically rises over the day, with a slow and incomplete recovery during rest pauses. ADL are notably difficult for these elderly individuals. Lying down can induce a sharp reoccurrence or increase of dyspnea and create a fear of sleeping, which further adds to the severe fatigue experienced with minimal activity by an individual with myocardial degeneration.

The ankle edema of cardiac failure needs to be distinguished from problems of venous drainage. Improper application of modalities, such as an intermittent compression boot or elevation of the lower extremities above the horizontal plane, could be detrimental to the elderly individual in cardiac failure, whereas they would be quite effective in positively modifying the problems encountered with venous-return pathologies. The PTA should contact the PT if ever in doubt and not make the determination alone.

Adverse reactions to exercise in the individual with congestive heart failure (cardiac failure) include an absence of the anticipated rise of systemic blood pressure, accumulation of a substantial oxygen debt, and a slow recovery of heart rate and ventilation after cessation of the effort. Stroke volume decreases rather than increases as the intensity of work is augmented. Cardiac contractility is also impaired.

The intensity of activity must be held below the level at which left ventricular failure begins to occur. Once failure has developed, there is little alternative to a combination of traditional medical therapy and rest until the heart is again operating on the favorable (compensated) portion of its pressure/volume reserve. Clinically, the patient may be on fluid restriction, bed rest, and being weighed daily to monitor fluid retention. Beta blocking agents may worsen the tendency to cardiac failure, as will alcohol abuse. Exercise should focus on functional ADL rather than more aggressive exercise programs. Progression should be based on individual tolerance of exercise levels.[36]

In dilated cardiomyopathies, the heart is not strong enough to move blood against the pressure in the blood vessels. As a result, fluid builds up in the pulmonary circulation causing pulmonary edema, difficulty breathing, low blood oxygen, and further stress on the metabolic need of the contracting cardiac muscle. Medical intervention is directed toward strengthening the heart's contraction using medications such as digoxin. More effective emptying of the heart can be achieved if the pressure against which the heart has to move blood is decreased; this is called *afterload reduction*. Agents that reduce afterload include nitrates, peripheral vasodilators, and other blood pressure lowering agents. Diuretics, which reduce the amount of fluid systemically (termed a *preload reduction*), also help to reduce pulmonary edema and improve cardiac efficiency.[37]

Conductive System Disease of the Heart

Conduction system diseases are those that affect the rate and rhythm of the heart's contractions. The susceptibility to both atrial and ventricular arrhythmias is increased in the elderly, even though they may appear to be clinically healthy.[38] The spread of the electrical current, which results in the coordinated contraction of the heart muscle, is initiated in the 2 pacemaker sites in the heart and carried initially along specialized pathways that spread the wave throughout the heart, called the *conduction system*. These pacemakers and pathways can be damaged by many different things, including those that result in cardiomyopathies and myocardial infarction.

The most common consequences of pacemaker dysfunction are extremely rapid (tachycardic) contractions, poorly coordinated (dysrhythmic) contractions, or extremely slow (bradycardic) contractions, which are less effective in moving blood and result in diminished cardiac output. Low cardiac output can result in confusion, fatigue, poor exercise tolerance, and congestive heart failure. Rapid reductions in cardiac output can cause a condition called *syncope*, which results in dizziness and fainting.[39]

Tachycardias and poorly coordinated rhythms, such as atrial fibrillation, are usually treated with medication to control the rate and convert the rhythm back to normal. Occasionally, electrical cardioversion is required. Bradycardia is usually managed by surgical implantation of an artificial pacemaker, which can be set to trigger a heartbeat at a predetermined rate. Age, per se, is not a contraindication to pacemaker therapy and the surgery is minor and well tolerated.[40]

Valve Diseases of the Heart

The heart valves, which function to keep the blood flowing in one direction, tend to withstand many micro-traumas throughout the course of life. Defects of the heart valves are of 2 types in older adults: *valvular stenosis*, or narrowing of the valve, which restricts blood flow[41]; and *valve insufficiency*, which results in regurgitation or backward flow of blood when the valve doesn't close tightly enough during contraction.[42] Both conditions increase the workload on the heart and greatly reduce the heart's efficiency.

Two valves are most often involved as a result of the aging process—the mitral valve and the aortic valve. The mitral valve is positioned between the left atrium and ventricle; the aortic valve is located at the base to the left ventricle and moves the blood into systemic circulation. Rheumatic valve disease, from previous episodes of rheumatic fever, is the most common cause of mitral stenosis and insufficiency valve disease in the aged.[43] Congestive heart failure, arrhythmias, and embolization of blood clots from the heart to the brain and other organs are the most common complications of mitral valve disease. These patients require attentive medical management, including the use of anti-coagulants to prevent emboli, diuretics to control congestive heart failure, and digitalis or other medications to control the heart rate. Nutritional support is also often required to ensure compliance with a low sodium diet. Because of the potentially serious side effects from too much anti-coagulant (bleeding, hemorrhagic stroke) and digoxin (arrhythmias), their narrow range of effective dosages, and the deleterious effect of inadequate dosage, exercise must be gradually implemented and progressed slowly. Additional interventions should focus on skin protection and maintenance of maximal functional capabilities, with close monitoring of the patient's vital signs and subjective responses of perceived tolerance to increasing activity levels.

Surgical intervention to correct mitral stenosis needs to precede the development of fixed pulmonary hypertension and right heart failure. Valve replacement and valvulotomy (where the valve is widened but not replaced) are done through open heart surgery. Transluminal valvulotomy in which the valve is widened by using catheter-guided balloons offers significantly lower operative risk in selected patients. Almost all patients continue to require medication for the control of heart rate, prevention of emboli, and treatment of congestive heart failure. The response to gradually increasing levels of physical activity following surgery is usually favorable.[44]

Aortic valve disease is common in the aged and results from rheumatic valve disease, increasing damage to a congenitally malformed valve, or the progression of age-related injury to an otherwise normal valve. The latter results from the gradual build up of scar tissue and calcium on the valve leaflets as part of the normal aging of the valve. The most clinically significant lesion is stenosis of the aortic valve. This results in a progressive increase in the resistance to the flow of blood out of the heart. As a result, the heart pumps blood against increasingly great afterload.[45] Patients can experience angina even without CAD, because even normal coronary arteries are unable to deliver sufficient blood to meet the metabolic demands of the overtaxed heart muscle. As the stenosis increases, decreases in cardiac output result in fainting (syncope). Finally, when the heart is no longer able to compensate by hypertrophy for the increasing resistance to flow, congestive heart failure occurs. Rehabilitation efforts are directed toward maintaining the maximal functional capabilities through exercise programs that use ADL as the exercise mode.

Hypertension

Hypertension is another common condition affecting the cardiovascular system. Older adults with systolic blood pressures above 160 mm Hg and diastolic pressures above 95 mm Hg are at increased risk for stroke, congestive heart failure (hypertensive cardiomyopathy), and renal failure. Much of the cardiovascular morbidity and mortality in the elderly is related to hypertension.[46] Treatment to lower blood pressure significantly lowers the risks of developing these complications. Medical and dietary management are important in controlling hypertension. There is little evidence whether anti-hypertensive drug therapy alters the course of asymptomatic elderly individuals. Nevertheless, systolic hypertension doubles the risk of cardiovascular complications, so that the risk, expense, and inconvenience of drug therapy must be compared with the benefits of lower systolic blood pressure. Complications of anti-hypertensive therapy are more frequent in the elderly individual because of decreased renal function (which increases the incidence of drug toxicity) and less sensitive baroreceptor responses (which makes the patient more susceptible to the orthostatic complications of volume depletion). Gradually assuming the upright posture may avert dizziness and syncope.

Exercise has been shown to have positive effects in reducing high blood pressure and is discussed in Chapter 10. Control of hypertension has the potential to decrease cardiovascular morbidity and mortality.[47]

Peripheral Vascular Disease

The peripheral vascular system is the arterial and venous network once the vessels leave the heart. Peripheral vascular problems include diseases that affect the brain, kidneys, or any extremity. With age, the aorta and major elastic arteries become elongated and stiffer with an increased pulse wave velocity. Evidence of endothelial network (vessels that line organs and cavities) changes that resemble atherosclerosis occurs with advancing age, decreasing circulation to organs and peripheral body parts. Due to changes in the vessel as described, the baroreflex, which fine tunes the heart and vessel response to sense position, is altered and peripheral vessel reflexes are blunted. This increases the likelihood that an older person will become dizzy with position changes. The cumulative affects of cardiovascular and reflex changes brought about by aging may have significant implications for circulatory homeostasis in health and disease.[48]

Peripheral vascular disease (PVD) is frequently the result of poor circulation to the extremities, untreated hypertension, cigarette smoking, diabetes mellitus, and elevated serum cholesterol. Atherosclerosis and other forms of PVD can lead to partial or complete obstruction of the main arterial supply to the limbs. The consequences include intermittent claudication with walking and skin lesions, which could lead to functional losses and ultimately to amputation.[49] When early intervention to reduce risk factors is unsuccessful, management proceeds through the modification of diet to reduce weight and cholesterol, medications to enhance blood flow and reduce blood pressure, and behavior modifications to reduce cigarette consumption.

Intermittent claudication, one of the primary symptoms in PVD, is muscular pain, which is analogous to angina pain and reflects an acute lack of oxygen to the working muscles.[50] The level of discomfort depends on the level of peripheral vascular obstruction. Pulse pressure is also a factor.

The strength of the pulse reflects the elasticity (or stiffness) of the vessels, and is often predictive of the prognosis of the disease. A diminished or absent pulse reflects a severely compromised vascular system.[51]

Temperature and color also reflects the health of the circulatory system. When there is poor circulation, the extremities are often cool or cold to the touch and have a deep red to bluish-purple appearance. If the circulatory system is healthy, the extremities are warm and pink.

With a severe circulatory problem, a minor orthopedic change, such as a hammer or claw toe, can develop an ulcer because of undue pressures that are undetected due to poor sensation, and can lead to a gangrenous lesion as a result of the absence of an adequate blood supply in the affected extremity. Immobility created by a gangrenous lesion can lead to depression and renal complications, and death is frequently the result of a coronary thrombosis or hemorrhage.

Amputation is required for the relief of pain and to stop the spread of infection (gangrene) in those patients for whom other surgical procedures are impossible. There is about a 5% incidence of amputations per year in patients with both diabetes and PVD. Because the patient's ability to ambulate is greatly affected by the level at which the amputation is performed, the most distal site is preferred. However, the amputation must be performed at a level where there is sufficient blood supply to ensure adequate healing. Progressive amputations often occur as a result of inadequate blood supply and poor incision healing. The result is that the patient is exposed to the risks of surgery again and again.

Exercise is particularly helpful in treating PVD from a preventative perspective. Walking has been found to be quite effective in improving peripheral circulation. When the patient is not able to ambulate long enough to benefit from this form of exercise, Buerger-Allen exercises (see protocol in Chapter 10) improve the vitality of the peripheral vascular system and impact on back and lower extremity flexibility and strength. These exercises also serve to decrease the debilitating effects of postural hypotension by facilitating adjustment to postural positional changes.[52]

Surgical intervention is effective in cases of symptomatic PVD that results in pain, claudication, or nonhealing ulcers. As in CAD, partial obstructions of peripheral arteries, most commonly in the lower extremities, can be treated with bypass grafting or by dilating the obstructed section of the artery using vessel angioplasty.

Prevention is the first line of defense. When efforts fail to preserve a limb, the challenge of treating an individual following amputation is great. The loss of a limb is a traumatic and life-changing event. Often the process of grieving must begin before the actual surgery and is aided by contributions from social services, psychiatry, nursing, and rehabilitative services. Depression is a major impediment to the successful rehabilitation of patients and must be addressed if intensive nursing and physical therapy are to be successful.[53] Detailed exercise protocol following an amputation will be presented in Chapter 10.

Pulmonary Manifestations of Aging

The most common diseases of the pulmonary system with age include respiratory infections (pneumonias), tuberculosis, chronic obstructive pulmonary disease, and chronic resistive diseases, such as bronchial asthma. The course of these diseases is different in the elderly, not only due to the physiologic process of aging but also the presence of comorbidities.[54] This is a very important variable in designing treatment programs for older respiratory patients.

The respiratory system functions to ensure the exchange of oxygen and carbon dioxide between the air and the blood within the lungs. This system can be thought of as having several related but separate components:

- Movement of air into and out of the lungs
- Exchange of oxygen and carbon dioxide
- Defense of the lung from infection.

Changes with age affect every aspect of the respiratory system, resulting in functional losses in the elderly. The chest wall becomes a less efficient bellows with age. The anteroposterior diameter of the chest increases and the rib cage becomes more rigid as progressive curvature of the spine, calcification of rib cartilage, and osteoporosis limit the compliance of the chest wall. The chest muscles atrophy with age and also contribute to the gradual decline in the efficiency with which air is moved into and out of the lungs. The collapse of small airways due to the loss of elasticity of lung tissue with age results in increasing resistance to air flow. As a result, the amount of physical effort that must go into breathing increases a great deal.[55] Monitoring and documenting respiration rate and perceived maximal exertion are important measurements that physical therapists will use to determine treatment progression.

Although the bronchi are not usually affected by normal aging, the surface area of the alveoli decreases by 4% with each decade of life. The alveolar wall is also thinner and contains fewer capillaries for the delivery of blood. The size of the alveoli increases due to the loss of elasticity and recoil. It is the loss of recoil that creates an increased susceptibility to airway collapse, the major factor contributing to the altered distribution of air within the lungs.

Ideally, each area of the lung where blood is available for gas exchange would be ventilated, giving a perfect match of ventilation and perfusion. With age, larger areas of the lung are perfused but not ventilated because of airway collapse and redistribution of blood flow. This results in the return of un-oxygenated blood to the general circulation and decreased efficiency of the respiratory system. Pulmonary circulation may also decline with age, further reducing the capacity of the system to respond to the demand for the increased supply of oxygen to tissues.[56]

Infections in the elderly patient are a challenge since the classical signs of infection are absent or ill-defined. Changing mechanics within the lung and chest wall also make the lung more susceptible to infection with age. The gag reflex is diminished, increasing the risk of aspiration. Concurrently, the cough reflex is also diminished and the effectiveness of the cough is reduced because of reduced chest wall compliance and chest muscle strength. Ciliary action, which normally moves secretions up and out of the lungs, also declines, particularly in smokers. These factors combine to compromise the lungs' ability to defend against infection. Some drugs play important roles in depressing the respiratory system. Sedatives and analgesics, such as alcohol and narcotics, are known to depress respiration and dull the cough and gag reflexes, thus predisposing the elderly person to the risks of hypoxia and aspiration pneumonia.[57]

Pneumonia

Pneumonia is the most common infectious cause of death in the elderly and the most common infection requiring hospitalization. It is often the means of death for patients with other serious conditions such as diabetes, cancer, stroke, congestive heart failure, dementia, and renal failure. The increased incidence of pneumonia with aging is due in part to the weakening of the local pulmonary defenses. However, the high mortality of pneumonia is largely due to its more subtle presentation in the elderly.[58]

Typical symptoms such as a productive cough, fever, and pleuritic chest pain are frequently absent. More subtle symptoms such as confusion, alteration of sleep-wake cycles, increased congestive heart failure, anorexia, and "failure to thrive" are more likely to occur. Misdiagnosis and late diagnosis are common and contribute to the high mortality of pneumonia in the aged.[59]

Successful treatment of pneumonia requires early recognition and institution of proper antibiotic therapy. The identification of the causative bacteria in the examination of a sputum sample is the single most important diagnostic test for determining initial antibiotic therapy. Unfortunately, such samples are often difficult to obtain in a dehydrated and confused elderly patient. As a result, therapy is often empirical and not as specifically directed or effective as possible. Hydration, nutritional support, chest physical therapy, and treatment of complicating illnesses are often required in addition to antibiotics.

Chronic Obstructive and Resistive Pulmonary Disease

Conditions that cause obstruction to air flow within the lungs are called *obstructive airway diseases*. They share the common characteristic of increased resistance to air flow within the airways.[60] *Asthma* is a reversible resistive airway disease characterized by episodic increases in airway resistance due to spasm, and narrowing of airways in response to infection, allergic reactions, and environmental conditions.[61] *Chronic obstructive pulmonary disease* (COPD) denotes conditions of increased airway resistance that are irreversible because of permanent structural damage resulting from cigarette smoking, infections, and toxic exposures.

Emphysema is a term used to describe the permanent destruction of alveoli with the resulting expansion of the remaining alveoli. A consequence of emphysema is to reduce the area in which gas exchange can occur. This results in perfusion/ventilation mismatch and hypoxia. Emphysema is associated with increased airway resistance due to collapse of small airways.[62]

Chronic bronchitis is a different disease process in which there is chronic inflammation of the small airways resulting in increased mucous, airway plugging, and destruction of small airways. As a consequence, airflow is reduced because of permanent narrowing of the small airways. There is often a reversible component of the airway obstruction superimposed on the chronic changes. Cigarette smoking is the leading cause of chronic bronchitis and multiplies the deleterious effects of other environmental agents such as asbestos, silica, coal dust, and fibers. Frequently, emphysema and chronic bronchitis coexist.[63]

Patients with obstructive airway diseases usually manifest disabilities that result either from hypoxia (low oxygen content), hypercapnia (excess of carbon dioxide in blood), or dyspnea (labored breathing). Both hypoxia and hypercapnia can cause confusion, fatigue, and worsening heart failure. Breathlessness, or dyspnea, is usually the most limiting symptom of COPD. Functional impairment due to COPD can be severe, and COPD is often fatal. Over half of the patients die within 2 years of their first episode of respiratory failure. These patients require extensive therapeutic and supportive interventions.[64]

The treatment goal of individuals with COPD, chronic bronchitis, emphysema, and asthma is to maintain optimum functioning for as long as possible. This usually involves chest physical therapy, medication, oxygen therapy, and environmental changes designed to reduce exertion. The depression that accompanies chronic illness of all types can be significant in respiratory patients, many of whom feel that they have brought it on themselves by their personal lifestyle choices (eg, smoking). Because of its complexity, pulmonary disease is an excellent example of a health problem that requires an interdisciplinary approach for appropriate management.

Neuromuscular Manifestations of Aging

Cerebrovascular Diseases

Cerebrovascular diseases could easily be placed under "Cardiovascular Manifestations of Aging;" however, since the ultimate functional outcomes result in significant neuromuscular deficits, this pathology will be covered in this section of this chapter.

Cerebrovascular disease commonly results in focal brain dysfunction. There are different types of cerebrovascular disease, each with a different pathophysiological mechanism, prognosis, and treatment. The mechanisms include the rupture of small blood vessels from hypertension, abrupt blockage of vessels by emboli from the heart or plaques in the large arteries leading to the brain, and spontaneous formation of blood clots within the blood vessels due to local increases in coagulability. The pathophysiology of cerebrovascular disease is the interruption of blood flow to brain tissue with resultant cell damage or death from ischemia. Decreases in the heart's ability to pump blood can lead to ischemia, as can blockage of the blood vessels to or within the brain from plaques, emboli, or inflammation of the lining of the blood vessels. Uncontrolled hypertension, diabetes mellitus, smoking, and elevated cholesterol contribute to cerebrovascular disease directly by affecting the entire circulatory system.[65]

Preventive interventions must be specifically directed at the underlying pathophysiology. Hypertension can be controlled by medication, diet, and exercise.[66] The prevention of emboli usually requires the use of anti-coagulants such as aspirin and other blood thinners. The risk of bleeding, both into the brain and into other organs, increases with the use of these agents and often limits their use in certain patients. If emboli result from cardiac arrhythmias, prevention results from a return to normal sinus rhythm through the use of electrical cardioversion or anti-arrhythmic medications. Because of the heightened risk of intracerebral bleeding, anti-coagulants are avoided in the presence of hypertension and in cerebrovascular accidents resulting from bleeding into brain tissue.

Recurrent, small cerebrovascular accidents can result in multi-infarct dementia. More commonly, however, limited areas of the brain are damaged and result in more focal disabilities. These can include loss of motor or sensory function over the right or left side of the body, and alterations in vision, speech, and the ability to interpret sensory inputs. The extent of the deficit following a stroke depends on the location and function of the injured part of the brain, the degree of damage, and the availability of unaffected regions of the brain that can assume the lost function. Residual effects can be so subtle as to be functionally negligible or so extensive that only the most basic brain functions, the control of respiration and blood pressure, are preserved.

Specific interventions with older stroke patients will be covered in depth in Chapter 10. PTs and PTAs play roles in preventive and palliative interventions post-stroke, in addition to rehabilitation therapy. Neurological recovery is ongoing, and the effectiveness of physical therapy can be significant in patients with cerebrovascular insults many months beyond the initial insult. Specialized techniques for the treatment of stroke will be covered in Chapter 10.

Central Nervous System Diseases

There is evidence that a major factor leading to sarcopenia (ie, age-associated loss of muscle mass) is the reduction of motor neurons, which results in lower electrical activity of the muscle fibers.[67] CNS impairment is a leading cause of functional disability in the aged. The normal process of aging results in the gradual decrease of size and number of cells in all locations within the CNS. The size and weight of the brain declines with age as demonstrated by autopsy and computed tomography (CT) scan results. Metabolic activity declines as measured by oxygen consumption and blood flow, and the rate of conduction of peripheral nerves declines steadily. Of great interest, however, is the observation that the changes of normal aging do not result in significant neurological impairment. Although there is a steady diminution of the components of the CNS over time, there is no associated neurological deficit that can be ascribed solely to aging.[68]

The CNS is highly plastic and adaptable. It plays a major role in compensation. However, signs of neurological dysfunction may be detected in older persons otherwise free of neurological disease, simply due to disuse. It has to do with the concept of *use it or lose it.*

The development of chronic, severe, cognitive impairment occurs in nearly 30% of individuals over 80. The functional impairments resulting from CNS dysfunction can be severe. It is useful to think of them as resulting from changes in cognition (such as judgment, comprehension, memory), changes in sensory input (blindness, deafness, neuropathy), and changes in ability to execute actions (paralysis, gait disorders, loss of coordination, incontinence, aphasia). Alterations of capacity in any of these spheres can result from and cause changes in physical and functional performance as well as independence and quality of life.[69]

The transcortical tracts are the final neurological pathway involved in cognitive functioning, movement, sensation, and sensory integration of movement. Neurological dysfunction is often associated with poor lower extremity function, falls, and reduced physical activity. Reduced physical activity, regardless of the reason, can accelerate neurological damage. Many specific diseases and conditions also result in cognitive and neurological dysfunction. Some conditions are preventable and early intervention essential. Exercise is a key element to maintaining neuromuscular functioning and CNS integrity. Once started, many neurological problems are relentlessly progressive and do not respond to disease-specific interventions. The following is a brief and greatly simplified survey of the more common types of neurological disease in the aging human.

Confusion and Delirium in the Elderly

There is no evidence that the clinical picture of *delirium* in elderly people differs from younger people. However, without identification and intervention, it may run a more chronic course. Many symptoms of confusion, delirium, and dementia overlap, making identification much more complex. Cognitive disorders of all types account for nearly two-thirds of nursing home admissions and make up a significant majority of those elderly persons who are incapacitated by illness. Severe cognitive dysfunction may not impair an individual's longevity, especially with meticulous attention to treatable complicating illnesses. As a result, the aged with cognitive dysfunction make up the largest group of functionally disabled individuals.[70]

The fact that delirium has a negative impact on function is a very important consideration. Confusion, restlessness, agitation, poor attention span, reversal of sleep/wake cycles, hallucinations, and paranoia can all be manifestations of delirium and result in limited function.[71] Subtle changes resulting from correctable toxic and metabolic abnormalities are recognized as potentially reversible. Appropriate interventions are frequently delayed with the medical bias that confusion is a *normal* part of aging. It is particularly important for these reversible conditions to be identified by the health care team. Failure to intervene in a timely manner can result in permanent cognitive dysfunction. Equally as important is the risk that inappropriate treatment will result in further functional impairment or a greatly increased risk of injury. Pathological brain dysfunction resulting from toxic and metabolic causes usually has a good prognosis for recovery when the underlying abnormality is corrected[72] (Table 4-1).

Interventions are directed at identifying and correcting the underlying metabolic problems. During a confused state, the individual is more prone to accidental injury, complications such as aspiration pneumonia, and further cognitive dysfunction due to inappropriate use of sedatives that may aggravate rather than relieve agitation. Acute toxic and metabolic delirium may coexist with chronic progressive forms of brain dysfunction, such as Alzheimer's disease.[73]

Dementias

Dementias are characterized by slow onset of increasing intellectual impairment, including disorientation, memory loss, and diminished ability to reason and make sound judgments, loss of social skills, and the development of regressed or antisocial behavior. Depression is often superimposed on dementia as a reaction to the perceived loss of intellectual skills and leads to further cognitive impairment.[74]

Table 4-1

COMMON CAUSES OF TOXIC AND METABOLIC CONFUSION AND DELIRIUM IN THE ELDERLY

DRUGS

Alcohol

Psychotropics (tranquilizers, anti-psychotics, anti-depressants)

Over-the-counter sleep, cold, and allergy medications

Analgesics

Anti-hypertensives

Beta blockers (propranolol)

Anti-Parkinsonian medications

Anti-convulsants (phenobarbital, phenylantoin, carbamazepine)

Digoxin

Amphetamines

H_2 blockers (cimetidine)

METABOLIC ABNORMALITIES

Hypoglycemia

Hyponatremia

Hypocalcemia

Hypothermia

Hypothyroidism

Hypoxia

Vitamin B_{12} deficiency

Cortisol deficiency

Hepatic failure (elevated ammonia)

Elevated cortisol

Renal failure (elevated blood urea nitrogen level, creatine)

Pulmonary failure (elevated carbon dioxide)

Alzheimer's disease and multi-infarct dementia are the 2 most common forms of irreversible dementia. Alzheimer's disease is usually slowly progressive and begins insidiously. Patients typically begin with short-term memory deficits that progress to severely regressed behavior, inability to learn or remember new tasks, and loss of ability to perform ADL.[75] Multi-infarct dementia is usually of more rapid onset, in younger individuals, and progresses in a step-wise fashion with abrupt worsening and subsequent plateaus of function. Frequently, there are focal neurological deficits such as paresis and parethesias. Often, the individual is hypertensive or diabetic and shows evidence of generalized atherosclerosis.[76]

It is important to distinguish between Alzheimer's disease and dementia disorders, such as vascular dementia, because the prevention of recurrent cerebral infarction may arrest the progression of multi-infarct dementia. Vascular insults without intervention lead to irreversible brain damage, resulting from repetitive ischemic injury caused by emboli or bleeding.[77] Normalization of blood pressure is the most effective intervention known. Other types of reversible dementia, such as those resulting from hypothyroidism, vitamin B_{12} deficiency, and normal pressure hydrocephalus, can become "fixed" and unresponsive to treatment unless identified and treated at an early stage. Early identification of these "correctable" dementias is essential.

Unfortunately, no such therapeutic imperative exists for Alzheimer's disease, which is of unclear etiology and without treatment at this time.

Regardless of the etiology of dementia, once reversible causes have been ruled out, the main tasks of the clinical team are to minister to the patient's emotional needs, assist in the act of grieving for lost function, alter the environment so that the patient's remaining skills can be used, augment the patient's capacity to successfully undertake ADL, educate the family, provide emotional and physical support for the family and caretakers, and provide the patient and family with a realistic prognosis. Any superimposed illness can cause a rapid and prolonged decline in mental status that may totally resolve as the underlying illness is treated.

Parkinson's Disease

Parkinson's disease is a chronic and progressive neurologic disorder characterized by specific motor deficits resulting from the degeneration of dopamine-producing neurons in the substantia nigra. There is characteristic increased limb rigidity, stooped posture, shuffling gait, decreased mental acuity, difficulty initiating movement, and tremor, which is usually symmetrical, rhythmic, and abolished by intentional movement. Early in its course, Parkinsonism may display an asymmetrical tremor, slight increase in muscle tone with associated decrease in spontaneous movement, masking of the face with loss of spontaneous expression, and generalized rigidity in muscle tone. Patients' inability to move freely and to perform everyday tasks restricts their independence and leads to increased reliance on caregivers and assistive devices. As these restrictions on voluntary movement progress, they result in significant functional impairment. Associated incontinence and constipation further complicate the management of these individuals.[78] Emotional and psychological well-being is also negatively affected.

In Parkinson's disease, drug treatment and intensive physical therapy are frequently helpful. These interventions do not change the relentless progression of functional impairments. Drug therapy is directed at the amelioration of symptoms at the lowest effective dose. Drugs are of 3 general classes: those that are anti-cholenergic, those that mimic the effects of dopamine (such as bromocryptine), and those that replete dopamine (L-dopa).[79] As the disease progresses, the response to drugs typically decreases and many motor complications develop that impact health-related quality of life.

Physical therapy to maintain strength, improve posture, prevent contractures, and maintain the maximal functional capabilities of the individual with Parkinsonism is crucial. Despite the progressive nature of this illness, many patients can maintain full function for several decades with a combination of physical therapy and drug intervention.[80] Physical therapy improves balance in patients with Parkinson's disease and as a result can significantly improve quality of life.[81] In fact, a sustained improvement of motor skills in Parkinson's patients has been found to be achievable with a comprehensive long-term rehabilitation program.[82]

Peripheral Nervous Systems

Aging of the peripheral nervous system is associated with several morphologic and functional changes, including a decrease in the number and size of peripheral nerve fibers with a decrease in nerve conduction velocity. These changes contribute to age-related decreases in muscle strength, sensory discrimination, and autonomic responses. There is often a clinically significant decrease in touch and vibration sense. The peripheral nerves, however, are easily affected by nutritional deficiencies, toxins, and endocrine disorders. The resulting neuropathies can cause marked loss of position sense with resulting instability and falling, chronic pain, and dysesthesia.[83]

Inflammation and inadequate antioxidant defenses are associated with accelerated decline on nerve conduction velocity.[84] Nutritional deficiencies in vitamin E, folic acid, vitamin B_{12}, and alcohol-related deficiencies of thiamine, pyridoxine, and other B vitamins can lead to neuropathy. Toxic neuropathies can result from heavy metal exposure, such as lead and arsenic, medications, or from uremia (the presence of urinary elements in blood causing toxicity). Replacement of the deficiency and removal of the toxin are the cornerstones of therapy. Prognosis is good for resolution.

Diabetic neuropathy can significantly affect the peripheral neurological system in several forms. There is a distal sensory *polyneuropathy,* which affects the hands and feet with diminished sensation and burning pain, a proximal motor neuropathy resulting in proximal muscle wasting and weakness, and a diffuse autonomic neuropathy resulting in orthostatic hypotension, *neurogenic bladder*, *obstipation* (intractable constipation), and *bowel immotility*. In addition to these diffuse forms of neuropathy, single nerves can be affected. The resulting *mononeuropathies* can cause loss of ocular muscle function and painful nerve root and branch dysfunction wherever an involved nerve travels.[85]

Treatment is symptomatic and may involve analgesics, physical therapy, and possible splinting. Relief from painful *dysesthesias* may be obtained in some cases with the use of certain drugs (diphenylhydantoin, amitriptyline, or carbamazepine). Control of the blood sugar appears neither to prevent nor lessen diabetic neuropathy. Rarely, another endocrine disease, hypothyroidism, can present with neuropathy. It responds to thyroid hormone replacement.[86]

Neurosensory Manifestations of Aging

Information from the different senses is seamlessly integrated by the brain in order to modify our behaviors and enrich our perceptions. It is only through the appropriate integration of information from the different senses that accurate and safe management in your environment is accomplished.[87] The following is a brief review of neurosensory pathologies that may disrupt function in older adults.

Skin Pathologies

The skin is the largest organ of the body and functions to protect the interior of the organism from the effects of pathogens, toxins, environmental extremes, trauma, and ultraviolet irradiation.[88] Accumulated effects of repeated injury throughout life change the skin. The skin grows and heals more slowly. It becomes more sensitive to most toxins and is less able to resist injury. It becomes less effective as a barrier to infections. The specialized appendages such as sweat and sebum glands, pressure and touch sensors, and hair follicles atrophy, resulting in dryness, less ability to alter body temperature through sweating, and loss of hair. The small blood vessels in the skin diminish with age, a change that contributes to its lessened effectiveness as a barrier to infection, diminished reserve for repair, and altered ability to assist in thermoregulation.

Skin cancer is the most common malignancy known to the human race and its incidence increases exponentially with age. The 3 most important malignant tumors of the skin in the aged are basal cell carcinoma, squamous cell carcinoma, and malignant melanoma.

Basal cell carcinomas arise in areas of sun exposed skin and increase with the intensity and duration of sun exposure as well as genetic background. These types of nonmelanoma skin cancers account for approximately 50% of all cancers reported each year in the United States. The most common sites are the face, tops of the ears, neck, anterior chest, arms, and hands. Treatment is virtually always successful in eradicating the tumor unless there has been extensive local invasion of muscle and bone. These tumors rarely ever metastasize but can be locally invasive and deforming if not treated soon enough.

Squamous cell carcinomas arise from chronically irritated skin. Sun damage is the most common cause but other irritants include tobacco (lip and mouth), snuff (nose), coal tar, soot, and x-rays. Chronically traumatized scars following burns or surgery are other sites at risk. These cancers are locally invasive and frequently metastasize to regional lymph nodes, the brain, and lung and therefore carry a higher mortality rate than basal cell carcinomas. Early detection and excision result in higher cure rates. Extensive surgery with excision of all regional lymph nodes and radiation therapy are frequently employed to cure these tumors. They are poorly responsive to chemotherapy.

Malignant melanoma is also the result of sun damage. The incidence of this disease is doubling every 10 to 15 years. The highest age-specific incidence rates occur in the population over the age of 60. Because the prognosis for survival with melanoma is related to the depth of skin invasion at the time of excision, these melanomas have a good prognosis if removed early. The nodular melanoma, which is more aggressive in nature, comprises approximately 20% of malignant melanomas. Melanomas metastasize early and extensively to brain, lung, liver, and bone tissue.[89]

PTAs could have a major impact on the early detection of skin cancers by assessing skin status during treatment, not only for obvious ulcerations or lesions, but the more subtle presentations of skin changes as well. Keen observation by the PTA with immediate, subsequent reporting to the PT, could prevent a small skin break or ulceration from becoming a larger

problem. The PTA's attentiveness to skin status could mean the difference between amputation and preserving a limb.

Herpes Zoster

Herpes zoster results from the reactivation of a dormant virus (chicken pox) and affects the sensory nerve root. The result is an intensely painful skin eruption over the area innervated by one sensory nerve root. Two types of disabilities result from this infection. First, the eruption itself requires local care to prevent infection by bacteria. The pain associated with herpes zoster inhibits mobility, appetite, and sleep. Second, there is a high incidence of *post-herpetic neuralgia* in the elderly. Severe burning pain can persist for months. This neuralgia usually requires narcotics for relief, which significantly impede safe function. The importance of rehabilitative efforts with herpes zoster is in maintaining mobility through functional exercise and ambulation. Especially when neuralgia exists, the elderly individual's pain imposed restriction of activity can lead rapidly to the devastating effects of bed rest.[90]

Decubitus Ulcers

Decubitus ulcers result from prolonged pressure and shear force-induced damage to the skin. Usually occurring over bony prominences, pressure and shear forces impair circulation to the area resulting in ischemic changes in the tissue and resulting ulcer formation. They occur when there is forced immobility, diminished pain perception, and altered nutritional status. Chronic weight loss leads to a decrease in subcutaneous fat, fragile epidermis, decreased blood flow to the dermal vessels, and a depressed immune function. Decubitus ulcers are potentially serious in frail elderly who are chronically ill. The patients most susceptible are those who are among the most debilitated and confined to a bed or chair. Decubitus ulcers are easier to prevent than they are to cure.[91] The PTA plays an important role in educating patients and caregivers about pressure relief strategies to prevent skin breakdown in skin that has lost sensory input as a result of disease (eg, diabetes) or nutritional deficits (eg, B complex deficiencies).

Physical therapy is an integral part of wound care and intervention includes low-intensity current or non-thermal ultrasound, debridement, and activity to enhance circulation. Functional activity and therapeutic exercise should be employed to maintain physical condition and capabilities of avoiding prolonged pressure. As previously mentioned, the PTA plays a key role in implementing pressure relief strategies and educating elderly individuals and their primary caregivers in monitoring skin status.

Visual Pathologies With Aging

Visual impairment is associated with the increased incidence of falling in the older adult. Vision is the sense that human beings seem to depend on the most. Much of our communication is via visual images such as the written word, nonverbal communication such as facial expression and body language, billboards, and television. Vision allows for the identification of much that is in the environment. It is a major tool for environmental safety, independence, and mobility.[92]

With aging, several structural changes occur in the eye that may evolve into pathologies. Many of these changes begin at an early age and progress steadily but slowly over time. The slow nature of the progression allows for the gradual accommodation for continued function. However, at some point, the cumulative effects of the process will result in some loss of independence and mobility.

The lens ages early so that by the age of 50 most people will exhibit some signs of aging. With age, the lens becomes discolored, opaque, and rigid. The ligaments and muscles weaken, limiting the ability of the anterior-posterior diameter of the lens to expand. Gradually, the lens becomes set in size and flat. This condition, known as *presbyopia*, leads to a decline in both visual acuity and field. As the lens ages, thickens, becomes yellowed and somewhat opaque, the risk of *cataracts* also increases. Because the lens is clouded, light rays entering through the lens scatter as they move through the visual system. This is the primary cause of glare, which can be disorienting for the aged person. As the lens thickens, the chamber becomes shallower. The major danger in such a case is the onset of *glaucoma*,[93] a flattening of the lens, which causes glare. An early indication of glaucoma is when an individual complains of blurring of lights, especially at night, and the presence of streaks or "tails" created by lights in the environment.

With increasing age, less light reaches the retina because the pupil becomes smaller. There is a linear decrease in the amount of light reaching the retina from the age of 20 to the age of 60. This results in the need for increasing available light in order to see, and an increase in the time needed to adapt to sudden changes from bright to diminished light or darkness. It should be noted that the eye requires approximately double the illumination for each additional 13 years of adult life. The final level of vision in diminished lighting, after time allowed for accommodation, is less for the aged person than for the younger.

Color vision is also affected by age. While the mechanism is still not entirely understood, it is believed that the discoloration of the lens leads to color filtering and a decline of color intensity, especially with greens and blues. It is thought that as the lens yellows with age, the shorter light waves of the greens and blues are more completely filtered out, while the longer-waved half of the color spectrum retains the capacity to pass through the lens to the retina. Yellows, oranges, and reds have been found to stimulate the sympathetic nervous system responses in the elderly. Elderly individuals tend to develop a "taste" for brighter colored clothes.[94] Color coding is often a technique that is useful to older individuals to assist them in identifying objects.

Color contrast is also very important. Older eyes may not be able to determine subtle variations in colors. For instance, if 2 shades of blue are used and they are too closely related in shade, an older individual may not be able to distinguish the difference. Therefore, contrasting colors (eg, dark against light) is a helpful way to safety-proof the environment.

Over time there is atrophy of orbital fat, which occurs with the pattern of general wasting. This leads to the loss of the normal fat cushion behind the globe and may produce some recession of the eye. This leads to the characteristic sunken eye appearance and is accompanied by a deepening of the upper lid-fold and a slight obstruction of the peripheral visual fields. The skin of the upper lid also tends to relax causing the upper lid to drop onto the lashes resulting in some restriction of the lid, and leading to an upper lid *ptosis*. When severe, such a condition will limit vision for objects above eye level, such as traffic lights and stop signs.

The production of tears also declines with age. This leads to eye irritation and excessive tearing. The result is that there is no opportunity for the eyes to be bathed in tears. This causes chronic dryness. This condition can be exacerbated by *senile ectropion*, a physical state in which the lower lid is physically unable to cover the lower portion of the eye, further drying it out. The opposite situation may also occur, that of *senile entropion*, or a turning inward of the lower lid leading to irritation of the cornea and lower conjunctiva by the lashes.

The vitreous body also undergoes changes with aging. The gel-like substance undergoes some amount of shrinkage after the age of 60. The primary role of the vitreous is to support the retina. This role becomes compromised as the amount of fluid available decreases. By the age of 70 or 80, most people develop some degree of detachment of the vitreous body from the posterior aspect of the globe. This occurrence is often heralded by transient flashes of light or by a small number of dark floating opacities. These flashes are noted most often when turning in bed and not noted when sitting quietly. A sudden shower of dark spots or floating opacities are strongly suggestive of a retinal break and should be treated as an emergency in order to decrease the possibility of actual retinal detachment. Frequently, surgery will also be suggested prophylactically for the uninvolved eye.[95]

Hearing Pathologies With Aging

Presbycusis is the most common form of hearing loss with aging. It is characterized by a decrease in perception of higher frequency tones and a decrease in speech discrimination. There are changes in the structures in the ear as a function of age which lead to pathological changes. Briefly, these changes are atrophy and degeneration of hair cells and supporting cells in the basal coil of the cochlea leading to *sensory presbycusis*. The loss of auditory neurons causes *neural presbycusis*. Atrophy of the stria vascularis (a layer of fibrous vascular tissue covering the outer wall of the cochlear duct) in the scala media (stair-like structure that serves as a passage to the cochlea) with corresponding deficiencies in bioelectric and biochemical properties of the endolymphatic fluids can result in *metabolic presbycusis*. Atrophic changes in structures associated with vibration of the cochlear partition, a hearing pathology known as *cochlear conductive presbycusis*, occur in greater frequency in the elderly. The loss of minute vessels that supply the spiral ligament, stria vascularis, and tympanic (ear drum) lip causes *vascular presbycusis* and a loss of neurons from the cochlear nucleus leading to *central presbycusis*. While each of these entities has been separately identified and studied, it is important to note that they seldom occur independently of each other.[96]

The magnitude of presbycusis varies widely and it is hard to determine how much of the hearing loss is due to aging and how much is due to exposure to environmental noise, toxic drugs, or chronic age-related conditions such as hypertension. Beginning around age 55, older adults experience a loss in threshold sensitivity to pitch as the very high frequencies are lost. The higher frequency consonants, such as t, p, k, f, s, and ch, are no longer heard due to the sensitivity loss in the high frequency. This leads to a decrease in ability to understand speech where parts of words or whole words are lost because of higher tones as well as the interference of background noise. The use of hearing aids and surgical implants has provided good relief for some, but the process of presbycusis is such that these steps can only blunt the effects of the problem. Because most cases of presbycusis are of mixed etiology, intervention will not completely correct the loss. Thus, the clinical focus should be on improving and maintaining as much of the hearing capability as possible and assisting the aged person, and the family, to adapt to the limitations necessitated by substituting other forms of communication and environmental stimuli in order to compensate for the loss that remains. The PTA needs to be very mindful of the effects of hearing loss on all aspects of the aged person's life. Failure to consider the effects of hearing loss when evaluating such problems as depression, confusion, possible attention span deficits, and a variety of other clinical problems may lead to less than adequate clinical intervention.[97]

Tinnitus is the diagnosis given to a variety of "ear noise" disorders and refers to a chronic ringing, buzzing, tinkling, humming, or other noise in the ears that only the individual can hear. It results in the perception of sound in the absence of an apparent acoustic stimulus. The prevalence increases with age and the elderly suffer from this condition to varying degrees. It is a very annoying problem; patients often report constant or intermittent noises such as buzzing, ringing, or hissing that result in a distortion of accurate reception of environmental sounds and voices. Treatable causes of tinnitus include high blood pressure, wax in the ear canal, or some medications like aspirin, antibiotics, or anti-depressants. If a cause can be identified then tinnitus may be cured. If patients complain of tinnitus, considerations for a quiet treatment environment should be made to decrease the bombardment of external noise sources superimposed on the internal sources.[98]

Unfortunately, older adults are not routinely screened for hearing loss. Signs of hearing impairment include:

- Other people are hard to understand
- The person doesn't speak clearly (it sounds as if he or she is mumbling)
- Background noise makes it even harder to hear
- A background hissing or ringing is heard
- Social events are less enjoyable
- The individual complains of straining to understand what others are saying.

Proprioceptive and Vestibular Dysfunction

Proprioception or *kinesthesia* is affected by changes in the neurosensory mechanisms. Although a greater degree of sensory-perceptual loss results from local system changes such as impaired vision from increased lens density, cerebral cortex cell loss may result in less cellular availability for sensory interpretation. This is important when evaluating an elderly individual's gait pattern and balance. PVD and diabetes may further complicate proprioceptive and kinesthetic input.

The ability to replicate passive motion at any joint and the ability to detect motion is diminished with increasing age. Older subjects detect motion less well at low frequencies of movement, though they still accurately report joint motion sensation. Perhaps proprioceptive loss is joint specific. It appears to decline in the lower extremities with advancing age and is an important consideration when working with the elderly. Loss of proprioception is usually an irreversible deficit and contributes a great deal to falls in the elderly.[99] Although the prospect of reversing proprioceptive deficits is low, the elderly individual can be taught to compensate for a decrease in position sense by visual input. Peripheral sensation is the most important sensory system in the maintenance of upright posture. To compensate for the deterioration in sensory input and processing ability, elderly individuals often develop a strategy of stiffening and freezing their lower legs during upright standing. It is felt that this is an attempt to shift sensory input to increased muscle input by cocontraction during standing.[100]

Vestibular functions show some deterioration with age. Degeneration occurs in the sensory receptors in both the otoliths and semicircular canals affecting the vestibular system. The function of this system is to monitor head position and to detect head movements. When an individual is deprived of visual and lower extremity somatosensory information, the vestibular system is left to control balance. Healthy young adults are able to balance without meaningful visual or support surface information. Healthy elderly, with normal amounts of vestibular degeneration, lose their balance and are at risk for falls when vestibular input is the only spatial orientation information available.[101] Diseases of the neuromuscular system further compound this problem. Balance problems or the fear of falling may severely compromise ambulatory capabilities in the elderly. Patients with vestibular lesions can be potentially treated with specific exercises to improve vestibular function or can be taught compensatory techniques using vision. Treatment of vestibular problems will be addressed in Chapter 10.

Sensory Changes in Smell With Aging

There is a close association between the sense of smell and human behavior. The olfactory memory is a very powerful one that can elicit strong emotions. The sense of smell is also important in recognizing what is occurring in the environment. The effects of aging alone on the ability to smell are minimal, and the decline of the sense of smell is probably related to an underlying pathology. Pathologically there does appear to be a decline in fiber in the olfactory bulb. By the age of 80 almost three-fourths of the fibers

are lost. Postmenopausal women exhibit decreased ability to smell, which is thought to be the result of a decline in estrogen levels following menopause. Eating is perhaps the most directly affected activity when olfactory acuity is involved. In order to detect the flavor of food, one must be able to smell it. Thus, the aged person with a loss of smell may complain that food is tasteless. For the person with olfactory loss, hot foods are more easily perceived than are cold foods. As with all of the senses, smell serves as an environmental safety indicator. The inability to smell will raise certain safety concerns that can be addressed by alternative methods, such as ensuring that there are smoke detectors in the house to compensate for the loss of ability to smell smoke.[102]

Sensory Changes in Taste With Aging

Taste sensitivities change throughout life with age-related alterations in both detection and recognition thresholds of taste. Oral somatic sensations do not change significantly.[103] The sense of taste is closely associated with the senses of smell and vision. How food looks and smells enhances or detracts from its taste. Any pathology affecting the tongue will also affect the ability to perceive the sensation (bitter, sweet, salty, or sour). A decline in taste sensitivity occurs with age. Cigarette and pipe smoking is a factor in the decline of taste. The decline in flow of saliva caused by certain medications of clinical dehydration also affects taste. The aged person seems to have an increased sensitivity to bitterness, and a decreased sensitivity to sweetness and saltiness.[104]

Compensation for these losses revolves around recognizing how to enhance the senses that are involved by making food visually more appealing, serving hot foods hot, increasing the use of herbs and spices to enhance the taste, creating an enjoyable social and physical environment, and the aggressive maintenance of good oral hygiene.

Gastrointestinal Pathologies With Aging

Age-related changes in function are apparent in the GI system, and these changes can lead to pathological states because of poor nutrition. This is important to physical therapy, because without an adequate energy source, functional capabilities of any individual become restrained and limited. GI complaints are extremely common in the aged. GI disease accounts for over one-quarter of hospital admissions.[4]

Dysphagia is difficulty in swallowing. It commonly results from neuromuscular disorders such as cerebrovascular accident, Parkinson's disease, diabetes, and other neuropathies. Malnutrition results from decreased intake; aspiration of oral contents is a common accompaniment that frequently leads to pneumonia. There is a fairly high incidence of swallowing problems involving the mouth, pharynx, and upper esophageal sphincter in the elderly population. It is common to classify dysphagia according to the lesions causing the abnormal movement of food through the mouth, pharynx, and upper esophageal sphincter as *oropharyngeal dysphagia*; and those abnormalities producing difficulty with the passage of ingested material through the smooth muscle portion of the esophagus as *esophageal dysphagia*.[105]

Oropharyngeal dysphagia is characterized by difficulty initiating swallowing and impaired ability to transfer food from the mouth into the upper portion of the esophagus. Cerebrovascular accidents and Parkinson's disease frequently result in dysphagia. Pathologies that affect the motor end plates such as *myasthenia gravis* can inhibit proper muscle functioning. Muscle problems such as those seen in metabolic myopathy (eg, thyroid disease, steroid therapy), primary myositis, or amyloidosis can create swallowing difficulties. Tumors or surgical scarring can cause local obstruction to the passage of food, and motility disorders like abnormal upper esophageal sphincter relaxation or pharyngeal/upper esophageal sphincter incoordination can cause oropharyngeal dysphagia.[106]

True esophageal dysphagia, where the transport of the ingested material down the esophagus is impaired, is common in the elderly. Carcinoma of the esophagus, which occurs with increasing frequency in the elderly, usually presents with dysphagia. The most common symptom is the sensation of food "hanging up" in the esophagus. It has a poor prognosis for cure and usually requires extensive palliative treatment.[107] Hiatal hernia can be another cause of dysphagia. It is important to understand that *achalasia* (failure to relax the smooth muscles of the GI tract) can initially present in the elderly, and other motility disorders such as diffuse esophageal spasm and scleroderma do occur in these individuals. Another cause of esophageal dysphagia that is unique to the elderly population is *dysphagia aortica*, in which the transport of material down the esophagus is impaired by a markedly tortuous and enlarged aorta or heart.

The role of the PT in treating dysphagia is to coordinate the team efforts of speech pathology, dietary, and nursing to provide a comprehensive positioning and feeding program (as discussed in Chapter 6).

The PT is involved in evaluating and treating head and trunk control, neck range of motion, neck weakness, sitting balance, and abnormal postural reflex activity interfering with head control and/or sitting balance, gross facial muscle test, ability to handle secretions, voluntary deep breathing ability, breath control and voluntary cough, and gross motor upper extremity ability. The PTA may be providing interventions on any or all of these as directed by the PT. Specific emphasis needs to be placed on wheelchair and bed positioning and respiratory status.

Ulcers affect about 20% of the older adult population. An ulcer is an area of the stomach that has been eroded by digestive juices and stomach acid. Normally, the lining of the stomach and duodenum are protected from the digestive juices from the stomach. The most common symptom of an ulcer is a burning pain in the abdomen. The pain can last minutes to hours, occurs often between meals, and can be relieved by eating something. Ulcer disease in the elderly commonly presents with atypical symptoms. *Dyspepsia* can be a manifestation and a common complaint in older adults diagnosed with Gastroesophageal Reflux Disease (GERD) or peptic ulcer.[108] Complications of obstruction, bleeding, and perforation are more common in the aged than in younger individuals with GI ulcers. Medical management is effective in uncomplicated cases and rests on the use of antacids, avoidance of drugs including aspirin and other nonsteroidal and steroidal anti-inflammatory agents.[109] Surgical repair may be necessary. The difficulties encountered in rehabilitation of the aged with ulcer disease are centered on the poor nutritional status and resulting decline in activity level. Focus needs to be on the maintenance of maximal functional capabilities and adequate nutrition.

Atrophic gastritis is a stomach disorder that is unique to the elderly. It involves a shrinking and inflammation of the inner lining of the stomach. While it may not cause any symptoms, it can increase the risk for stomach cancer. While this was once thought to be a normal process of aging, more recent evidence indicates that it is caused by prolonged infestation of *heliocobactor pylori* (H. pylori) and *campylobacter pylori* (C. pylori), which is common in older adults.[110]

Pernicious anemia results from a common age-related decline in the absorption of vitamin B_{12}. This usually occurs in the setting of chronic inflammation of the lining of the stomach called *atrophic gastritis*. Not only can impaired B_{12} absorption cause significant disease (eg, dementia, neuropathy, anemia, etc), but it is associated with a higher incidence of carcinoma of the stomach. Replacement of vitamin B_{12} through monthly injections effectively prevents or corrects the deficiency, in addition to monitoring B_{12} intake through dietary means. The most clinically significant findings in patients with pernicious anemia are low energy levels, confusion, and peripheral neuropathies resulting in proprioceptive problems.[111]

Achlorhydria refers to an insufficient production of stomach acid. It may be caused by atrophic gastritis. Achlorhydria is the most common cause of B_{12} deficiency. The stomach must secrete adequate amounts of gastric acid and a protein known as intrinsic factor as well as produce the digestive enzyme pepsin for B_{12} absorption to occur. Changes in the GI tract can affect absorption of vitamin B_{12}. Since the liver is able to store large amounts of B_{12} it can take up to 5 years before symptoms of deficiency appear. However, it is important to recognize symptoms early since any neurological damage may be irreversible. Symptoms of B_{12} deficiency can be misdiagnosed since they can look like Alzheimer's disease or other dementias. Symptoms include dementia and confusion, extreme fatigue, and tingling and weakness in the arms and legs.[112]

Gastrointestinal malignancies account for the second largest number of cancer deaths, lung cancer being the leading cause. The esophagus, stomach, pancreas, and large intestine are the most common sites. Cancer of the stomach is more common with advancing age. Cancer of the pancreas has a similar 5-year survival rate, but its peak incidence is in the sixth decade. Late diagnosis due to atypical, vague, or misleading symptoms (such as depression or altered mental status) is the rule. Cancer of the colon accounts for half of all GI malignancies. Because they are usually less "clinically silent" than the other malignancies, intervention is usually earlier and more successful. Rectal bleeding, anemia, weight loss, and altered bowel habits are the common presenting complaints. However, weakness, depression, fatigue, anorexia, and decreased functional competence are early nonspecific clues to colon cancer. Unless the elderly person's condition makes it likely that death is imminent from another cause, surgery is often required for cure or to prevent intestinal obstruction. Five-year survival rates vary widely depending on the extent of the tumor at the time of initial treatment, but complete cures and long remissions are common.[113]

Constipation is increasingly common with advancing age. Although bowel transit times are normal in otherwise healthy adults, many other age-related factors can contribute to having fewer than 3 stools per week. Inactivity, inadequate dietary fiber, inadequate fluids, drug side effects (eg, narcotics, iron, sedatives, anti-cholinergics), over-sedation, confusion, and prior laxative abuse can all contribute to

constipation. Alterations in the intestine due to local disease such as hemorrhoids, strictures, diverticulitis, and cancer can also contribute to constipation. Correction of contributory factors, use of regular periodic laxatives, and patient education are usually effective. Activity and exercise is one of the best remedies for constipation.[114]

Urinary incontinence is created by a weakness in the pelvic floor musculature and predisposes significant numbers of elderly individuals to institutionalization. Urinary incontinence is a condition in which involuntary loss of urine is a social or hygienic problem. Four types of urinary incontinence have been defined. *Stress incontinence* is the involuntary loss of urine with increases in intra-abdominal pressures, such as during a cough, sneeze, laugh, or exercise. It is due to a weakness in the pelvic floor coupled with weakness in the bladder outlet or urethral sphincter. *Urge incontinence* is a leakage of urine resulting from an inability to delay voiding after sensation of bladder fullness is perceived. This can occur due to overconcentration of the urine (usually a result of dehydration or concentration of excess drugs or vitamins in the urine) and is also associated with urinary tract infection, tumors, outlet obstruction, or CNS disorders such as stroke, dementia, Parkinsonism, or spinal cord injury or disease. *Overflow incontinence* is a leakage of urine resulting from mechanical forces such as obstruction by the prostate, a cystocele (ie, dropping of the bladder externally), or could have a neurogenic basis such as in spinal cord lesions or multiple sclerosis. *Functional incontinence* is associated with the inability to get to the toilet, or once there, the inability to manage clothing. This is often related to poor physical function and endurance, environmental barriers, or impairment in cognition.[115] Specific treatment interventions will be more thoroughly discussed in Chapter 10.

Renal disease has a high morbidity and mortality in the elderly, in addition to significantly decreasing the quality of life. Acute cessation of renal function can occur at any age, but the diminished blood supply of the aging kidney renders it more susceptible to injury. Hypotension is the usual precipitating cause and can result from dehydration, overmedication, surgery, or sepsis. Acute injury from certain antibiotics or from contrast dye used in radiology can also result in acute renal shut down. Acute renal failure is associated with the rapid build up of toxic waste products and drugs, fluid overload, and elevation of serum potassium. Any of these complications can be fatal if not managed correctly. In addition, the immune system is impaired; patients with acute renal failure frequently die with infections.[116]

Chronic renal failure is marked by the slow deterioration of renal function and is usually detected when the presence of another illness stresses the renal system and elevated blood urea nitrogen (BUN), hyponatremia, or increased fluid retention lead to an evaluation of renal function.[117] The functional effects of chronic renal failure result primarily from anemia and congestive heart failure. Patients with renal disease severe enough to cause significant chronic mental status changes have a poor prognosis and often require dialysis or transplantation.[118]

The clinical implications of problems in the kidney in relation to exercise and activity tolerance center on the electrolyte balance and the potential inability of the kidney to facilitate homeostasis.[119] Increasing energy expenditure through exercise is positively correlated with an improvement in mortality and morbidity through a number of mechanisms. Despite these benefits, there has been some reluctance, especially in the elderly with renal failure, in recommending fitness programs because of the fear that exercising too intensely will provoke cardiac arrhythmias, myocardial infarction, or increased blood pressure. Regular eccentric training can increase protein turnover (37% higher muscle catabolism) in older people and can require a higher protein intake; combined with a calorie-appropriate diet, regular exercise maintains a reasonable body weight, delays loss of lean muscle mass, and promotes good physical performance. Activity level is a predictor of survival for people ages 60 to 90 years.[120]

Endocrine and Metabolic Diseases With Aging

The endocrine system encompasses a diverse group of organs and specialized glands that produce hormones. Hormones are chemical messengers that instruct those cells with complementary receptors to perform a specific metabolic act. The thyroid gland elaborates thyroxin, which in turn modulates the overall metabolic rate of cells within the organism. Parathyroid glands elaborate parathyroid hormone, which is central to regulation of calcium metabolism. The islet cells of the pancreas produce insulin, which helps regulate glucose metabolism. Three hormones help modulate the fluid and electrolyte balance of the body: the posterior pituitary gland makes antidiuretic hormone (ADH), the kidneys produce renin, and the adrenal glands produce aldosterone.

Although many other hormones exist, excess and deficiency of the previously listed hormones account for most of the clinically significant endocrine diseases encountered in the aged. With aging, there appears to be a reduction in the sensitivity of the target cells to the hormone messenger. This is due to a lessening of the number of hormone receptors found on the target cells.[121]

Clinically, significant disease can result from both excess and deficiency of thyroid hormone. In both hyperthyroidism and hypothyroidism, the presentation of the syndrome can be very different in the aged than it is in younger patients. As is the rule in most illnesses in the aged, the presentation is usually more subtle and the symptoms and signs less specific. *Hypothyroidism* is common in the aged and results from failure of the thyroid gland to elaborate sufficient thyroid hormone despite maximum stimulation of the gland by the thyroid stimulating hormone (TSH). Vague symptoms abound: dry skin, chronic muscle and joint pains, lethargy, confusion, weight gain, edema, depression, apathy, sensitivity to sedatives, and cold intolerance. More subtle abnormalities such as pseudo dementia, depression, and lethargy are more common in ambulatory patients. Treatment involves the gradual replacement of thyroid hormone on a daily basis until the TSH value becomes normal.[122]

Hyperthyroidism is the overproduction of thyroxin. Common manifestations include the new development of glucose intolerance (diabetes mellitus), congestive heart failure, atrial fibrillation, muscle weakness, weight loss, diarrhea, and agitation. Subclinical levels of hyperthyroidism may also present with depression, apathy, failure to thrive, and constipation. Although their symptoms are similar to patients with hypothyroidism, correction of the elevated thyroid hormone level abolishes the symptoms.[123]

Surgical removal of the thyroid gland is rare and is usually reserved for situations in which the enlarged gland compromises the patient's airway. The use of radioactive iodine, which is selectively concentrated in the gland, produces the most lasting reduction in hormone levels. It is so effective that virtually all patients treated with this modality develop hypothyroidism requiring hormone replacement. Medications that block the production of thyroid hormone are effective alternatives to radioactive iodine. Their use is complicated by the development of bone marrow suppression and a significant relapse rate when the medication is withdrawn. However, in the majority of cases, both types of treatment produce excellent results.

ADH increases the reabsorption of water from the kidney, and its release is stimulated by a decrease in circulating fluid volume or an increase in osmolarity. It is an important part of the endocrine system, which maintains fluid balance. Under certain circumstances, the pituitary makes excessive amounts of ADH, which results in the *syndrome of inappropriate ADH secretion* (SIADH). Several intracranial processes such as stroke, meningitis, and subdural hematoma, and intrathoracic conditions, such as pneumonia, tuberculosis, and bronchiectasis, can cause SIADH. SIADH results in excess water retention, which in turn causes a severe dilution of serum sodium, which results in lethargy, confusion, and seizures. It usually responds to restricting free water and correcting the precipitating factors.[124]

There is an age-related increase in the prevalence of *glucose intolerance*. The number of insulin receptors found on cell membranes decreases with age. Reflecting this change, the incidence of glucose intolerance increases with age, reaching nearly 25% by age 80. In the aged, it is important to identify glucose intolerance not only to prevent the complications of untreated diabetes (neuropathy, retinopathy, nephropathy, and accelerated atherosclerosis), but, even more, to identify those individuals at risk for non-ketotic hyperosmolar coma or severe hyperglycemia, which can be precipitated by infection, dehydration, or other physiologic stress.[125]

Dehydration and hypotension are more significant clinical problems than hyperglycemia. Treatment consists of fluid replacement and very low dose insulin therapy to slowly bring down the elevated blood sugar. Prevention of this syndrome involves the early identification of diabetic patients who are slipping into the cycle of infection, decreased oral intake, dehydration, increased blood sugar, and the resulting acceleration of dehydration through the forced excretion of water when the kidneys cannot reabsorb all of the glucose presented to it and glucose is lost in the urine. Rehydration and treatment of the primary illness will usually prevent the development of non-ketotic hyperosmolar coma.[126]

Diabetes mellitus is a chronic disease that affects approximately 12 million people in the United States. Insulin is needed for glucose to be transferred from the blood to the muscle and fat cells. People who suffer from diabetes cannot produce enough insulin (type I) or cannot properly use the insulin they do produce (type II), causing hyperglycemia. The complex nature of diabetes creates a broad spectrum of physical complications and reactions that can make the condition extremely dangerous. Diabetes is the leading cause of blindness and can cause glaucoma and cataracts. Diabetics are twice as likely to have heart attacks and strokes, 5 times more prone to foot ulceration with the development of gangrene, and 17 times more prone to kidney disease when compared to the general population. Complications of diabetes also affect the mouth; the reproductive, nervous, vascular, and muscular system; the skin; and reduce an individual's defense mechanisms in the presence of infection.[127]

Symptoms of diabetes include increased urination, increased thirst, increased hunger, fatigue or lethargy, weight loss, and numbness or tingling in the feet and hands. Although no clear understanding of the cause of diabetes has been found and there is no cure, the disease has been found to be controllable by achieving and maintaining normal blood glucose levels. This requires a carefully balanced utilization of 4 critical components—diet, exercise, education for self-monitoring, and drug therapy. Diet control is critical to diabetes control, especially in type II diabetes. Patients with diabetes should be encouraged to eat less, to consume fewer calories, and to eat less fat and simple sugars.[128]

Exercise improves blood glucose control, improves circulation, reduces cardiovascular risk, and keeps the patient fit. Daily exercise increases the tissue sensitivity to insulin for 2 to 3 days, thereby decreasing the need for insulin injection.[129] Drug therapy for diabetes consists of oral agents (type II only) and insulin. Insulin is obtained from animal sources, such as cows and pigs, or from a biosynthesis process that results in insulin products that are the same as human insulin. The synthesized insulin has gained popularity in recent years because it causes the formation of fewer insulin antibodies and is less likely to cause allergic reactions. Insulin requirements may change in patients who become ill, especially with vomiting or fever. Signs of hyperglycemia may be caused by a missed insulin dose, overeating, not following the diabetic diet, or fever and infection; they include excessive thirst and/or urination, dry mouth, drowsiness, flushed dry skin, fruit-like breath odor, stomachache, nausea, vomiting, and difficulty breathing. Signs of hypoglycemia may be caused by too much insulin, missing a snack or meal, sickness, too much exercise, drinking alcoholic beverages, or taking medications that contain alcohol. Symptoms include anxiety, chills, cold sweats, cool pale skin, confusion, drowsiness, excessive hunger, headache, nausea, nervousness, shakiness, vision changes, and unusual tiredness or fatigue. If these symptoms occur, the consumption of a sugar containing food (eg, orange juice, honey, etc) should reverse the symptoms.[130]

MULTISYSTEM INVOLVEMENT

Unlike younger populations, the biggest challenge to rehabilitation efforts is the fact that most of the elderly we treat have more than 1 diagnosis. The national average for people over the age of 75 is 6 diagnoses and 6 drugs per person. Often systems must be prioritized in therapeutically approaching the primary diagnosis. For example, if a patient is being referred for therapy with a total knee replacement, but also has cardiac disease, the cardiovascular system needs to be a primary focus in regaining functional capabilities of the lower extremity. Specific treatment strategies using the systems approach will be covered in Chapter 10.

CONCLUSION

Aging is a major risk factor for degenerative pathologies including heart disease, cancer, neurodegeneration, type II diabetes, osteoporosis, sarcopenia, and vision problems. The incidence of disease increases as one ages. Although an apparent paradox, it appears that the most effective way to delay or even to avert diseases is to manage activity, nutrition, hydration, and stress throughout life. The fitter individual tends to live a longer, healthier life. Disease states seem to be the result of micro-insults over one's lifetime, which are universal in all systems of the body, although the end-state pathology may be different and progression may evolve at varying speeds.

We are more responsible for the way we age than we used to think. With all the information available today, we now understand that chronological age is not a reliable indicator of a person's ability to function. Many problems that are commonly seen in older people are preventable and/or treatable. Few of the problems seen in old age are actually caused by the aging process: most are caused by diseases, inactivity and poor fitness, environmental exposures and stresses, and social changes.

PEARLS

- PTAs need to closely monitor the patients they are working with for signs and symptoms of underlying pathology that the elderly may attribute to "getting old."

- Many communities offer some type of exercise class geared toward the elderly person. PTAs should be aware of these programs and may be able to help promote better compliance of patients through encouraging participation in such programs. If there is not such a class available in the community, the PTA should develop and propose a plan to his or her facility or to the management at the local health club.

- Be sure you know which type of arthritis the patient has so you can follow through with the correct intervention and provide appropriate patient education. Often patients will be unsure of the specific differences in treatment and care of the different forms of arthritis.

- Any time exercise training is provided to elderly patients, it is important to remember that their signs and symptoms of exercise intolerance will vary from those of younger and generally healthy individuals. Pay close attention to any shortness of breath (dyspnea) rather than waiting for angina to develop. PTAs also need to be aware of cardiac medications the patient may be on as these will decrease the accuracy of using heart rate and blood pressure to gauge the patient's response to exercise.

- It is critical to understand the underlying cardiac pathology prior to initiating intervention with patients to avoid inaccurate measurements or measurement tools, inappropriate interventions (intermittent compression in the case of congestive heart failure), and an exercise level inappropriate for the individual.

- Be aware of the different presentations of pathology in the elderly. PTAs can help alert appropriate staff to potential complications and pathology by being aware of and reporting subtle changes in patient's normal behavior and activity levels.

- PTAs could have a major impact on the early detection of skin cancers by assessing skin status during treatment, not only for obvious ulcerations or lesions, but the more subtle presentations of skin changes as well.

- PTAs should pay attention to the elderly patient's reports of visual changes and help him or her recognize when advice of an eye doctor is needed. PTAs should also recognize that physical exertion can exacerbate acute symptoms, as well as interfere with recent repairs of the eye, and should be avoided.

Take Home Pearls

For effective intervention and management of elderly patients/clients PTAs must:

- Keep in mind that their elderly patients may present with differing signs and symptoms of pathology than their younger patients

- Remember that even in their later years elderly patients can still benefit from a regular exercise/activity routine that is designed to meet their abilities and needs

- Prepare exercise programs that take into account the multiple system involvement with which elderly patients may present.

REFERENCES

1. Schenker N, Parker J. From single-race reporting to multiple-race reporting: using imputation methods to bridge the transition. *Stat Med.* 2003;2:1571-1587.
2. Schoenborn CA, Adam PF, Sundik EJ, et al. Health behaviors of adults: United States, 2005-2007. *National Vital Health Statistics*, Hyattsville, MD: 2010;10:1-132.
3. Ingram DD, Parker JD, Schenker N, et al. United States census 2000 population with bridged race categories. *Vital Health Stat.* 2003;2:1-47.
4. Heron M, Hoyert DL, Murphy SL, et al. Deaths: Final data for 2006. *National Vital Statistics Reports*, Hyattsville, MD: 2009;57:1-135.
5. Navarro A, Lopez-Cepero JM, Sanchez del Pino MJ. Skeletal muscle and aging. *Front Biosci.* 2001;6:D26-D44.
6. Renault V, Thornell LE, Eriksson PO, Butler-Browne G, Mouly V, Thorne LE. Regenerative potential of human skeletal muscle during aging. *Aging Cell.* 2002;1:132-139.
7. Finch CE. A perspective on sporadic inclusion-body myositis: the role of aging and inflammatory processes. *Neurology.* 2006;66(suppl 1):S1-S6.
8. Alford AI, Hankenson KD. Matricellular proteins: extracellular modulators of bone development, remodeling, and regeneration. *Bone.* 2006;38:749-757.
9. Bogoch ER, Elliot-Gibson V, Beaton DE, Jamal SA, Josse RG, Murray TM. Effective initiation of osteoporosis diagnosis and treatment for patients with a frailty fracture in an orthopedic environment. *J Bone Joint Surg Am.* 2006;88:25-34.
10. Pietschmann P, Kerschan-Schindl K. Osteoporosis: gender-specific aspects. *Wien Med Wochenschr.* 2004;154:411-415.
11. Taylor JC, Sterkel B, Utley M, Shipley M, Newman S, Horton M. Opinions and experiences in general practive on osteoporosis prevention, diagnosis and management. *Osteopor Int.* 2001;12:844-848.
12. Stafford RS, Drieling RL, Johns R, Ma J. National patterns of calcium use in osteoporosis in the United States. *J Reprod Med.* 2005;50(11 suppl):885-890.
13. Ahmed MS, Matsumura B, Cristian A. Age-related changes in muscles and joints. *Phys Med Rehabil Clin N Am.* 2005;16:19-39.
14. Loeser RF, Shakoor N. Aging or osteoarthritis: which is the problem? *Rheum Dis Clin North Am.* 2003;29:653-673.
15. Marin JA, Buckwalter JA. Aging, articular cartilage chondrocyte senescence and osteoarthritis. *Biogerontology.* 2002;3:257-264.
16. Savelberg HH, Meijer K. The effect of age and joint angle on the proportionality of extensor and flexor strength at the knee joint. *J Gerontol A Biol Sci Med. Sci.* 2004;59:1120-1128.
17. Bennell K, Hinman R. Exercise as a treatment for osteoarthritis. *Curr Opin Rheumatol.* 2005;17:634-640.
18. Olivieri I, Palazzi C, Peruz G, Padula A. Management issues with elderly-onset rheumatoid arthritis: an update. *Drugs Aging.* 2005;22:809-822.
19. Gossec L, Pavy S, Pham T, et al. Nonpharmacological treatments in early rheumatoid arthritis: clinical practice guidelines based on published evidence and expert opinion. *Joint Bone Spine.* 2006;73:396-402.
20. Mayoux-Benhamou MA. Fatigue and rheumatoid arthritis. *Ann Readapt Med Phys.* 2006;49:385-388.
21. Lakatta EG. Age-associated cardiovascular changes in health: impact on cardiovascular disease in older persons. *Heart Fail Rev.* 2002;7:29-49.
22. Ferrarai AU, Radaelli A, Centola M. Invited review: aging and the cardiovascular system. *J Appl Physiol.* 2003;95:2591-2597.
23. Duri D, Jakovljevi V, Stojkovi M, Duri A, Petrovi B. Clinical assessment of major artery vasomotor endothelial function: methodology and importance for evaluating aging as a cardiovascular risk factor. *Med Pregl.* 2003;56(suppl 1):9-12.
24. Nietlispach F, Hug B, Jansen C, et al. Echocardiographic quantification of atherosclerosis leads to cost-effective treatment with statins. *Swiss Med Wkly.* 2005;135:62-68.
25. Mack WJ, Hameed AB, Xiang M, et al. Does elevated body mass modify the influence of postmenopausal estrogen replacement on atherosclerosis progression: results from the estrogen in the prevention of atherosclerosis trial. *Atherosclerosis.* 2003;168:91-98.
26. Burkauskiene A. Age-related changes in the structure of myocardial collagen network of auricle of the right atrium in health persons and ischemic heart disease patients. *Medicina.* 2005;41:145-154.
27. Bales AC. Medical management of chronic ischemic heart disease. Selecting specific drug therapies, modifying risk factors. *Postgrad Med.* 2004;115:39-46.
28. Miller WL, Tointon SK, Hodge DO, Nelson SM, Rodheffer RJ, Gibbons RJ. Long-term outcome and the use of revascularization in patients with heart failure, suspected ischemic heart disease, and large reversible myocardial perfusion defects. *Am Heart J.* 2002;143:904-909.
29. Rosana GM, Vitale C, Onorati D, Fini M. Quality of life in elderly patients with ischemic cardiopathy. *Ital Heart J.* 2004;5(suppl 2):16S-22S.
30. Graham MM, Ghali WA, Faris PD, Galbraith PD, Norris CM, Knudtson ML. Survival after coronary revascularization in the elderly. *Circulation.* 2002;105:2378-2384.
31. Yamasaki N, Kitaoka H, Matsumura Y, Furuno T, Nishinaga M, Doi Y. Heart failure in the elderly. *Intern Med.* 2003;42:383-388.
32. Chimenti C, Kajstura J, Torella D, et al. Senescence and death of primitive cells and myocytes lead to premature cardiac aging and heart failure. *Circ Res.* 2003;93:604-613.
33. Skarabal MZ, Stading JA, Hilleman DE. Advances in the treatment of congestive heart failure: new approaches for an old disease. *Pharmacotherapy.* 2000;20:787-804.
34. Keteyian SJ, Brawner CA, Schairer JR, et al. Effects of exercise training on chronotropic incompetence in patients with heart failure. *Am Heart J.* 1999;138:233-240.
35. Matsumura Y, Elliott PM, Virdee MS, Sorajja P, Doi Y, McKenna WJ. Left ventricular diastolic function assessed using Doppler tissue imaging in patients with hypertrophic cardiomyopathy: relation to symptoms and exercise capacity. *Heart.* 2002;87:247-251.
36. Myers J, Wagner D, Schertler T, et al. Effects of exercise training on left ventricular volumes and function in patients with non ischemic cardiomyopathy: application of magnetic resonance myocardial taggeing. *Am Heart J.* 2002;144:719-725.
37. Dec GW, DeSanctis RW. Cardiomyopathies: dilated cardiomyopaty. *Cardiovascular Medicine, XIV Cardiomyopathies.* http://www.acpmedicine.com/. Accessed April 1, 2010.
38. Wenger NK, Helmy T, Patel AD, Hanna IR. Approaching cardiac arrhythmias in the elderly patient. *Medscape General Medicine.* 2005;7:24-32.
39. Ansalone G, Russo M. Treatment of arrhythmias and syncope in the elderly with heart failure. *Ital Heart J.* 2004;(suppl 10):52S-59S.

40. Tsuneda T, Inoue H. Arrhythmias in the elderly population and their management. *Nippon Ronen Igakkai Zasshi.* 2005;42:261-270.

41. Demer LL. Cholesterol in vascular and valvular calcification. *Circulation.* 2001;104:1881-1883.

42. Otto S, Baum T, Keller F. Sex-dependence of the relative number of elastic fibres in human heart valves. *Ann Anat.* 2006;188:153-158.

43. Shikano M, Nakatani S, Kim J, et al. Impaired left ventricular systolic function in mitral stenosis. *J Cardiol.* 2003;42:75-79.

44. Shiokawa Y, Kado H, Yasui H. The surgical treatment of congenital valve disease. *Nippon Geka Gakkai Zasshi.* 2001;102:342-347.

45. Segal BL. Valvular heart disease. Part 1. Diagnosis and surgical management of aortic valve disease in older adults. *Geriatrics.* 2003;58:31-35.

46. Izzo JL. Aging and systolic hypertension: cluster patterns and problem-solving strategies to aswer the genetic riddle. *Hypertension.* 2001;37:1067-1068.

47. Najjar SS, Scuteri A, Lakatta EG. Arterial aging: is it an immutable cardiovascular risk factor? *Hypertension.* 2005;46:454-462.

48. Plante GE. Vascular response to stress in health and disease. *Metabolism.* 2002;51(6 suppl 1):25-30.

49. Frieden RA. The geriatric amputee. *Phys Med Rehabil Clin N Am.* 2005;16:179-195.

50. Bauer TA, Brass EP, Hiatt WR. Impaired muscle oxygen use at onset of exercise in peripheral arterial disease. *J Vasc Surg.* 2004;40:488-493.

51. Nichols WW, Singh BM. Augmentation index as a mesure of peripheral vascular disease state. *Curr Opin Cardiol.* 2002;17:543-551.

52. Oka RK, Altman M, Giacomini JC, Szuba A, Cooke JP. Exercise patterns and cardiovascular fitness of patients with peripheral arterial disease. *J Vasc Nurs.* 2004;22:109-114.

53. Doyle J, Creager MA. Pharmacotherapy and behavioral intervention for peripheral arterial disease. *Rev Cardiovasc Med.* 2003;4:18-24.

54. Makowka A, Zimmer-Nowicka J, Nowicki M. Respiratory tract diseases in the elderly. *Pol Arch Med Wewm.* 2004;(112, special issue):147-160.

55. Kammoun S, Rekik WK, Ayoub A. The aging lung: structural and functional modifications related to aging. *Tunis Med.* 2001;79:10-14.

56. Vanpee D, Swine C, Delwiche JP, Delaunois L. Evaluation of flow limitation in elderly patients unable to perform a forced expiratory maneuver. *Aging Clin Exp Res.* 2002;14:208-211.

57. Balleste CR, Gonzalez G, Ramirez-Ronda CH, et al. Potentially serious infections in the aging person: diagnosis, treatment, and prevention. *PR Health Sci J.* 2004;23:19-24.

58. Kikawada M, Iwamoto T, Takasaki M. Aspiration and infection in the elderly: epidemiology, diagnosis and management. *Drugs Aging.* 2005;22:115-130.

59. Janssens JP, Krause KH. Pneumonia in the very old. *Lancet Infect Dis.* 2004;4:112-124.

60. Donma O, Donma MM. Relationship of senescence of pulmonary system to chronic obstructive pulmonary disease in the advanced life. *Med Hypotheses.* 2002;59:208-211.

61. Barua P, O-Mahony MS. Overcoming gaps in the management of asthma in older patients: new insights. *Drugs Aging.* 2005;22:1029-1059.

62. Muller KC, Welker L, Paasch K, et al. Lung fibroblasts from patients with emphysema show markers of senescence in vitro. *Respir Res.* 2006;7

63. Tsang KW. Solutions for difficult diagnostic cases of acute exacerbations of chronic bronchitis. Chemotherapy. 2001;47(suppl 4):28-38.

64. Yohannes AM, Hardy CC. Treatment of chronic obstructive pulmonary disease in older patients: a practical guide. *Drugs Aging.* 2003;20:209-228.Boisseau MR. Roles of mechanical blood forces in vascular diseases. A clinical overview. *Clin Hemorheol Microcirc.* 2005;33:201-207.

65. Wyss JM, Carlson SH. The role of the nervous system in hypertension. *Crr Hypertens Rep.* 2001;3:255-262.

66. Sowers MR, Crutchfield M, Richards K, Wilkin MK, Furniss A, Jannausch M, et al. Sarcopenia is related to physical functioning and leg strength in middle-aged women. *J Gerontol A Biol Sci Med Sci.* 2005;60:486-490.

67. Walston J, Hadley EV, Ferrucci L, et al. Research agenda for frailty in older adults. *J Am Geriatr Soc.* 2006;54:991-1001.

68. Vandervoort AA. Aging of the human neuromuscular system. *Muscle Nerve.* 2002;25:17-25.

69. Leentjens AFG, van der Mast RC. Delirium in elderly people: an update. *Curr Opin Psychiatry.* 2005;18:325-330.

70. Rahkonen T, Makela H, Paanila S. Delirium in elderly people without predisposing disorders: etiology and 1-year prognosis after discharge. *Int Psychogeriatr.* 2000;12:473-481.

71. McCusker J, Cole M, Dendukuri N. Delirium in older medical inpatients and subsequent cognitive and functional status: a prospective study. *CMAJ.* 2001;165:575-583.

72. Cole MG, McCusker J, Dendukuri N, Han L. Symptoms of delirium in elderly medical patients with or without dementia. *J Neuropsychiatry Clin Neurosci.* 2002;14:167-175.

73. Lam CK, Lim PP, Low BL, Ng LL, Chiam PC, Sahadevan S. Depression in dementia: a comparative and validation study. *Int J Geriatr Psychiatry.* 2004;19:422-428.

74. Gillette-Guyonnet S, Andrieu S, Coretes F, et al. Outcome of Alzheimer's disease: potential impact of choinesterase inhibitors. *J Gerontol Med Sci.* 2006;61A:516-520.

75. Roman GC. Vascular dementia may be the most common form of dementia in the elderly. *J Neurol Sci.* 2002;203-204:7-10.

76. De Jong D, Jansen R, Kremer B, Verbeek MM. Cerebrospinal fluid Amyloid 42/phosphorylated Tau ration discriminates between Alzheimer's disease and vascular dementia. *J Gerontol Med Sci.* 2006;61A:755-758.

77. Moyer P. New guidelines update diagnosis and treatment of parkinson's disease. *Neurology.* 2006;66(suppl 1-2):968-1002.

78. Scheife RT, Schumock GT, Burstein A, Gottwald D, Luer MS. Impact of Parkinon's disease and its pharmacologic treatment on quality of life and economic outcomes. *Amer J Health-Sys Pharm.* 2000;57:953-962.

79. De Goede CJ, Keus SH, Kwakkel G, Wagenaar RC. The effect of physical therapy in Parkinson's disease: a research synthesis. *Arch Phys Med Rehabil.* 2001;82:509-515.

80. Stankovic I. The effect of physical therapy on balance of patients with Parkinson's disease. *Int J Rehabil Res.* 2004; 27:53-57.

81. Pellecchia MT, Grasso A, Biancardi LG, Squillante M, Bonavita V, Barone P. Physical therapy in Parkinson's disease: an open long-term rehabilitation trial. *J Neurol.* 2004;251:595-598.

82. Vrancken AF, Franssen H, Wokke JH, Teunissen LL, Notermans NC. Chronic idiopathic axonal polyneuropathy and successful aging of the peripheral nervous system in elderly people. *Arch Neurol.* 2002;59:533-540.

83. Di Iorio A, Cherubini A, Volpato S, et al. Markers of inflammation, vitamin /E and peripheral nervous system function: the InCHIANTI study. *Neurobiol Aging.* 2006;27:1280-1288.

84. Resnick HE, Stansberry KB, Harris TB, et al. Diabetes, peripheral neuropathy, and old age disability. *Muscle Nerve.* 2002;25:43-50.

85. Hess JR, Brenner MJ, Myckatyn TM, Hunter DA, Mackinnon SE. Influence of aging on regeneration in end-to-end neurorrhaphy. *Ann Plast Surg.* 2006;57:217-222.

86. Laurienti PJ, Burdette JH, Maldjian JA, Wallace MT. Enhanced multisensory integration in older adults. *Neurobiol Aging.* 2006;27:1155-1163.

87. Coffey JF, Searles GE. Malignant photo damage. *Geriatrics Aging.* 2005;8:56-61.

88. Burns EA, Leventhal EA. Aging, immunity, and cancer. *Cancer Control.* 2000;76:513-522.

89. Cottam JA, Shenefelt PD, Sinnott JT, Stevens GL, Cancio M, Sakalosky PE. Common skin infections in the elderly. *Infect Med.* 1999;16:280-290.

90. Brillhart B. Preventive skin care for older adults. *Geriatrics Aging.* 2006;9:334-339.

91. Buckley JG, Elliott DB. Ophthalmic interventions to help prevent falls. *Geriatrics Aging.* 2006;9:276,278-280.

92. West CG, Gildengorin G, Haegerstrom-Portnoy G, Lott LA, Schneck ME, Brabyn JA. Vision and driving self-restriction in older adults. *J Am Geriatr Soc.* 2003;51:1348-1355.

93. Foster CS. Highlights of the association for research in vision and ophthalmology. *Medscape Opthalmology.* 2004;5:1-9.

94. Rizzo M. Clinical assessment of complex visual dysfunction in the elderly. *Semin Neurol.* 2000;20:75-87.

95. Scholtz AW, Kammen-Jolly K, Felder E, Hussl B, Rask-Andersen H, Schrott-Fischer A. Selective aspects of human pathology in high-tone hearing loss of the aging inner ear. *Hear Res.* 2001;157:77-86.

96. Tremblay KL, Piskosz M, Souza P. Effects of age and age-related hearing loss on the neural representation of speech cues. *Clin Neurophysiol.* 2003;114:1332-1343.

97. Ahmad N, Seidman M. Tinnitus in the older adult: epidemiology, pathophysiology and treatment options. *Drugs Aging.* 2004;21:297-305.

98. Brumagne S, Cordo P, Verschueren S. Proprioceptive weighting changes in persons with low back pain and elderly persons during upright standing. *Neurosci Lett.* 2004;366:63-66.

100. Benjuya N, Melzer I, Kaplanski J. Aging-induced shifts from a reliance on sensory input to muscle cocontration during balanced standing. *J Gerontol A Biol Sci Med Sci.* 2004;59:166-171.

101. Schweigart G, Chien RD, Mergner T. Neck proprioception compensates for age-related deterioration of vestibular self-motion perception. *Exp Brain Res.* 2002;147:89-97.

102. Finkel D, Pedersen NL, Larsson M. Olfactory functioning and cognitive abilities: a twin study. *J Gerontol B Psychol Sci Soc Sci.* 2001;56:P226-P233.

103. Fukunaga A. Age-related changes in renewal of taste bud cells and expression of taste cell-specific proteins in mice. *Kokubyo Gakkai Zasshai.* 2005;72:84-89.

104. Davenport RJ. The flavor of aging. *Sci Aging Knowledge Environ.* 2004; nsl. http://sagete.science.mag/cgi/content/full/2004/12/nsl.

105. Tamura F, Ayano R, Haishima H, Ishida R, Mizukami M, Mukai Y. Distribution of causes and treatment of dysphasia at dysphasia/dysphasia rehabilitation clinic of Showa University Dental Hospital: 1999-2002. *Int J Orofacial Myology.* 2004;30:53-62.

106. Gaziano JE. Evaluation and management of oropharyngeal dysphagia in head and neck cancer. *Cancer Control.* 2002;9:400-409.

107. Boyce HW. Palliation of dysphagia of esophageal cancer by endoscopic lumen restoration techniques. *Cancer Control.* 1999;6:73-83.

108. Shaib Y, El-Serag HB. The prevalence and risk factors of functional dyspepsia in a multiethnic population in the United States. *Am J Gastroenterol.* 2004;99:2210-2216.

109. Katz PO, Liker HR, Fendrick AM, Scheiman JM. Gastrointestinal mucosal protection and cardiovascular risk–contemporary approach to acid reflux and non-steroidal anti-inflammatory drug therapy. *Medscape Gastroenterology.* 2005. CMEMedscape. http://cme.medscape.com/viewarticle/511721. Accessed April 1, 2010.

110. Rembiasz K, Konturek PC, Karcz D, Konturek SJ, Ochmanski W, Bielanski W, et al. Biomarkers in various types of atrophic gastritis and their diagnostic usefulness. *Dig Dis Sci.* 2005;50:474-482.

111. Aitelli C, Wasson L, Page R. Pernicious Anemia: presentations mimicking acute leukemia. *South Med J.* 2004;97:295-297.

112. Bredenoord AJ, Baron A, Smout AJ. Symptomatic gastro-oesophageal reflux in a patient with achlorhydria. *Gut.* 2006;55:1045-1055.

113. Balducci L. Anemia, cancer, and aging. *Cancer Control.* 2003;10:478-486.

114. Camilleri M, Lee JS, Viramontes B, Bharuch AE, Tangalos EG. Insights into the pathophysiology and mechanisms of constipation, irritable bowel syndrome, and diverticulosis of older people. *J Am Geriatr Soc.* 2000;48:1142-1150.

115. Lekan-Rutledge D. Urinary incontinence strategies for frain elderly women. *Urol Nurs.* 2004;24:281-283,287-302.

116. Rajan AR. Management of Diabetic Renal Disease: New Paradigms. ENDO 2002, The 84th Annual Meeting of the Endocrine Society. http://www.medscape.com/viewarticle/440105. Accessed April 1, 2010.

117. Kang DH, Nakagawa T. Uric acid and chronic renal disease: possible implication of hyperuricemia on progression of renal disease. *Semin Nephrol.* 2005;25:43-49.

118. Morita S, Fukuhara S, Akizawa T, et al. Prognostic factors for a composite end-point of renal outcomes in patients with chronic kidney disease. *Ther Apher Dial.* 2006;10:72-77.

119. Knap B, Buturovi-Ponikvar J, Ponikvar R, Bren AF. Regular exercise as a part of treatment for patients with end-stage renal disease. *Ther Apher Dial.* 2005;9:211-213.

120. Zauska A, Zauska WT, Bednarek-Skublewska A, Ksiazek A. Nutrition and hydration status improve with exercise training using stationary cycling during hemodialysis (HD) in patients with end-stage renal disease (ESRD). *Ann Univ Mariae Curie Sklodowska [Med].* 2002;57:342-346.

121. Veldhuis JD. Endocrinology of aging. *Medscape Diabetes & Endocrinology.* 2000;2:1-21.

122. Guha B, Krishnaswamy G, Peiris A. The diagnosis and management of hypothyroidism. *South Med J.* 2002;95:475-480.

123. Yang F, Teng W, Shan Z, et al. Epidemiological survey on the relationship between different iodine intakes and the prevalence of hyperthyroidism. *Eur J Endocrinol.* 2002;146:613-618.

124. Veldhuis JD. Endocrinology of aging. *Medscape Diabetes & Endocrinology.* 2000;2:1-21.

125. Jack L, Boseman L, Vinicor F. Aging Americans and diabetes. A public health and clinical response. *Geriatrics.* 2004;59:14-17.

126. Sjostrand F, Nystrom T, Hahn RG. Intravenous hydration with a 2.5% glucose solution in type II diabetes. *Clin Sci Lond.* 2006;111:127-134.

127. Gavin JR, Alberti KG, Davidson MB, et al. Report of the Expert Committee on the Diagnosis and Classification of Diabetes Mellitus. *Diabetes Care.* 1999;22(suppl 1):s5-s19.

128. Schaefer-Graf UM, Buchanan TA, Xiang AH, Peters RK, Kjos SL. Clinical predictors for a high risk for the development of diabetes mellitus. *Am J Obstet Gynecol.* 2002;186:751-756.

129. Klein S, Sheard NF, Pi-Sunyer X, et al. Weight management through lifestyle modification for the prevention and management of type II diabetes: rationale and strategies. *Diabetes Care.* 2004;27:2067-2073.

130. Greenfield JR, Samaras K, Jenkins AB, Kelly PJ, Spector TD, Campbell LV. Moderate alcohol consumption, estrogen replacement therapy, and physical activity are associated with increased insulin sensitivity: is abdominal adiposity the mediator? *Diabetes Care.* 2003;26:2734-2740.

Psychosocial Theories and Considerations of Aging

Psychosocial theories have to do with the interaction of an individual with the environment from an emotional and spiritual realm as well as his or her social roles, life situations and experiences, and engagement in his or her current life circumstances. Psychosocial theories describe the interaction of the individual with his or her world. Psychosocial theories of aging provide the basis of all relevant practice interventions, public policies, programs, and research. They evolve and change over time based on new knowledge, cultural and environmental changes, and psychological and social conditions that affect the well-being of older adults.[1]

Aging involves more than the physical components discussed in Chapter 3. The way we age may actually have a lot to do with our outlook and the way we as individuals perceive the aging process. Psychosocial aspects including psychological, emotional, spiritual, and social elements often directly affect physical health. The impact of life experience, health, disability, and perception of life satisfaction can alter an older individual's physical well-being.[2] Depression, for instance, may have significant implications for how an older individual manages in rehabilitation therapies. Successful outcomes following a medical episode, such as a hip fracture, may be directly affected by the elderly person's emotional state and mental abilities, as well as his or her emotional outlook and perceived health status.[3]

Although the PTA does not receive extensive education in the area of psychosocial sciences, the awareness of factors beyond the physical impairments or disabilities and how they might change the course of rehabilitation are important considerations when working with a geriatric population. For example, a patient who is motivated to be actively involved in therapy and is optimistic that physical capabilities will be regained is going to fare much better in the rehabilitation setting than the person whose attitude toward the possibility of regaining function is pessimistic. Often elderly patients are too depressed or unmotivated to deal with rehabilitation efforts and exhibit a "what's the use?" attitude. Since the ultimate goal of rehabilitation is to obtain maximal functional capabilities, the elderly individual's means of coping with his or her illness will play a powerful role in the success of therapy intervention.

This chapter will explore current psychosocial theories on aging and cognitive changes in late life that impact adaptation to the many losses and changes encountered in the developmental phase called "old age." Considerations such as loss, grief, and the experience of death and dying will also be presented.

Psychosocial Theories of Aging

Aging is another developmental period of the circle of life. In fact, if old age is defined as 65 years of age and

Bottomley J. *Geriatric Rehabilitation: A Textbook for the Physical Therapist Assistant* (pp 95-118).

older (as it is in the United States), many individuals will spend as much as 40 years in this period of life.

In the early 1900s, life expectancy (for both sexes) was 47 years. Now an individual has a mean life expectancy of approximately 84 years on average (for both sexes), another lifetime beyond retirement at the age of 65 years. This is a period in which adjustments to changes in social roles, employment status, financial stability, loss of family and friends through relocation and death, as well as one's own perception of aging, "the golden years," and his or her own eminent death will be powerful elements in one's psychosocial response to the process of aging. If the unprecedented increase in life expectancy has a downside, it is the exposure of risk to chronic age-related diseases and disorders.[4]

Additionally, physical and immunological resiliency is not as robust in older individuals.[5] As a result, they may often be limited by functional and physical impairments, which also impact their perspective on aging.

Developmental Lifespan Theories

In the past, attention focused on segments of the lifespan, usually childhood and adolescence. Many of the mainstream theories centered on psychological development of the child with almost complete exclusion of late adult life or old age. Today, these developmental views have been extended by other theorists to encompass all ages. New theories have evolved, such as the theory of thriving, a holistic lifespan perspective for studying people in their environments as they age.[6] The theories presented in this chapter divide the lifecycle into recognizable phases or states through which all persons pass in their journey from cradle to grave.[7]

Erikson's Developmental Theory

Erikson, aged himself when he developed his theory, established the first psychological profile of development that extended into old age. He theorized that the developmental process throughout life was a series of 8 stages through which one pregresses. The stages are hierarchical, with progression to the next phase dependent on the successful completion of preceding stages of development. The full development of one's ego is central to this theory. Each of these stages, listed in Table 5-1, represents a positive versus a negative choice toward the development of one's personality and ego. The last 2 stages are those that involve the phases important to the older person.[8]

A successful life choice of *generativity* consists of guiding, parenting, and monitoring the next generation. If an adult person does not experience generativity then stagnation will predominate. *Stagnation* is evidenced by anger, hurt, and self-absorption. The

Table 5-1

ERIKSON'S STAGES OF PERSONALITY AND EGO DEVELOPMENT

PERIOD IN LIFE	ERIKSON'S STAGE
0 to 12 months	Trust vs mistrust
2 to 4 years	Autonomy vs shame
4 to 5 years	Initiative vs guilt
6 to 11 years	Industry vs inferiority
12 to 18 years	Identity vs identity confusion
Young adulthood	Intimacy vs isolation
Adulthood	Generativity vs stagnation
Late life	Integrity vs despair

Adapted from Erikson EH. *Identity, youth and crisis.* New York: Norton; 1968.

final stage of Erikson's portrayal of old age comprises the most years (40) of all the life stages; here he suggests that the older person must accept his or her life with the sense that if "I had to do it all over again, I'd do it pretty much the same." This represents the choice of *integrity*.[9] With this choice, the person experiences an active concern with life, even in the face of death, and learns to experience his or her own wisdom. *Despair* creates the opposite. The older individual regrets things that were not accomplished, has feelings of despair, self-disgust, and a fear of death. In order to successfully age, an older individual must achieve wisdom and integrity and the sense that his or her life has been meaningful and appropriate. Such ego integration allows for participation in life and acceptance of responsibility for leadership and legacy.[10]

Jung's Developmental Theory

Jung's theory on development designates adult stages based on experience from his own clinical theory and practice (Jung was one of the first to do so). His theory described the youth period, from puberty to middle age, as a stage in which the person is concerned with sexual instincts, broadening horizons, and conquering feelings of inferiority. The adult stages, between the ages 35 to 40, involve the transport of the youthful self into the middle years. During this stage, Jung theorized that the person's convictions strengthen until they become somewhat more rigid at the age of 50. In later years, Jung suggests that activity levels decrease and that men become more expressive and nurturing, and women become more "instrumental," providing care and continuation of the generations they have nurtured in their lives.[11] Jung also suggests that the later years are those in which the older person confronts his or her own death. Success in this involves the acceptance of his or her imminent death as a part of the cycle of life, not something to be feared.[12]

Maslow's Developmental Theory

In 1962, Maslow published his first articles establishing a theory of quality of life. His theory is based on the development toward happiness and true being grounded on the concept of human needs. Maslow's hierarchy of human needs is not a theory singular to aging, but a framework for exploring growth, development, and motivation[13] (see Figure 5-1). Maslow's hierarchy of needs takes on the form of a pyramid, each need then builds on the other. The lowest level, *biological and physiological integrity*, is where the person is trying to feed him- or herself and stay warm and clothed. At the second level, *safety and security*, the person protects him- or herself against the elements and against other people. This cannot be achieved

unless the person is first fed and clothed. In the third level, *belonging or love needs*, the person begins to seek love from other persons, such as a parent or significant other. When the person feels the love needs met, he or she can then progress to the next level, *self-esteem*, where the person cherishes him- or herself, respects his or her own values and ideas, and feels good about who he or she is. Finally, the level of *self-actualization* is where the person is no longer worried about the lower needs but is now able to give to others and has reached a higher level where he or she is able to transcend the lower self-esteem needs. He or she can nurture and feed others, develop his or her own ideas, and actually live his or her own values and ideas in the community. According to Maslow, very few people in society are self-actualized.[14]

It seems that this concept of self-actualization plays an important role in rehabilitation. As most chronic diseases do not disappear, patients seek improvement in their lives' journeys by seeking to fulfill life despite their disabilities.

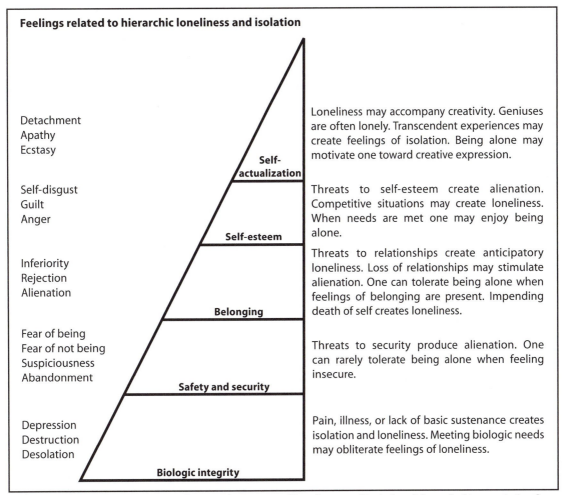

Figure 5-1. Maslow's Developmental Pyramid—Factors of loneliness and isolation. Adapted with permission from Maslow A. *Motivation and Personality*. New York: Harper & Row; 1954.

One must successfully fulfill the lower needs before ascending to the higher needs. When one is in a particular level, his or her energies are consumed at that level. Maslow theorizes that one rarely stays at a higher level, but rather, reverts to lower levels when the lower needs are not met. For example, a recently widowed woman may feel isolated or lonely, may fear that her basic needs for food and clothing will not be met, and be unable to experience the higher levels of self-esteem or self-actualization until her grief has subsided. This theory is particularly useful in the area of motivation. Since older persons are more likely to have physical decline, their needs will descend to the lower levels of the hierarchy. Therefore, motivation strategies should be aimed at the level of the person's needs. For example, if the person is unstable when walking, then strategies to encourage exercises in this area should appeal to his or her sense of "safety and security." If, however, the same person is more concerned about hunger during a treatment session, he or she will be unable to focus on the exercises toward safety. Maslow's hierarchy has been adapted to palliative (soothing or calming) care and the levels defined as (1) distressing symptoms such as pain or dyspnea; (2) fears for physical safety, of dying, or of abandonment; (3) affection, love, and acceptance in the face of devastating illness; (4) esteem, respect, and appreciation for the person; (5) self-actualization and transcendence.[15] This theory provides a comprehensive approach for the assessment of patients' needs and the design of interventions to achieve goals that start with comfort and potentially extend to the experience of transcendence.[16]

Levinson's Theory of Late Life

While Erikson focuses on ego and personality development, Levinson's theory of late life is concerned with the social tasks and roles that must be managed at each developmental stage of the person's life.[17] These theories approach the stages or "seasons" of adulthood as a developmental process involving occupation, love relationships, marriage and family, relation to self, use of solitude, and roles in various social contexts (ie, relationships with individuals, groups, and institutions that have significance for life). According to adult developmental theories, these components make up the underlying structure or pattern of a person's life. Levinson refers to this pattern as the person's "life structure." Two basic types of developmental periods are hypothesized as determining life structure: *structure building* and *structure change*.

Levinson identifies a "novice" phase of adult development that consists of 3 seasons: early adult transition (a structure-changing phase), entering the adult world (structure building), and transition (during which structure changing again takes place). The most important developmental "tasks" of early adulthood, according to Levinson's theory, are entering an occupation, developing mentor relationships, and forming a love or marriage relationship. During the transition phase, the primary task is reappraisal of the first part of adulthood and redirection and change as determined by this reexamination of earlier life choices. The transition may be relatively easy or very difficult, but it is characteristic of this phase to either make new life choices or reaffirm old choices. The next phase is the settling down phase. Here the individual establishes his or her niche in society (eg, occupation, family, community) and works toward advancement. This is followed by the mid-life transition phase. Levinson offers some examples of polarities such as young/old, destructive/creative, masculine/feminine, and attachment/separateness. The most important task is coming to terms with real or impending biologic decline, accompanied by the recognition of one's own mortality, as well as the societal attitudes that denigrate or devalue the status of middle age in favor of youth. The next phase is another structure-building period. Having faced the polarities of the mid-life transition, the person now makes new choices or reaffirms old ones. As an individual moves to the end of this period, yet another structure-changing phase is entered as the person once again reevaluates his or her life upon entry into "old age."

Disengagement Theory

Neugarten and Havighurst noted that successful adaptation to age was related to personality and not necessarily age. They propose the following 4 personality types:

1. *Integrated*: Shows a high degree of competence in daily activities and a complex inner life; this personality type is generally the best adapter.

2. *Passive dependent*: Seeks others to satisfy his or her emotional needs.

3. *Armored*: Attempts to control his or her environment and impulses; tends to be a high achiever.

4. *Unintegrated*: Shows poor emotional control and intellectual competency; this type of personality tends to have the poorest adaptation in late life.[18]

The last 3 personality types led to the disengagement theory of aging. Although controversial, Cummings and Henry postulated that older people and society disengage or mutually withdraw from each other.[19] The disengagement theory purports that aging individuals become less involved with others, become more self-satisfied, and prepare themselves and society to face the inevitability of their death. Cummings and Henry describe changes that result in an older person becoming less tied to the social system. As the elderly shift their attention and progressively withdraw from adult roles, such as working, society relinquishes the elderly from those social roles, and a mutual withdrawal process occurs. Changes in the amount of interaction result in a more isolated lifestyle according to this theory. Cumming and Henry suggest that the process of social and psychological withdrawal is a model for aging that is both intrinsic and inevitable, and that it is not only a correlate of successful aging but a condition of it.

Continuity and Activity Theories

The continuity and activity theories are 2 theories that were developed in response to the disengagement theory and provide a much more optimistic view of aging. The *continuity theory* proposes that activities in old age reflect a continuation of earlier life patterns,[18,20] while the *activity theory* states that successful adaptation in late life is associated with maintaining as high a level of activity as possible. The older person finds substitute activities to replace work and family roles. The individual, in both cases, develops an active rather than a passive role toward his or her daily life and maintains a high level of social involvement. He or she engages rather than disengages.[21]

COGNITIVE CHANGES IN LATE LIFE

Several important components of cognition are thought to be affected by age, including memory, learning affect, and reasoning. Each of these components of cognition will be discussed in terms of normal aging and pathological mechanisms.

Memory

Memory has been studied extensively, yet no definitive conclusions have been reached as to whether memory is affected by the aging process. Some studies show a decline in memory with age, while others show no change.[22,23] Studies do agree that older persons tend to have poorer techniques for organizing new information.[24] Older persons perform better on more familiar memory tasks.[25]

Poor nutrition, drugs, insomnia (sleeplessness), and inactivity can result in poorer information retrieval and significantly increase cognitive processing times.[26] Often, depression is the underlying cause of complaints of memory loss, not actual memory loss, and once depression is treated, problems with short-term memory are reversed.[27,28] For the most part, researchers agree that a true memory loss is associated with a pathological process resulting in dementia, rather than a normal part of aging.

Intelligence and Learning

Measurement of intelligence is impossible. What is measured is the "performance" of a person's intelligence on cognitive tasks. Performance can easily be influenced by health, motivation, medications, nutrition, sleep patterns, and sensory changes (eg, hearing, vision, etc). Cultural and educational variations can also influence an individual's "apparent" intellectual performance.[29]

Intelligence is broken into fluid and crystallized "intelligences." *Fluid intelligence* is the individual's ability to use short-term memory, create concepts, perceive complex relationships, and undertake abstract reasoning. *Crystallized intelligence* is life-long learning patterns that are influenced by sociocultural and educational components. This type of intelligence involves the ability to perceive relations (eg, right/wrong, love/hate, etc), engage in formal reasoning, and understand "principles" (eg, perspectives, opinions, etc).[30]

The implications of these 2 types of intelligences from a clinical perspective are many. The PTA can expect the intellectual ranges in older persons to be varied. Poor performance may not mean poor learning; rather it may be the result of disinterest, depression, or any of the factors discussed above.

Areas of new learning should seek to integrate previous learning and be consistent with the needs of the individual. Especially in rehabilitation, learning new activities or ways of functioning with a disability can lead to a great deal of frustration for the older person if the individual does not need or see the value of that task in his or her ADL. Therefore, it is better to tap into an activity that is of interest to him or her and has value in his or her daily life. For instance, someone who enjoyed golfing can be set up to putt to gain upper extremity and trunk range of motion, flexibility, and strength, in addition to challenging balance.

Focus needs to be placed on one task at a time. Cognitive and motor practice of each component of that task needs to be step by step. In other words, one step needs to be successfully learned before proceeding to the next step. Make the learning experience as concrete as possible using supportive instruction and assisting in organizing the new information. Reduce distractions such as noise and environmental stimulation. The concentrated use of all of the senses toward the accomplishment of a new task will facilitate learning.[31]

Affect and reasoning do not change with aging[32] although pathological dementias, drug complications, depression, sleeplessness, inactivity, or poor nutrition may affect these areas. Later in this chapter, there will be a more thorough exploration of these areas of "intelligence" and their relationship to dementia.

Depression

"Depression has been termed the common cold of the elderly."[33] Aging does not cause depression per se, but circumstantial life variables such as retirement, loss of loved ones, cognitive impairment, incontinence, and chronic conditions and disabilities, to name a few, may result in depressive symptoms.[34,35] Often depression goes undiagnosed because the elder individual sees "depression" as a character flaw and will not admit to feeling "blue." Instead of admitting their depression, elders frequently bury their depression in somatic complaints. For instance, rather than saying they didn't get out of bed because they were feeling sad, they indicate that they weren't feeling well and so stayed in bed.

Depression is an illness and is treatable. Depression is characterized by having symptoms (Table 5-2) for a period of at least 2 weeks. The PTA, as a result of daily interaction with the elderly individual, may be the first professional to see these themes and symptoms of depression emerge. Observation of any of these symptoms on an ongoing basis by the PTA during treatment sessions should be reported to the PT or occupational therapist who evaluated the individual and prescribed rehabilitative treatment and intervention. The elder can then be referred to the appropriate professionals for medical, nutritional, pharmacological, and mental status evaluations and psychological interviews as warranted. Additionally, anyone who interacts with the patient is in essence providing therapy for the individual's depression. Therefore, the PTA should be aware of the treatment plans and goals and the patient's perception of and motivation toward these anticipated outcomes. Using humor, positive reinforcement, kindness, and a nurturing approach will help the individual focus less on his or her illness and depression and more on the possibility of regaining lost function. As a result of daily interaction with the elderly individual, the PTA may be the key relationship the elder establishes that helps to motivate and inspire him or her, and breaks the depressive cycle.

Social Isolation

Social isolation can be divided into geographical isolation, presentation isolation, behavioral isolation, or attitudinal isolation.[36]

Table 5-2

SYMPTOMS OF DEPRESSION

Cognitive Symptoms	Poor concentration
	Low self-esteem
	Indecisiveness
	Guilt
	Hopelessness
	Inability to concentrate
	Suicidal ideations
Somatic Symptoms	Fatigue
	Altered sleep patterns
	Weight gain or loss
	Tearfulness
	Agitation
	Heart palpitations
	Overall weakness
Affective Symptoms	Sadness
	Anxiety
	Irritability
	Fear
	Anger
	Depersonalization
	Feelings of isolation (loneliness)

Geographical isolation results in territorial restriction and is usually a result of widowhood, urban crowding, rural life, or institutionalization. For example, in the urban situation, the older person may be faced with a fast-paced or depersonalized lifestyle that gives him or her little opportunity to be in contact with family and friends. Any relocation must be examined for the potential ramifications of the elder individual's access to socialization opportunities. Interventions may be helpful in resolving this type of isolation if it exists. Table 5-3 lists some formal and informal support systems that may be employed and are recommended to prevent the depression that accompanies this correctable form of isolation.[36]

Presentation isolation results from an unacceptable appearance. Unfortunately, in our society many judgments are made on superficial appearance, and as the body ages, its appearance no longer conforms to the given stereotype. Aging is often perceived as an illness and something to be avoided.

The wrinkling of skin or the graying of the hair is seen as a flaw rather than beautiful. Additionally, disfigurement accompanies many physical disabilities associated with aging. The PTA can help older persons to deal with presentation isolation in several ways:

1) Help them to establish new relationships with people that can accept them as they are now.

2) Teach them to avoid overexposure to individuals with negative views of aging.

3) Give lots of positive feedback on present strengths and appearances.

4) Ask questions to determine what the person really thinks about him- or herself.

5) Teach them to develop reasonable expectations.[37]

Behavioral isolation results from "unacceptable" actions. Behavioral isolation occurs when an older person displays behaviors that are perceived as unacceptable by him- or herself or by others. The most likely behaviors to fall into this category are eccentricity, confusion, incontinence, and deviant behavior (eg, anger toward everything and everyone resulting in physical aggressiveness). The PTA may be instrumental in helping an individual identify the behavior and seeking appropriate intervention for alleviating the problem. For instance, if urinary incontinence results in isolation, behavioral modification programs may be the answer to preventing incontinence.

Attitudinal isolation arises from cultural or personal bound values. Attitudinal isolation is strongly entrenched in society's response to the older person. Ageism and the belief that it is acceptable and expected for older persons to be lonely are held by the older person and society as a whole (often including health care professionals). The intervention for this type of isolation is for society as a whole to evaluate its prejudices and misconceptions and gain a more positive view of aging. The PTA must explore whether or not it is desirable for the older person to be alone. To do this, the PTA should understand the difference between loneliness and being alone. Loneliness is a state of longing and emptiness, whereas being alone is being apart, solitary, quiet, and undisturbed. Any 1 of the 4 types of isolation bars the older person from full acceptance by others. This will cause the elderly individual to feel alienated and out of step, and will affect self-esteem and the desire to stay active and healthy.

Institutionalization

Due to the organizational structure of institutions, an elder may be required to develop new coping

Table 5-3

SUPPORT SYSTEMS FOR GEOGRAPHICAL ISOLATION

Formal Support	Involvement in social issues for seniors
	Senior centers
	Volunteer activities
	Friends of the library
	National Retired Teacher's Association
	Retired senior volunteer program
	Foster grandparenting programs
	Grandparenting (child care)
Informal Support	Neighbors/friends and family
	Social groups
	Home or nursing home therapists
	Medical visits (office or home)
	Pets
	Fictional kin (books-on-tape, soap operas)
	Beauty salons, restaurants, shops, etc
	Housekeepers
	Retirement communities
	Churches

mechanisms that could have a profound impact on an individual's behavior. The classic text on the behavioral effects of institutionalization is *Asylums* by Goffman.[37] He identifies 5 aspects of a total institution (any institution where an individual spends 24 hours a day in residence):

1. A hierarchical authority exists with residents on the lowest rung. This type of authority results in situations where the staff is always right and the residents are punished or reprimanded.

2. Total institutions take control of personal habits. For example, mealtimes are regulated, as well as urination and defecation. This makes it difficult for the resident to satisfy personal needs in an efficient way.

3. Residents of institutions are often made to feel humiliated. For example, many residents of institutions are not allowed to close their doors.

4. The setting often makes it impossible for the person to engage in face-saving behaviors. Any defensive behavior a resident may take after being rebuked may then become the focus of a new attack. For example, if a resident becomes angry because the doors must remain open, the staff may then begin to rebuke the resident for inappropriate anger.

5. The person's status within the institution is solely defined by his or her status within the institution and any outside roles are rarely counted. For example, a rehabilitation therapist who has worked hard for years to help people in an outside role will be treated the same as a criminal in an institution.

Interventions for helping the older person cope with institutionalization (short of changing the entire system) begin with the individual. The following list gives ways to help personalize the institutional setting:

- Develop meaningful relationships
- Give accurate information
- Involve the family
- Recognize accomplishments with plaques, posters, and so forth
- Recognize and address people by their preferred name
- Recognize birthdays on the appropriate day
- Provide memorials for residents who have died
- Conduct life reviews
- Establish contacts with plants, pets, and children
- Provide every person with some personal items
- Arrange room sharing only between compatible residents
- Provide legal aid to protect the residents' rights
- Provide choices in all matters.

Anxiety Disorders

Anxiety disorders in the older person are frequently underreported or missed.[38] The incidence of anxiety disorders increases with age and is more frequent in women than in men.[39] Anxiety disorders either present with symptoms of fear, worry, or nervousness; or as a somatic problem without any physical cause. Descriptions of various anxiety disorders are listed in Table 5-4.

While Table 5-4 is quite extensive, several symptoms are seen more frequently by rehabilitation professionals, including tremors, headaches, chest pain, weakness and fatigue, neck and back pain, dry mouth, dizziness, parasthesias, and nonproductive cough.[40] The presence of these symptoms does not mean that the older person has an anxiety disorder, because there may be physical causes as well as organic causes of anxiousness, such as caffeine, hypoglycemia, or thyroid disease. In addition, rehabilitation professionals should screen for the symptoms of depression already described, as depression may cause some of the symptoms of anxiety disorders.

Chronic Illness

The importance of coping with chronic illness is imperative for successful aging. Chronic illness may be mild with minimal need for adaptation or lifestyle changes; however, a chronic illness may be extremely physically and emotionally limiting requiring major functional and environmental modifications. Serious illness or a devastating life event can cause profound changes in a person's appreciation of life, and often result in a shift of goals, relationships, and values.

Death, Dying, and Grief

Many people think of aging as a time of loss. Some of the most common losses include the loss of mobility, productivity, usefulness, body image, time left to live, health, income, and social status. These and other losses occur throughout life; however, their frequency increases with old age, and their cumulative effect increases the emotional impact as a person ages.

Death is a part of the lifecycle. The fear of death diminishes as one ages due to the increased exposure to dying, though some elderly individuals feel they are not ready to die and have not found fulfillment in their lives.[41]

Much has been written about the process of dying. Kubler-Ross is most well known for her work in this area and she provides the stages of dying as (1) denial, (2) anger, (3) bargaining, (4) depression, and (5) acceptance.[41] In interpreting these stages, it is important to note that not all people go through all of the stages. The role of the PTA in working with the dying patient includes the awareness of these stages and support to enhance the older person's ability to die with dignity and achieve final growth. The most common unmet needs are freedom from pain, loneliness, conservation of energy, and maintenance of self-esteem. PTAs, due to their routine involvement with these patients, can provide modalities and treatment interventions that offer modification and hopeful relief of pain; a listening, caring

Table 5-4

ANXIETY DISORDERS AND THEIR CENTRAL FEATURES

DISORDER	CENTRAL FEATURES
Adjustment disorder with anxious mood	Nervousness/anxiety in reaction to identifiable psychosocial stressor
Anxiety states	Persistent or recurrent anxiety not provoked by identifiable stimulus, generally noninstitutional
Obsessive-compulsive disorder	Intrusive thoughts and/or repetitive behaviors performed under a sense of pressure; Attempts to resist increased anxiety
Post-traumatic stress disorder	Acute and delayed reactions to a traumatic event; Involves "reliving" the experience, emotional numbing, and development of somatic symptoms
Panic disorder	Sudden, unpredictable panic attacks involving intense apprehension and physical symptoms
Generalized anxiety disorder	Generalized, persistent anxiety for more than 1 month; Includes 3 of the following: motor tension, autonomic hyperactivity, apprehension, hypervigilance
Phobic disorders	Persistent, irrational fear or anxiety provoked by stimulus object, activity, or situation; Avoidance of stimulus; Fear recognized by patient as irrational or excessive
Agoraphobia	Feared stimulus: being alone or in a public place where escape would be difficult or help hard to find; Occurs with or without panic attacks
Social phobia	Fear stimulus: social situations involving possible embarrassment or humiliation
Simple phobia	Fear stimulus: situations similar to a previous terrifying experience

Adapted from Turnball J, Turnball S. Management of specific anxiety disorders in the elderly. *Geriatrics.* 1985;40:75-81.

presence focusing on the immediate future and present opportunities; modification of environmental factors to reduce excessive energy expenditure; and boosts to self-esteem. The latter can be accomplished by paying close attention to physical comfort; using sensory feedback as much as possible in visual, auditory, and tactile realms; and by simply listening in a nonbiased, nonvalue-laden manner, respecting that dying is a very individual experience.

Dementia

Dementia or cognitive impairment is the major cause of disability in older persons. The prevalence of dementia increases with advancing age, with an estimated 5% of those over the age of 65 having some degree of cognitive impairment. For those over the age of 75, the estimate jumps to 20% and, in nursing home settings, it is estimated that the prevalence reaches 50%.[42] Dementia can be subdivided into the following categories:

1. *Acute disorders.* These are potentially reversible impairments that include delirium, depression, multiple causes, and accidents.

2. *Chronic disorders.* These are irreversible cognitive impairments that include Alzheimer's disease, vascular disease, and subcortical disorders.

3. *Presenile dementias*: These diseases tend to be rarer and to occur in younger population. They are not reversible.

Acute cognitive disorders have multiple causes. Among these causes are drugs, translocation, infection, neoplasm, trauma, malnutrition, toxic states, metabolic imbalances, and depression. The most common reversible causes of dementia are drugs, depression, and metabolic changes.

The symptoms of acute cognitive impairment (except for the acute delirium caused by depression) are characterized by a rapidly developing confusion in which the individual displays clouded, fluctuating consciousness accompanied by agitation. Additionally, the person may be hypersensitive to light or sound and suffer from visual, auditory, or tactile hallucinations, have short-term memory impairment, illogical and disjointed thoughts, be disoriented to time, and hypo-alert or hyper-alert.

The manifestation of delirium due to depression differs in several major aspects. The depressed patient will have a slower onset of these symptoms, a longer history of somatic complaints, and a lower self-esteem. The depressed patient will tend to be on the hypo side of alertness and the greatest cognitive decline will be in the realm of the inability to process information.

The chronic causes of dementia most often seen in the elderly include: Alzheimer's disease (which accounts for an estimated 50% of the chronic disorders), vascular disease, and subcortical disorders.[43] Alzheimer's disease results from neuronal degeneration from neurofibrillary tangles and plaques, and shows a slow, gradual, and steady decline in cognitive abilities. In chronic dementia from vascular or multi-infarct diseases, the cognitive decline is the result of small cerebral infarcts, arteriosclerotic disease, major cerebrovascular accidents, vertebrobasilar insufficiency, diabetic deterioration of blood vessels, carotid atherosclerosis, and diffuse cerebrovascular ischemia. The decline is characterized by a stepwise decline related to each infarct.

All chronic dementias will show signs of cognitive impairment over a course of several months. There is a slow loss of short-term memory with accompanying anxiety or depression. Unlike the acute dementias, the level of consciousness does not fluctuate.

Some general guidelines for working with the cognitively impaired elderly are as follows:

1. *Simplify.* Simplify instructions, programs, and environment.

2. *Explain.* This should be done thoroughly, frequently, constantly, and repetitively.

3. *Reorient.* Remind the patient of the time, place, and activity. Have clocks, calendars, and pictures easily visable to assist in orientation (eg, a picture of a dresser labeled "dresser" taped to the dresser).

4. *Slow down.* Take the amount of time needed in all aspects of intervention.

5. *Avoid change.* Don't change the environment, personnel, or programming, if possible.

6. *Encourage familiarity.* Use familiar objects and people; exercises should mimic familiar activities.

7. *Touch.* Convey caring and support to a patient who is going through an uncontrollable change and may be frightened.

8. *Encourage independence.* Use simple commands and label items for ease of recognition.

9. *Respect individual dignity.* Encourage the patient to discuss and demonstrate previous successes and accomplishments. Photographs are helpful in establishing memorable moments. Respect modesty and dignity.

10. *Educate and support the family.* Be prepared to confront denial in the family and patient.

11. *Listen to the patient.* Even if the patient is not making sense, he or she may be trying to communicate a specific message.

12. *Take care of yourself.* Working with cognitively impaired patients can be emotionally exhausting.

BELIEF SYSTEMS REGARDING AGING

Subjective Well-Being

There is a close theoretical relationship between age identity (ie, how old a person feels he or she is) and subjective well-being. Feeling younger than one's actual age is considered a self-enhancing illusion and contributes to subjective well-being, even beyond other factors such as health and socioeconomic status. As the United States is youth oriented compared with other countries and cultures, one would expect American adults to be more adaptive. Research indicates that this is not the case. It would be expected that feeling younger than one's actual age would be related to higher levels of life satisfaction and lead to an optimistic affect and outlook. However, country-specific analyses indicate that age identity and a negative affect hold only for the United States.[44] Cultural context clearly needs to be included in any discussion of gerontological theories and research.

Ageism

The perception of aging has changed throughout history. In colonial times in the United States, old age was honored and individuals were esteemed as leaders in the new world. The industrial revolution corrupted this social standing and older workers were increasingly viewed as redundant and expendable. *Ageism* was the term Butler coined to denote a prejudice against a person, or group of persons, due to their age.[45] The problems inherent in ageism are particularly pronounced in the health care arena. Older patients may be seen as complaining, uninteresting, or helpless. Often, services are denied to an older person based on age alone. It has been shown that there are less aggressive rehabilitation services and goal setting practices for older patients.[46] In fact, studies of health professionals' attitudes toward elders indicate that they tend to have worse ageist attitudes when compared to the rest of our society. There have been proposals to ration health care to elders, yet age is not often a reliable indicator of functional capability or future. It is important that treatment be based on an individual level and not based on age (refer to the Appendix at the end of the chapter).

Many studies have focused on quantifying an older individual's attitude about aging and what contributes to his or her health and sense of well-being. A model of healthy aging emerges.[47] To older people, health means going and doing something meaningful. Four things were identified as important for having good health:

1. having something worthwhile to do
2. having a balance between abilities and challenges
3. having appropriate external resources
4. having the right attitudinal characteristics (eg, positive vs negative attitude).

By reframing healthy aging in older people's own terms, knowing the 4 components for having good health, and encouraging interdisciplinary support of individuals' desired goals and outcomes, the PTA can have a very positive influence on helping older individuals stay healthy and active.

STRESS AND ADAPTATION

Retirement, illness, and changes in living conditions are all possible lifestyle adaptations in late life. A simple way of viewing some of these lifestyle adaptations is through the stress mechanism. *Stress* is defined as the response of the body to any demand made on it.[48] At any age, stress is a part of life. Young and old alike have to face difficult situations and overcome obstacles.

While young adults struggle to establish a career, achieve financial security, or juggle work and family demands, older people may face failing health and dwindling finances, or simply the challenges of retaining their independence. Unfortunately, the body's natural defenses against stress gradually break down with age. Stress comes in 2 basic forms, physical and emotional, and both can be especially taxing for older people.

The impacts of physical stress are clear. As people reach old age, wounds heal more slowly and colds become harder to shake. A 75-year-old heart can be slow to respond to the demands of exercise; and when an 80 year old walks into a chilly room, it will take an extra long time for his or her body temperature to adjust. Emotional stress is more subtle, but if it is chronic, the eventual consequences can be as

harmful. At any age, stressed-out brains sound an alarm that releases potentially harmful hormones such as cortisol and adrenaline. Ideally, the brain turns down the alarm when stress hormones get too high. Stress hormones provide energy and focus in the short term, but too much stress over too many years can throw a person's system off balance. Overloads of stress hormones have been linked to many health problems, including heart disease, high blood pressure, and weakened immune function. For older people already at heightened risk for these illnesses, managing stress is particularly important.

Over time, the brain can slowly lose its skills at regulating hormone levels. As a result, older people who feel worried or anxious tend to produce larger amounts of stress hormones, and the alarm doesn't shut down as quickly. According to a 2005 study published in *Psychoneuroendocrinology*,[48] women are especially susceptible to an overload of stress hormones as they age. The study found that the impact of age on cortisol levels is nearly 3 times stronger for women than for men.

On a physical level, stress increases the secretion of adrenalin and cortisol and lowers the body's sensitivity to insulin and its tolerance to carbohydrates.[49] These physiological changes can cause an increase in blood pressure, as well as a decrease in the immune system's ability to combat various diseases. Chronic stress in older people may result in a decreased caloric intake, a lowered body weight, and a lowered lymphocyte count. In addition, older individuals who have experienced this stress response will show an increased systolic pressure and mean arterial pressure, and some degree of left ventricular hypertrophy.

Stress doesn't just make a person feel older. In a very real sense, it can speed up aging. A 2004 study published in the *Proceedings of the National Academy of Sciences* found that stress can add years to the age of individual immune system cells.[49] The study focused on telomere (see Chapter 2) caps on the end of chromosomes. Whenever a cell divides, the telomeres in that cell get a little shorter and a little more time runs off the clock; when the telomere becomes too short, time runs out. The cell can no longer divide or replenish itself. This is a key process of aging, and it is one of the reasons humans can't live forever. Researchers checked both the telomeres and the stress levels of 58 healthy premenopausal women and found a stunning result: on average, the immune system cells of highly stressed women had aged by an extra 10 years. The study didn't explain how stress adds years to cells making up the immune system. As the study authors write, "the exact mechanisms that connect the mind to the cell are unknown." Researchers have a theory though: stress hormones could be somehow shortening telomeres and cutting the lifespan of cells.[49]

A complex array of symptoms may indicate stress. For example, on the physiological level, an increase in skin temperature, blood pressure, temperature, heart rate, respiration, and autonomic system activity all indicate stress. Impairment in problem-solving ability, social responsiveness, judgment, reality interpretation, and thoughts are all cognitive changes. Motor changes affected by stress are tremor, speech disturbance, and muscle tension. Finally, an older person under stress may display anger, guilt, depression, or anxiety. Frequent cues to stress in the elderly are decreased productivity, lack of awareness to the outside environment, decreased interest, rumination, preoccupation, lack of concentration, irritability and angry outbursts, withdrawal, tendency to cry, suspiciousness, and becoming critical of self and others.[50]

Physical Therapist Assistant's Role in Managing Stress

In working with the older adult, it is important for the PTA to be empathetic to the role that stress plays in the therapeutic environment. Since older persons may have experienced an accumulation of stressors, the intervention itself should impose as few changes as possible. There are several factors that affect coping patterns of older persons. The first factor is social support. Older persons who believe that they are loved, esteemed, and mutually obligated to a support system have better coping mechanisms. The older person's inner resources have also been found to improve coping responses, and the most important of these are flexibility, past experiences with successful coping, nonavoidance, and resumption of daily activities as soon as possible. Finally, older persons with improved problem-solving ability respond better to stressful events than poor problem solvers.[51]

Management of stress could include physical techniques such as progressive neuromuscular relaxation, biofeedback, physical activity, and breathing control. These techniques are all readily available to the PTA. It should be assumed that the majority of older adults in the rehabilitation setting are experiencing some level of stress. Awareness of this and support of the elderly individual in the therapeutic environment is crucial for successful intervention.

Retirement

Retirement is an example of a lifestyle adaptation that can prove to be good or bad. Retirement presents an emotion-laden change because work fulfills many social needs and bestows a status. Work fixes associations and relationships with other people, and regulates activity. The retiree often misses the association with work-related relationships and loses structure in daily activities. Work offers a meaningful life experience, which without preretirement and retirement planning may be felt as a loss. With planning, many older adults see retirement as a new chapter in their lives. This period may open many opportunities that were not available with the restrictive schedule of employment.[52]

CONCLUSION

As PTs and PTAs work to foster healthy aging, they must also seek ways to prevent the disabling disorders that keep many older persons from enjoying their longevity. The high prevalence of chronic illness and functional limitation among older persons underscores the need for strategically directed health and social services. Successful patient management must extend beyond diagnosis and disease treatment and include promotion of function and prevention of decline.

Achieving this goal requires a seamless continuum of management and interdisciplinary caregiving. There also must be a focus on improving the understanding of the entire aging experience. This chapter has reviewed the psychosocial theories of aging, the cognitive changes in late life, as well as multiple situations requiring coping mechanisms as a person ages. Important problems, such as depression and dementia, were discussed with treatment implications for the PTA. Finally, it looked at aspects of lifestyle adaptation and society's belief system toward aging and older persons. The reader should now have a more holistic view for managing his or her aging patients.

PEARLS

- The PTA can directly affect a patient's ability and desire to participate in therapy, eg, coordinating with the nursing staff so that pain medication is given prior to treatment time, enhancing a patient's willingness to participate in therapy.

- Because of the direct hands-on care the PTA provides, he or she may be the first to observe signs of depression (see Table 5-2).

- Developing a rehabilitation program that is clearly functional for the patient can help with performance and patient success. For example, an older person, who has no interest or need to stack cones while standing, may see more purpose in challenging balance by getting clothes out of a closet or reaching for a kitchen item on a higher shelf.

- Have the patient perform tasks in a situation that is, or very closely resembles, a functional activity he or she will need when he or she returns to his or her previous living situation (eg, practice transfers to a bed rather than a treatment table; have the patient walk through an area that resembles the smaller areas found in homes vs a long clear hallway found in many rehabilitation situations).

- Several interaction techniques that the PTA can use in treating the patient who has depression include listening, focusing on the elder's issue, not comparing his or her situation to a like-situation in your life, and empathizing with his or her expression of emotions.

  o The PTA who really listens to and structures the rehabilitation experience to meet his or her patient's needs and goals will be successful in treating the whole patient versus just his or her physical being.

  o Ask questions and really listen to the answers of your patients so individuals can be treated in a way that will meet their needs with dignity and respect.

  o Keep an eye out for behavioral or functional changes that may indicate depression, dementia, or other health problems. Report them immediately to the PT.

  o Make sure the patient can readily see the purpose of treatment approaches and identify with how the interventions being used apply to his or her life.

  o Ensure patient success with each treatment session by adjusting the intensity and difficulty level of interventions.

- The PTA can promote *patient-centered care* on an individual level by being truly present (versus carrying on a conversation with others in the area), referring to personal stories that a patient has shared, and allowing the patient a choice in when and where therapy occurs.

- In settings such as home and occasionally long-term care, the PTA may be *the* health care provider interacting with the elder with the most consistency and longest sessions. Therefore, it is essential to be continually assessing changes in cognition, documenting these changes, and notifying the PT accordingly.

- It is important to recognize negative variations in behaviors during treatment as possible reactions to stress and not take it personally.

  o The rehabilitation team needs to remain value neutral (eg, not belittle or criticize) and identify strategies to assist the patient in accomplishing his or her goals, despite moodiness or aberrant behavior.

  o Sometimes, something as simple as acknowledging and responding to a patient's complaint of being cold by getting a blanket or conducting therapy in a warmer room may reduce stress and result in a more productive treatment session.

- Quickly identifying and reporting psychosocial issues can prevent functional loss and loss of valuable rehabilitation time.

REFERENCES

1. Fokin VA, Fokin IV. Social theory of aging in the USA: development and current status. *Adv Gerontol.* 2002;9:22-29.
2. Putnam M. Linking aging theory and disability models: increasing the potential to explore aging with physical impairment. *Gerontologist.* 2002;42:799-806.
3. Holahan CK, Suzuki R. Adulthood predictors of health promoting behavior in later aging. *Int J Aging Hum Dev.* 2004;58:289-313.
4. Cassel CK. Successful aging. How increased life expectancy and medical advances are changing geriatric care. *Geriatrics.* 2001;56:35-40.
5. Gilford DM, ed. *The Aging Population in the Twenty-First Century.* Washington, DC: National Academy Press; 1998.
6. Haight BK, Barba BE, Tesh AS, Courts NF. Thriving: a life span theory. *J Gerontol Nurs.* 2002;28:14-22.
7. McAuley JD, Jones MR, Holub S, Johnston HM, Miller NS. The time of our lives: life span development of timing and event tracking. *J Exp Psychol Gen.* 2006;135:348-367.
8. Erikson EH. *Identity, Youth & Crisis.* New York: Norton Press; 1968.
9. Norman SM, McCluskey-Fawcett K, Ashcraft L. Older women's development: a comparison of women in their 60s and 80s on a measure of Erikson's developmental tasks. *Int J Aging Hum Dev.* 2002;54:31-41.
10. Westermeyer JF. Predictors and characteristics of Erikson's life cycle model among men: a 32-year longitudinal study. *Int J Aging Hum Dev.* 2004;58:29-48.
11. Koss-Chioino JD. Jung, spirits and madness: lessons for cultural psychiatry. *Transcult Psychiatry.* 2003;40:164-180.
12. Jung CG. *The Stages of Life. The Structure and Dynamics of the Psyche.* New York: Pantheon Press; 1960.
13. Maslow A. *Motivation and Personality.* New York: Harper & Row; 1954.
14. Yang KS. Beyond Maslow's culture-bound linear theory: a preliminary statement of the double-Y model of basic human needs. *Nebr Symp Motiv.* 2003;49:175-255.
15. Zalenski RJ, Raspa R. Maslow's hierarchy of needs: a framework of achieving human potential in hospice. *J Paolliat Med.* 2006;9:1120-1127.

16. Ventegodt S, Merrick J, Andersen NJ. Quality of life theory III. Maslow revisited. *ScientificWorldJournal.* 2003;3:1050-1057.

17. Goukon A, Ohuchi T, Kikuchi T, Hirano M, Noguchi K, Hosokawa T. Developmental order driving the relationship between executive functions and theory of mind: a case study. *Psychol Rep.* 2006;98:662-670.

18. Havighurst R, Neugarten B, Tobin S. Disengagement and patterns of aging. In: Neugarten B, ed. *Middle Age and Aging.* Chicago: University of Chicago Press; 1975.

19. Cummings E, Henry W. *Growing Old: The Process of Disengagement.* New York: Basic Books; 1961.

20. Havighurst RJ. Flexibility and the social role of the retired. *Am J Sociol.* 1954;59:399.

21. Butler R, Lewis M. *Aging and Mental Health.* St. Louis, MO: Mosby-Year Book; 1982.

22. Criak F, Masani P. Age differences in the temporal integration of language. *Brit J Psychol.* 1967;58:291-299.

23. Hultoch D, Masson M, Small B. Adult age differences in direct and indirect test of memory. *J Gerontology.* 1981;46:22-30.

24. Saffran EM. Aphasia and the relationship of language and brain. *Semin Neurol.* 200;20:7-14.

25. Botwinck J. *Aging and Behavior.* 2nd ed. New York: Springer; 1978.

26. McEnte W, Crook T. Age associated memory impairment: a role for catecholamines. *Neurology.* 1990;40:526-530.

27. Saczynski JS, Rebok GW. Strategies for memory improvement in older adults. *Top Adv Pract Nurs.* 2004;4:2-8.

28. Gurland B. The comparative frequency of depression in various adult age groups. *J Gerontology.* 1976;31:283-292.

29. Labouvie-Vief G. Intelligence and cognition. In: Birren JE, Schaie KW, eds. *Handbook of the Psychology of Aging.* New York: Van Nostrand Reinhold; 1985.

30. Cattell RB. Theory of fluid and crystallized intelligence: a clinical experiment. *J Educ Psychol.* 1963;54:1.

31. Hayslip B, Kennelly KJ. Cognitive and non-cognitive factors affecting learning among older adults. In: Lumsden BD, ed. *The Older Adult as a Learner.* Washington, DC: Hemisphere; 1985.

32. Knox AB. *Adult Development and Learning.* San Francisco: Jossey-Bass; 1977.

33. Bettes S. Depression: the "common cold" of the elderly. *Generations.* 1979;3:15.

34. Gurland B. The comparative frequency of depression in various adult age groups. *J Gerontology.* 1976;31:283-292.

35. Crystal S, Sambamoothi U, Walkup JT, Akincigil A. Diagnosis and treatment of depression in the elderly medicare population: predictors, disparities, and trends. *J Amer Geriatr Soc.* 2003;51:11-30.

36. Ebersole P, Hess P. *Towards Healthy Aging: Human Needs and Nursing Response.* St. Louis, MO: Mosby; 1981.

37. Goffman E. *Asylums: Essays on the Social Situations of Mental Patients and Other Inmates.* Garden City, NY: Doubleday; 1961.

38. Shader R, Goodman M. Panic disorders: current perspectives. *J Clin Psychopharmacol.* 1982;2:2-15.

39. Carey G, Gottesman I, Robins E. Prevalence and rates for the neurosis: pitfalls in the evaluation of familiality. *Psychol Med.* 1980;10:437-443.

40. Turnball J, Turnball S. Management of specific anxiety disorders in the elderly. *Geriatrics.* 1985;40:75-81.

41. Kubler-Ross E. *The Final Stage of Growth.* New York: Touchstone; 1986.

42. Huang J, Meyer JS, Zhang Z, et al. Progression of mild cognitive impairment to Alzheimer's or vascular dementia versus normative aging. *Curr Alzheimer Res.* 2005;2:571-578.

43. Gerritsen D, Kuin Y, Steverink N. Personal experience of aging in the children of a parent with dementia. *Int J Aging Hum Dev.* 2004;58:147-165.

44. Westerhof GJ, Barrett AE. Age identity and subjective well-being: a comparison of the United States and Germany. *J Gerontol B Psychol Sci Soc Sci.* 2005;60:S129-136.

45. Butler R. Age-ism: another form of bigotry. *Gerontologist.* 1969;9:243.

46. Rybarczyk B, Haut A, Lacey RF, Fogg LF, Nicholas JJ. A multifactorial study of age bias among rehabilitation professionals. *Phys Ther.* 2001;82:625-632.

47. Bryant LL, Corbett KK, Kutner JS. In their own words: a model of healthy aging. *Soc Sci Med.* 2001;53:927-941,

48. Traustadottir T. The HPA axis response to stress in women: effects of aging and fitness. *Psychoneuroendocrinology.* 2005;30:392-402.

49. Epel ES. Accelerated telomere shortening in response to life stress. *Proc Natl Acad Sci USA.* 2004;101:17312-17315.

50. Sapolsky RM. *Why Zebras Don't Get Ulcers.* 3rd ed. New York: Henry Holt and Company; 2004.

51. Beisgen BA, Kraitchman MC. *Senior Centers: Opportunities for Successful Aging.* New York: Springer; 2003.

52. Butrica BA, Cori EU. *How Will Boomers Fare at Retirement? Final Report to AARP Public Policy Institute.* Washington, DC: The Urban Institute; 2004.

APPENDIX: FACTS ON AGING QUIZ

Prior to assigning this chapter, it can be a good exercise to have the PTA students take and then discuss this quiz. Explanations to each of the true/false answers are provided to enhance student discussions (note that answers are provided by this author, not the author of the quiz). This quiz tests information provided from the 4 previous chapters and is framed to determine any age bias that students may have. It is also a useful activity for a clinical instructors meeting, as many clinical instructors also have been socialized toward age bias in the provision of physical therapy. Answer true or false to the following questions:

Facts on Aging Quiz[1]

T F 1. The majority of old people (65 years or older) have Alzheimer's disease.

T F 2. As people grow older, their intelligence declines significantly.

T F 3. It is very difficult for older adults to learn new things.

T F 4. Personality changes with age.

T F 5. Memory loss is a normal part of aging.

T F 6. As adults grow older, reaction time increases.

T F 7. Clinical depression occurs more frequently in older than younger people.

T F 8. Older adults are at risk for HIV/AIDS.

T F 9. Alcoholism and alcohol abuse are significantly greater problems in the adult population over the age of 65 than under the age of 65.

T F 10. Older adults have more trouble sleeping than younger adults.

T F 11. Older adults have the highest suicide rate of any age group.

T F 12. High blood pressure increases with age.

T F 13. Older people perspire less, so they are more likely to suffer from hyperthermia.

T F 14. All women develop osteoporosis as they age.

T F 15. A person's height tends to decline in old age.

T F 16. Physical strength declines in old age.

T F 17. Most old people lose interest in and capacity for sexual relations.

T F 18. Bladder capacity decreases with age, which leads to frequent urination.

T F 19. Kidney function is not affected by age.

T F 20. Constipation increases as people get older.

T F 21. All 5 senses tend to decline with age.

T F 22. As people live longer, they face fewer acute conditions and more chronic health conditions.

T F 23. Retirement is often detrimental to health—ie, people frequently seem to become ill or die soon after retirement.

T F 24. Older adults are less anxious about death than are younger and middle-aged adults.

T F 25. People 65 years of age and older make up about 20% of the US population.

T F 26. Most older people are living in nursing homes.

T F 27. The modern family no longer takes care of its elderly.

T F 28. The life expectancy of men at age 65 is about the same as that of women.

T F 29. Remaining life expectancy of Black Americans at age 85 is about the same as White Americans.

T F 30. Social Security benefits automatically increase with inflation.

T F 31. Living below or near the poverty level is no longer a significant problem for most older Americans.

T F   32.   Most older drivers are quite capable of safely operating a motor vehicle.

T F   33.   Older workers cannot work as effectively as younger workers.

T F   34.   Most old people are set in their ways and unable to change.

T F   35.   The majority of old people are bored.

T F   36.   In general, most old people are pretty much alike.

T F   37.   Older adults (65+) have higher rates of criminal victimization than adults under 65.

T F   38.   Older people tend to become more religious as they grow older.

T F   39.   Older adults (65+) are more fearful of crime than are persons under 65.

T F   40.   Older people do not adapt as well as younger age groups when they relocate to a new environment.

T F   41.   Participation in voluntary organizations (churches and clubs) tends to decline among older adults.

T F   42.   Older people are much happier if they are allowed to disengage from society.

T F   43.   Geriatrics is a specialty in American medicine.

T F   44.   All medical schools now require students to take courses in geriatrics and gerontology.

T F   45.   Abuse of older adults is not a significant problem in the United States.

T F   46.   Grandparents today take less responsibility for rearing grandchildren than ever before.

T F   47.   Older persons take longer to recover from physical and psychological stress.

T F   48.   Most older adults consider their health to be good.

T F   49.   Older females exhibit better health care practices than older males.

T F   50.   Research has shown that old age truly begins at 65.

Adapted with permission from Palmore E. The facts on aging quiz: part two. *Gerontologist.* 1981;21:431-437.

Answers

False. 1.   Almost 90% of people who are 65 years of age do *not* have Alzheimer's disease.

False. 2.   Although there are some circumstances where the statement may hold true, current research evidence suggests that intellectual performance in healthy individuals holds up well into old age. The average magnitude of intellectual decline is typically small in the 60s and 70s and is probably of little significance for competent behavior. There is more average decline of most abilities observed once the 80s are reached, although even in this age range there are substantial individual differences. Little or no decline appears to be associated with being free of cardiovascular disease, little decline in perceptual speed, at least average socioeconomic status, a stimulating and engaged lifestyle, and having flexible attitudes and behaviors at mid-life. The good news is that research data now indicate that intellectual decline can be modified by modest interventions.

False. 3.   Although, on average, learning performance tends to decline with age, all age groups can learn. Research studies have shown that learning performances can be improved with instructions and practice, extra time to learn information or skills, and relevance of the learning task to interests and expertise. It is well established that those who regularly practice their learning skills maintain their learning efficiency over their lifespan.

False. 4.   Personality remains consistent in men and women throughout life. Personality impacts roles and life satisfaction. Particular traits in youth and middle age will not only persist but may be more pronounced in later life.

True. 5.   As one ages, there is modest memory loss, primarily in regard to short-term memory (recent events). Older adults are more likely to retain past or new information that is based on knowledge acquired or that builds on their life course or events. Retrieval of information may slow with age. The causes of these changes are unknown, but may include stress, loss, physical disease, medication effects, and depression. Lack of attention, fatigue, hearing loss, and misunderstanding are among factors impacting memory loss in persons of all ages. Strategies such as activity and exercise, association, visualization, environmental cueing, organization by category, and connection to a place may help to prompt memory. New research has revealed that 40% of persons diagnosed with mild cognitive impairment (beyond what is expected for a person of that age and education) are likely to develop Alzheimer's disease within 3 years.

True. 6.   Reaction time is the interval that elapses between the onset of a stimulus and the completion of a motor response, such as hitting the brake pedal of a car when the traffic light turns yellow or red. When processing ordinary stimuli, adults show large increases in response time with increasing age.

False. 7.   Depression does *not* occur more often in older adults than younger groups. However, it is the most frequent mental health problem of older adults. Depression may vary from feeling "blue" from grief over a loss, to a diagnosis of clinical depression by criteria as listed in the *Diagnostic and Statistical Manual of Mental Disorders-IV*. Accurate diagnosis and treatment options are often hindered by the resistance to mental health intervention and situational depression in older adults as they react to isolation, role change, illness, and medication effects.

True. 8.   Blood transfusions and unprotected sex put older adults at risk for HIV/AIDS as in other populations. It is estimated that as many as 10% of all persons diagnosed with HIV/AIDS are over 50 years of age.

False. 9.   There is no substantial support for this idea. A growing body of evidence suggests that, although the majority of older adults are not abstinent, the frequency and quantity of alcohol consumed tends to decrease with age. This is at least partially explained by changing patterns of sociability with age, age-related health problems, and complications associated with alcohol interacting with prescribed medications. Problems with drinking later in life appear usually to be a continuation of drinking patterns established in the earlier adult years and not with late-onset drinking. Therapeutic intervention is at least as effective with older adults as with adults generally.

True. 10.   Older adults are more prone to sleep complaints, such as insomnia due to changing sleep patterns of frequent awakenings, earlier rising, and emotional problems. The quality of sleep declines with age. It becomes particularly more difficult to stay asleep. Daily sedation, boredom, loneliness, illness, time changes, work schedules, physical changes, and alcohol or medication may affect sleep patterns. Sleep behaviors common to older adults may include increased napping, periods of sleep apnea (stopped breathing), more frequent awakenings, lengthened onset of sleep, increased time in bed, and increased total sleep time. Current research verifies that REM (sleep in which dreaming takes place) deep sleep in older adults may be half what it is in younger persons.

True. 11.   The national suicide rate is about 12 per 100,000 population, while it is 13 for those ages 65 to 74, and 23 per 100,000 for those over age 85. It has been estimated that 17% to 25% of all reported suicides occur in persons aged 65 and older.[2] However, older White males largely account for this high rate; for White women, and men and women of all other races, the suicide rate peaks earlier in the lifespan. Older adults also have a higher ratio of completed to attempted suicides than younger groups. The higher suicide rates might be explained by a variety of factors, including the loss of roles and status, chronic illnesses that diminish one's sense of control, and social isolation.

True and False. 12. There is evidence that high blood pressure increases with age; however, there is controversy over the criteria for high blood pressure. Studies and physicians differ in their definition of high blood pressure. Most consider a person's age plus 100 as a reasonable systolic reading with diastolic of 90 mm. The systolic (higher number) measure is the pressure when the heart is stressed as it contracts and is recorded when the pressure cuff is first released after being tightened. The diastolic (lower number) is the blood pressure when the heart is at rest and is derived when the blood pressure returns to normal after the first rush of blood upon release of the cuff. It is has been found that the young and old have the same blood pressure, so 140/90mm Hg is a standard benchmark.[3] It is thought that more than 50% of persons over 65 years in industrialized society have a greater blood pressure than 140/90mm Hg.

True. 13. Perspiration and quenching of thirst help to combat overheating. Older adults perspire less, are less aware of thirst, and are less able to feel or adapt to extremes in temperature than younger persons. Less sensitive skin sensors, less insulation of fatty deposits under the skin, and the less efficient functioning of the hypothalamus (the temperature regulating mechanism in the brain) occur in older adults. Prolonged time for older adults to return to core temperature after exposure to extreme heat or cold begins at age 70 years and increases thereafter. Education and taking precautions may prevent most deaths related to temperature extremes. Increased fluid intake, gradual accommodation to climate change, rest, minimizing exertion during heat, use of fans or air conditioning, wearing hats and loose clothing, and avoidance of alcohol are some strategies for hyperthermia.

False. 14. There is a gradual loss of boney tissue, which causes brittle bones that fracture more easily in both men and women as they age. Osteoporosis develops more often in women when calcium is lost (following hormonal changes after menopause) or insufficiently taken and absorbed. Deficiency in bone mineral density occurs in 50% of women over 50 years of age to 57% of women 70 years or older, but decreases to 45% for those over 80 years. Women rarely develop osteoporosis until age 70. A test of bone density (absorptiometry) can measure bone mass by x-ray or computer analyzed e-ray. Prevention of osteoporosis begins with adequate calcium intake in one's teens and thereafter with increased attention after menopause. Weight-bearing exercise, hormone replacement therapy, decreased alcohol, protein, salt and caffeine consumption, smoking cessation, and adequate vitamin D intake may minimize bone loss. Hormone replacement therapy may offer some protection against heart disease, cognitive impairment, and bone loss, but also may present risks for cervical cancer. Risk factors of osteoporosis include excess alcohol, little physical activity, deficient calcium intake, no pregnancies, no breastfeeding, fair complexion, blond or red hair, and of European nationality.

True. 15. Due to osteoporosis, osteoarthritis, and a lifetime of wear and tear, upper vertebrae are weakened, joint spaces and buffering tissues wear, and muscles are lost. These changes foster decreased padding between vertebral discs, which accounts for a loss of height. The height changes and imbalances contribute to pain and stress on the lower back with advanced age.

True. 16. Muscle mass declines, cartilage erodes, membranes fibrose (harden), and fluid thickens. These contribute to stiffness, gait problems, lessened mobility, and limited range of motion. From age 30, muscle mass declines to almost 50% in old age. Research shows that weight-bearing exercise, aerobics, and weight resistance can restore muscle strength, increase stamina, stabilize balance, and minimize falls.

False. 17. Recent studies validate that more than 70% of men and women continue sexual activity after 65 years. Men and women over 70 are still considered potentially "sexy." Reasons for limited sexual activity include loss of partners, illness, and medications. Most older adults consider intimacy crucial to relationships and emotional well-being. Intimacy may be satisfied by means other than sexual relations such as touching, hugging, and holding.

True. 18. The muscle of the bladder loses elasticity and tone. Hence, the bladder holds almost 50% less urine (causing more frequent urination) and empties less completely. The warning period between the urge and actual urination is shortened or lost as one ages. Muscular disability, spinal cord effects on the bladder muscle, tumors, infection, and anatomic damage to the sphincters or bladder neck may cause incontinence in advancing age. Other risks for incontinence in old age include chronic disease, cognitive impairment, medications, smoking, pelvic muscle weakness, low fluid intake, and environment.

False. 19. The *amount* of blood flow through the kidney and ability of the kidney to filter blood is about *half* that of younger ages. This is caused by the age-related structural and anatomic changes within the kidney. Some studies show that as much as one-third of older adults have no change in their urine creatinine (creatinine clearance is a measure of how well the kidney is able to filter the blood, the glomeruler filtration rate, or GFR). However, other studies show decline that begins at 40 years. Age-related kidney changes create more risks for fluid and electrolyte imbalance and renal damage from medications or diagnostic contrast materials. Disease, surgery, or fever may stress and interfere with the kidney's ability to regulate and excrete fluids and electrolytes particularly in older adults.

False. 20. Cultural notions about "daily regularity" held by the current cohort of older adults makes the myths of constipation and the elderly seem more important and credible. However, age-related changes in the gastrointestinal system are *less* responsible for constipation in older adults than factors such as activity, diet, and medication. Decreased intake and absorption of vitamins, proteins, and other important nutrients, and dental issues present greater health threats to older adults. Despite a decrease in gastrointestinal muscle strength and motility, lax sphincters, and lowered digestive juices, the gastrointestinal system is better able to compensate for the harmful effects of these changes.

True. 21. While there is considerable individual variation, on average sensory processes (vision, hearing, taste, smell, and touch) do not work as well as people get older. Another way to say it is that the threshold at which we take in stimuli increases with age. The eye lens, for example, is less able to change shape, adjust to close and far objects, and the size of the pupil narrows so as to let in less light. Hearing loss begins at age 20, and for many involves the growing inability to hear higher frequencies as sensory receptors in the ear and nerve cells in the auditory pathway to the brain are lost. Taste buds become less sensitive with aging and after age 80 more than 75% of older adults show major impairment in their sense of smell. Many of these normal changes can be compensated for through increasingly sophisticated assistive devices (hearing aids, glasses, etc) and through modifications of the older person's environment.

True. 22. The incidence of acute or temporary conditions, such as infections or the common cold, decreases with age, although those that do occur can be more debilitating and require more care. Older people are much more likely than the young to suffer from chronic conditions. These are long-term (more than 3 months), often permanent, and leave a residual disability that may require long-term management or care rather than cure. More than 80% of persons age 65 and over have at least 1 chronic condition, with multiple health problems being common. Arthritis is the most commonly occurring chronic condition.

False. 23. Health decline is related to age or previous health problems, not retirement per se. Retirement may actually improve functional health by reducing stress on the individual.

True. 24. Although death in industrialized society has come to be associated primarily with old age, studies generally indicate that death anxiety in adults decreases as age increases. Among the factors that may contribute to lower anxiety are a sense that goals have been fulfilled, living longer than expected, coming to terms with finitude, and dealing with the deaths of friends. The general finding that older adults are less fearful of death than middle-aged counterparts should not obscure the fact that some subgroups may have considerable preoccupation and concern about death and dying. Some fear the process of dying much more than death itself.

False. 25. People over age 65 currently make up about 13% of the population. However, as the "baby boom" generation begins to turn 65 in 2011, the proportion of older adults will grow dramatically. It is estimated that by 2030 adults over 65 will compose 20% of the population.

False. 26. According to the US Bureau of the Census,[4] slightly over 5% of the 65-year-old population occupy nursing homes, congregate care, assisted living, and board-and-care homes, and about 4.2% are in nursing homes at any given time. The rate of nursing home use increases with age from 1.4% for the young-old to 24.5% of the oldest-old. Almost 50% of those 95 and older live in nursing homes.

False. 27.   Evidence from several studies and national surveys indicates that families are the major care providers for impaired older adults. Families provide 70% to 80% of the in-home care for older relatives with chronic impairments. Family members have cared for the typical older adult who reaches a long-term care setting for a significant amount of time first. Research has shown that adult children are the primary caregivers for older widowed women and older unmarried men, and they are the secondary caregivers in situations where the spouse of an older person is still alive. Parent care has become a predictable and nearly universal experience across the life course, although most people are not adequately prepared for it.

False. 28.   Remaining life expectancy at age 65 is about 4.5 years less for men than women. Women have an average remaining life expectancy of 19.4 years compared to 15.0 years for men. Overall life expectancy at birth is about 7 years greater for women (80.4) than men (73.5).

True. 29.   Although the remaining life expectancy of Black American men and women at age 65 is about 2 years less than that of White men and women at age 65, by the time they reach 85 their life expectancies are nearly the same. One possible explanation for this convergence effect is that Black men and women who make it to the oldest ages do so in spite of many disadvantages and are "survivors", who have developed physiological and social psychological survival advantages.

True. 30.   Social Security benefits are periodically automatically adjusted to inflation. Current law ties this increase to the consumer price index (CPI) or the rise in the general wage level, whichever is lower.

False. 31.   While the proportion of older people (age 65 and older) living below the poverty level has declined significantly since 1960 to about 10.5%, this index rather dramatically underestimates need. The poverty level is based on an estimate of the cost of items in the Department of Agriculture's least costly nutritionally adequate food plan, and multiplied by 3 (suggesting that food costs represent one-third of a budget). This is probably not a fair representation of living costs in many areas of the country, particularly urban areas.[5] Therefore, gerontologists and economists also look at the proportion near poverty level (up to 150% of poverty level) and find that nearly one-quarter of older adults fall below this line. These older people tend to be disproportionately women and unmarried (including widowed, Black or Hispanic Americans, living alone).

True. 32.   Some older adults do have visual, motor, or cognitive impairments that make them dangerous drivers. Many drive more slowly and cautiously, or avoid driving in conditions they consider threatening in order to compensate for these changes. Until approximately age 85, older adults have fewer driver fatalities per million drivers than men 20 years old, although they do have more accidents per miles driven. Unsafe speed and alcohol use are leading factors in accidents for young drivers, while right-of-way violations are the leading cause of accidents involving older drivers. This implies a breakdown in such cognitive-perceptual components as estimating the speed of oncoming cars or reacting too slowly to unexpected events. Older drivers' skills can be improved considerably by specific driver training such as through the American Association of Retired Persons' "55 ALIVE/Mature Driving" program.

False. 33.   Negative perceptions of older workers persist because of health issues, diminished energy, discomfort with technology, closeness to retirement, and reaction to change in the work place—all associated with older adults. To the contrary, research identified characteristics of low turnover, less voluntary absenteeism, and fewer injuries in older workers. Recent high ratings of older workers from employers cite loyalty, dependability, emotional stability, congeniality with coworkers, and consistent and accurate work outcomes. While more are retiring earlier and spending fewer years working, older workers will be in greater demand with dwindling entrants into the work force.

False. 34.   The majority of older people are not set in their ways and unable to change. There is some evidence that older people tend to become more stable in their attitudes, but it is clear that most older people *do* change. To survive, they must adapt to many events of later life such as retirement, children leaving home, widowhood, moving to new homes, and serious illness. Their political and social attitudes also tend to shift with those of the rest of society, although at a somewhat slower rate than younger people.

False. 35.   Older persons are involved in many and diverse activities. After retirement, many participate as volunteers in churches, schools, or other nonprofit organizations and report themselves to be "very busy." As they age, most persons are likely to continue the level of activity to which they were accustomed in middle age.

False. 36.   Older adults are at least as diverse as any other age group in the population, and in many dimensions they may actually be more diverse. People vary greatly in their health, social role, and coping experiences. As the older population becomes more and more ethnically diverse, differences could be even greater. It is very misleading to talk about older adults as "the elderly," as this term may obscure the great heterogeneity of this age group.

False. 37.   Although the media may leave the impression that older adults are a major target of violent crime, annual data from the National Crime Victimization Surveys consistently indicate that violent crime, personal theft, and household victimization rates for persons ages 65 and older are the lowest of any age group.[6] Data indicate that this holds true for virtually all categories of criminal victimization: rape, robbery, aggravated assault, simple assault, and personal larceny without contact. Only for the category of personal larceny with contact (eg, purse snatching, pocket picking) is the victimization rate higher for persons ages 65 and over compared to those ages 25 to 64. Nevertheless, the health and financial consequences may be greater for the older victim.

False. 38.   Studies have found *no* increase in average religious interest, satisfaction, or activities among older people as they age. The present generation of older persons (cohort) tends to be more religious than younger generations due to their upbringing, that is, they have been more religious all their lives rather than becoming more religious as they aged. However, research has indicated that religion does seem to become more important with age and older adults do rely on their faith to cope with losses.

False. 39.   Although several surveys show that fear of crime exists among some older adults, there is no substantial evidence that older people are more likely to be afraid of crime than younger people. One survey examined different types of victimization and found no increase in fear among older adults in any of the types. Studies that have shown an increase in fear of crime in later life possibly have used measures of questionable validity.

False. 40.   While some older people may experience a period of prolonged adjustment, there is no evidence that there is special harmfulness in elderly relocation. Studies of community residents and of institutional movers have found an approximately normal distribution of outcomes—some positive, some negative, but mostly neutral or mixed, and small in degree. For many, relocation brings a better fit between personal needs and the demands of the physical and social environment. Research generally has demonstrated that adjustment to residential relocation is determined, at least in part, by perceived predictability and controllability, and by the similarity between the originating and receiving environments.

False. 41.   Women in their 30s and 40s comprise the greatest *number* of volunteers. However, 40% of older adults volunteer. Older adults may be less likely to belong to organizations than younger persons, but are more consistent in their activities and loyal to groups from middle age until their 60s. Volunteerism is correlated with life satisfaction, usefulness, physical and mental well-being, and a sense of accomplishment. Persons with higher education and income levels, histories of volunteerism, and broad interests are more likely to volunteer. Health problems, lack of transportation, and limited income may limit volunteer activities.

False. 42.   This view is based on an early theory called disengagement theory, which said that it is normal and expectable that the older person and society withdraw from each other so as to minimize the disruption caused by the older person's death. Although many people obviously do scale back certain activities, particularly if health deteriorates, there is substantial evidence that many who remain active and engaged have higher levels of function and happiness. For many, staying involved physically, cognitively, socially, and spiritually in the social group is a basis for happiness.

True. 43.   Geriatrics refers to the clinical aspects of aging and the comprehensive health care of older persons. Study of geriatrics actually began in the early 1900s, although formal training in geriatrics is relatively new. A Certificate of Added Qualifications (CAQ) in geriatric medicine or geriatric psychiatry is offered through the certifying boards in family practice, internal medicine, osteopathic medicine, and psychiatry for physicians who have completed a fellowship program in geriatrics.

False. 44.   Although a number of medical schools require course work in geriatrics/gerontology, many still have only elective courses or no courses at all. Some medical schools have received incentives in the form of materials, support, and grants to develop and institutionalize formal curricula from such organizations as the Association of American Medical Colleges, the American Geriatrics Society, and the Association for Gerontology in Higher Education, as well as foundations such as the John Hartford Foundation. Top-ranked medical schools for geriatrics training include Harvard University, Duke University, Johns Hopkins University, Mount Sinai School of Medicine, University of California—Los Angeles, University of Washington, University of Michigan, Wake Forest University, University of Pennsylvania, and Yale University.

False. 45.   The low number of reported cases of elder abuse belie the magnitude of elder abuse in this country. The latest figures estimate more than 551,000 reported cases of abuse (physical, verbal, and sexual types of neglect or abuse) to persons over the age of 60 per year[7] (there are more than 30 million Americans over 60 years). Actual reported cases represent a fraction of what is thought to occur due to perceived fearful consequences and inconsistent and inefficient report mechanisms. Self-neglect and exploitative types of abuse were not part of the above study, and yet, are more common. Men and women are equally culpable in the perpetration of abuse.

False. 46.   The longevity revolution has increased the number of 3-, 4-, and 5-generation families. This, along with a growing incidence of divorce and remarriage, drug and alcohol addiction, AIDS, incarceration, and unemployment within the parental generation has resulted in grandparents stepping into the surrogate parent role with increasing frequency. Census figures estimate the number of grandchildren living with their grandparents (about one-third without a parent present) to be as high as 5.5 million, with Black Americans being slightly more than 3 times more likely than their White counterparts to be in this type of living arrangement. There are grandparent-headed households in every socioeconomic and ethnic group.[8]

True. 47.   Older adults experience multiple losses of loved ones and friends, illness, relocation, retirement, income, and change and decline in abilities. It may take an older adult longer to adjust to a major change or recover from prolonged and intense physical and emotional stress. The recovery of an older body from a traumatic event may be delayed due to age-related decreases in cardiac output and heart rate, and more vulnerability to disease with a less effective immune system. However, the many older adults who have developed active and healthy lifestyles may be able to resist or mitigate some of the negative effects of stress or illness due to their physiological fitness. Likewise, coping skills that have been honed during a lifetime may lessen the damage of psychological stresses and ease adjustments to loss and change.

True. 48.   The majority of older adults perceive their health to be good to excellent, as they do not compare their current condition to former states, but rather to their peers who are their same age and older and are "worse off." The "ratings" are not a medical assessment. While chronic disease, frailty, and disability are correlated with advanced age, the *Myths and Realities of Aging 2000* study discovered that 84% of all Americans would *like* to live to 90 years, and half of persons over 65 years described their lives as "the best years of my life."[9] Disease and disability are being delayed and functional levels are improving, especially in persons over 80 years. Less than 10% of noninstitutionalized persons 70 years and over are unable to perform one or more ADL. Disability increases to 22% for those 85 years and older.

True. 49.   In general, women throughout adulthood are more likely to attend to minor symptoms than are men. Men are more likely to have been socialized even as children to be stoical, and consequently are less likely to see a doctor for nonferrous health problems. When they do get sick, men are likely to have more hospital visits and longer hospital stays. Women, on the other hand, are more likely to have had regular contact with the health care system through childbirth, attending to their children's health, and having regular screening procedures for cervical and breast cancer. Although women report more chronic conditions than men in later life, the severity of their problems tends to be less than that of same age men, probably due to their earlier health care practices—hence, the phrase "women get sicker, but men die quicker."

False. 50.   Old age is a social construct. Meanings, definitions, and experiences of aging vary across cultures and throughout history. What people consider to be "old" has changed significantly just within the past 100 years in the United States as people live longer and healthier. Being identified as "old" is related not only to chronological age, but also health, functional ability, social roles, and self-perception. Age 65 is an arbitrary marker that has been associated with eligibility for governmental programs such as Social Security and Medicare (although the age of eligibility for Social Security is gradually being raised to 67 by 2027).

REFERENCES

1. Palmore E. The facts on aging quiz: part two. *Gerontologist.* 1981;21:431-437.
2. Hooyman NR, Kiyak HA. *Social Gerontology: A Multidisciplinary Perspective.* 5th ed. Boston: Allyn and Bacon, 1999.
3. Department of Health and Human Services Annual Report on the State of the Nation's Health. *Aging Research and Training News.* November 1999;113.
4. US Bureau of the Census.
5. US Department of Agriculture.
6. National Crime Victimization Survey.
7. Abuse Study cited in answer 45.
8. US Bureau of the Census.
9. National Council on the Aging. *Myths and Realities of Aging 2000.* Washington, DC: International Longevity Center-USA, Ltd., Jewish Home and Hospital; 2000.

BIBLIOGRAPHY

Atchley RC. *Social Forces and Aging: An Introduction to Social Gerontology.* 9th ed. Belmont, CA: Wadsworth; 2000.

Ebersole P, Hess P. *Toward Healthy Aging: Human Needs and Nursing Response.* 5th ed. St. Louis, MO: Mosby; 1998.

Federal Interagency Forum on Aging Related Statistics. *Older Americans 2000: Key Indicators of Well Being.* Washington, DC; 2000.

Freedman V. Functional limitation among older Americans. *Am J Public Health.* 1998;88(10):1457.

Maddox GL, ed. *The Encyclopedia of Aging.* 2nd ed. New York: Springer; 1995.

Miller RB, Dodder RA. A revision of Palmore's facts on aging quiz. *Gerontol.* 1980;20:673-679.

Morgan L, Kunkel S. *Aging: The Social Context.* Thousand Oaks, CA: Pine Forge Press; 1998.

Palmore E. Facts on aging: a short quiz. *Gerontol.* 1977;17:315-320.

Nutritional Considerations With Aging

Nutrition and aging go hand in hand. How the body is nourished throughout the lifecycle will affect the way one ultimately ages. Since the beginning of the human species, people have hunted, grown, and eaten food for survival. With the evolution of science and research, wisdom has been gained indicating that not only quantity, but an appropriate quality and balance of food products is required to live a healthy life. Research concludes that particular nutrient patterns play a role in wellness, health promotion, disease prevention, and rehabilitation.

Nutrition plays a vital role in all phases of the lifecycle for growth and development, maintenance of health, disease prevention, and recuperation from illness.[1] Nutrients sustain metabolism of all cells, tissues, body systems, and in the interactions that function to maintain homeostasis of the body at rest and during activity. There are at least 50 nutritional compounds and elements that are essential for proper cellular functioning. If even one of these essential nutrients is deficient or excessive, the sequence of cellular events is disrupted and can lead to disease and sometimes death.

There is a decreased need for calories as we age, but not for nutrients; thus, there is a challenge to ensure a healthy diet but avoid excessive weight gain (exercise, once again, helps to maintain weight). There are several age-related changes in the digestive tract that have an impact on nutrition (discussed in Chapter 3), and along with these changes we need to understand the psychosocial context as it affects good nutrition. For example, the statement,

"Mom doesn't eat much anymore, it must be her age" only offers one view of the problem; the PTA must look at what other factors can cause poor appetite, such as:

- Poor dental health affecting the ability to chew
- Loneliness, lack of desire to prepare food and eat by oneself
- Change in taste may make food seem bland
- Drug interaction or side effects causing a loss of appetite
- Decreased saliva production causing chewing difficulty
- Meal times are not good times for the individual
- Diseases affecting digestion (ie, causing pain, discomfort)
- Poor eyesight affecting ability to distinguish food or resulting in embarassment when food is spilled
- Decreased sense of smell removing some of the anticipatory delight
- Mental confusion.

All of these possible causes can be addressed with techniques to overcome the difficulty.

This chapter will address common deficiencies and risk factors for poor nutrition in an aged population. How nutritional deficiencies affect function will be presented, as well as functional problems that may lead to feeding problems. Current guidelines

Bottomley J. *Geriatric Rehabilitation: A Textbook for the Physical Therapist Assistant* (pp 119-148).
© 2010 SLACK Incorporated

for good nutrition in the elderly and the impact of inadequate nutrition on the physical, emotional, and cognitive well-being of the elderly will also be addressed. Components of nutritional programs for the elderly will be presented to provide the necessary guidelines for nutritional intervention programs from a rehabilitation perspective. The goal of a comprehensive team approach, in any care setting that supports nutritional feeding programs, is to promote health, prevent or reduce risks of certain diseases, support other medical interventions, and improve the quality of life in old age.

AGE-RELATED CHANGES THAT AFFECT NUTRITION WITH AGE

The biological, anatomical, and physiological changes that occur with aging will be discussed in this chapter as they relate to the nutritional status of the elderly. There are extraneous factors complicating the nutritional and homeostatic capabilities of the body such as advancing age, frequency of disease and disabilities, multiple medications, and hereditary and genetic predispositions. The decline in physiological functioning shows considerable variation from one individual to the next and is dependent to a large extent on lifelong activity and nutritional patterns.[2] Table 6-1 summarizes the common physiological changes accompanying aging, their potential functional outcome, and the probable clinical manifestations that may affect the nutritional status of an elderly individual.

Nutritional status is influenced by a range of medical, physiological, psychological, social, and situational variables. Adequate nutrition and physical activity are aspects of a health-promoting lifestyle. Encouraging better nutrition and partaking in exercise on a regular basis is a cost-effective way of decreasing the incidence and progression of age-related disease. A primary factor that affects nutritional intake and directly impacts physical functional capabilities is general deconditioning from inactivity and disuse. Lower energy levels may impact the ability to tolerate sitting throughout the consumption of a meal. Physical limitations may lead to an inability to handle eating utensils or get food to the mouth. Pathologies that may affect swallowing or oral-motor function could lead to an inability to safely manage various food substances. Additionally, a loss in cognition could lead to poor interpretation of food items or a problem with remembering what utensils are and their purpose, as well as a short attention span and lack of safety awareness.[3]

Visual problems can also lead to nutritional problems. The inability to read labels or see food items that are being prepared or consumed places an individual at risk for consuming potentially harmful food (ie, foods that cause allergies, foods that have gone past their expiration dates). Poor lighting in a food preparation area can result in accidents and make it impossible for a visually impaired elder to carry out a wide range of cooking tasks safely.[4] Other sensory changes, such as the loss of taste or smell, may result in a lack of interest in eating. Poor dentition, or the presence of dentures, makes eating a less than gratifying experience for many elders. Physical limitations, postural changes, metabolic or vestibular disorders, medications, visual disturbances, or cognitive impairments may contribute to the risk of falls, creating a substantial inability to safely manage the cooking or eating environment.[5] Physical disability can also contribute to the inability to open food containers or manage kitchen utensils and appliances safely. Obtaining food may be difficult due to an inability to get to a grocery store or, once there, the inability to safely navigate the store's environment.

Beyond physical, functional, sensory, or cognitive diabilities, the elderly individual may be depressed or socially isolated. Depression often decreases the motivation to prepare a meal and diminishes the desire to eat. Always eating alone can further diminish any desire to prepare or eat a meal. Financial restrictions often limit the amount and variety of foods purchased and consumed by elderly individuals.

Many chronic conditions lead to nutritional problems. Table 6-2 provides some of the frequently seen diagnoses in the elderly and their potential impact on nutrition.

NUTRITIONAL NEEDS OF THE ELDERLY

The progression of aging leads to a decreased margin of homeostatic reserve and a reduced ability to accommodate metabolic challenges, including nutritional stress. *Nutritional frailty* refers to the disability that occurs in old age owing to rapid, unintentional loss of body weight and loss of lean body mass (sarcopenia).[6] As we age and become less active, our basal metabolic rate decreases. Research indicates that, with lower levels of activity, fewer nutrients are actually absorbed by the system despite ingestion of adequate amounts. This is in part due to the homeostatic properties of cellular functioning, whereby the cell's "brain" thinks it does not need these nutrients because it is functioning at a lower level physiologically. Therefore, when

Table 6-1

PHYSIOLOGICAL CHANGES AND FUNCTIONAL NUTRITIONAL CONSIDERATIONS

PHYSIOLOGICAL CHANGES WITH AGING	POTENTIAL FUNCTIONAL OUTCOME	PROBABLE CLINICAL OUTCOME
Musculoskeletal		
Decreased number and size of muscle fibers	Decrease in lean body mass	Decreased muscular strength, and mobility
Decreased bone density	Osteoporosis	Increased risk of fractures
Decreased joint mobility and wear and tear of the joint	Narrowing of joint space	Impaired mobility, and pain
Central Nervous System		
Decreased sensory function	Decreased reaction to pain, touch, heat, and cold	Decreased perception leading to accidental injury
Impaired proprioception	Diminished mechanisms controlling balance	Increased susceptibility to falls
Cerebral atrophy, senile plaques, neurofibrillary tangles	Parkinson's-like symptoms, supranuclear palsy	Confusion, diminished response and perception, memory loss, decreased ADL, poor nutritional compliance
Skin		
Thinning of epithelial and subcutaneous layer	Tissue and vascular fragility	Increased susceptibility of skin tears, abrasions, bruises, and burns
Eye		
Sclerosis of lens	Cataract, decreased peripheral vision	Impaired peripheral vision, susceptibility to accidents
Degeneration of muscles of accommodation	Smaller pupils, stiffness of the lens	Impaired visual acuity, decreased socialization
Degenerative changes in vitreous, retina, and choroid	Decreased color vision and decreased night vision, eye fatigue	Susceptibility to accidents, increased risk of infection
Degeneration of intrinsic/ extrinsic ocular muscles	Impaired upward gaze, poor peripheral vision	Susceptibility to falling, unable to accurately interpret environment
Hearing		
Degeneration of organ of corti	Loss of high frequency tones	Decreased hearing, decreased socialization, poor learning
Smell		
Atrophy of olfactory mechanism	Impaired sense of smell	Decreased appreciation of food
Oral Cavity		
Decreased salivary flow	Dry mouth	Poor oral hygiene, gingivitis, impaired food bolus formation
Resorption of gums and surrounding bony tissue surrounding	Tooth loss, impaired force of bite	Preference for softer foods, malfunctioning dentures
Diminished taste bud sensory input	Increased salt and sugar consumption	Diet high in sugar and salt

(Continued)

Table 6-1 continued

PHYSIOLOGICAL CHANGES AND FUNCTIONAL NUTRITIONAL CONSIDERATIONS

PHYSIOLOGICAL CHANGES WITH AGING	POTENTIAL FUNCTIONAL OUTCOME	PROBABLE CLINICAL OUTCOME
Gastrointestinal		
Decrease in esophageal smooth muscle, dysfunction of lower esophageal sphincter	Decreased esophageal mobility	Difficulty swallowing, high-bulk foods, hiatal hernia
Decreased intestinal blood flow, decreased liver size	Impaired intestinal absorption and liver metabolism	Subclinical malnutrition
Decreased contractile function of smooth intestinal muscle	Decreased intestinal motility	Constipation
Decreased HCL secretion, decreased number of absorbing cells	Defective absorption of calcium and iron	Pernicious anemia, iron deficiency anemia, osteoporosis
Decreased gallbladder motility	Gallstones	Gastrointestinal upsets, fatty food intolerance
Renal		
Decrease in nephrons, atherosclerosis in combination with decreased cardiac output	Decreased ability to dilute and concentrate urine, diminished renal blood flow	Renal insufficiency, increased potential for dehydration
Endocrine imbalance	Inability to absorb trace nutrients	Malnutrition, renal failure
Pancreatic beta cells, function, and insulin end-organ responsiveness diminish	Progressive glucose intolerance with advancing age	Diabetes mellitus, susceptibility of hypoglycemia if on insulin or oral hypoglycemic drugs
Psychological		
Role changes	Retirement, loss of productivity, increased leisure time	Depression, decreased nutritional intake, decreased finances
Loss	Multiple physical, cognitive, financial, and social loss	Depression, isolation, decreased nutrient intake

the body is stressed, nutrients (such as protein for the production of amino acids required for energy, or calcium which is a crucial element for nerve conduction, cardiac muscle contraction, skeletal muscle contraction, and synaptic connections within the brain) are drawn from the body's warehouses. Protein is taken from the muscles and calcium from the bones, respectively.

The most significant change that accompanies advancing age is a decrease in the energy required to meet basal metabolic demands to maintain weight and compensate for energy expenditure from physical activity. This decrease in demand is related to the decrease in lean body mass or protein-rich type II muscle fibers as a result of increasingly lower levels of physical activity. The component that most affects energy needs is muscle protein. As the muscle mass shrinks, less energy is required to maintain its smaller

mass at rest. Along with muscle mass, other protein compartments also decline, including organ tissue, collagen, antigens and antibodies, enzymes, and hormones. These changes affect nutritional requirements.

Sarcopenia, a loss of muscle mass and strength, contributes to functional impairment. Weight loss is common due to a reduction in food intake; its possible etiology includes a host of physiological and non-physiological causes. The release of cytokines during chronic disease may also be an important determinant of frailty. In addition to being anorectic, cytokines also contribute to lipolysis (the breakdown of fat), muscle protein breakdown, and nitrogen loss.[7]

Because the changes are gradual and often small, at first glance they may not seem significant. However, small deficits over extended periods can have unexpected and functionally negative consequences. Therefore, throughout life, everyone needs

Table 6-2

CHRONIC CONDITIONS AND RELATED NUTRITIONAL PROBLEMS

CHRONIC CONDITION	RELATED NUTRITIONAL PROBLEMS
Alzheimer's disease; other dementias	Cachexia and emaciation due to poor eating habits and self-care
Celiac sprue	Malabsorption, malabsorption with secondary vitamin deficiencies; diarrhea; weight loss
Cerebrovascular accident	Suppressed cough reflex, increased risk of choking; dysphagia
Chronic mesenteric ischemia	Abdominal pain after eating; weight loss; malabsorption
Constipation	Prolonged transit time especially with immobility; decreased colonic motility
Colitis	Decreased elasticity of rectal wall; abdominal discomfort; fecal impaction
Coronary artery disease	Dyspnea; drugs lead to suppressed appetite and constipation
Diabetes mellitus	Glucose intolerance; poor energy utilization
Diverticular disease	Gastrointestinal pain, bowel discomfort, possible bleeding; infection; lack of appetite; weight loss
Emphysema	Dyspnea leading to lack of appetite and difficulty eating
Gallbladder disease	Gallstones; cholecystitis; pancreatitis; food restriction; some foods repugnant; undernutrition
Gastritis/duodenitis	Malabsorption of proteins, vitamin B_{12}, and iron; some food restrictions, other foods repugnant; undernutrition
Gastroenteritis	Malabsorption, protein and vitamin B complex deficiencies, poor absorption of calcium and all other nutrients; loss of appetite
Hiatal hernia	Gastroesophageal reflux; heartburn; dysphagia
Liver diseases	Foods repugnant; restricted protein; drug level changes
Obesity	Energy intakes usually low, need for essential nutrient intake
Osteoarthritis	Difficulty in food shopping and preparation
Osteoporosis	Dyspnea with vertebral collapse; distortion of thorax and abdominal compression; lack of appetite; difficulty eating; decreased intake
Peptic ulcer	Obstruction, bleeding, and perforation; dysphagia, dyspepsia, retrosternal discomfort; antacid overuse and undernutrition
Pernicious anemia	Vitamin B_{12} deficiency, spinal cord degeneration
Renal disease	Limited ability to handle protein, sodium, potassium, and water

to eat a well-balanced diet containing all of the essential nutrients and maintain a functional activity level that is sufficient to enhance the absorption of these dietary elements.

It is impossible to get all of the nutrients required for normal physiological functioning from just one food source. Therefore, ingesting a variety of foods is important to obtain an adequate balance. Nutrients that make up a well-balanced diet include protein, carbohydrate, fat, water, water-soluble vitamins, fat-soluble vitamins, and minerals.

Proteins contain approximately 4 calories per gram. An adequate intake of protein is important because it is an essential substrate (a material used to make new compounds) in maintaining muscle and organ mass, healing wounds, repairing fractures, and fighting infections. Despite losses in total body protein pools, recent studies indicate that protein requirements may actually be higher in older people because they do not absorb protein as efficiently as younger, more active individuals. In some older people, protein undernutrition is chronic—a problem that is often missed.

Proteins come from sources such as meat, poultry, fish, eggs, dairy products, and nitrogen-containing vegetables and legumes such as soybeans, lentils, and black beans. Many older individuals become at risk for protein undernutrition because of the high cost of foods rich in protein, lactose intolerance, or the GI disturbances associated with the consumption of food products from the vegetable and bean families. Additionally, although vegetables and legumes are generally not expensive, obtaining high-biologic value protein from mixtures of different legumes and vegetables requires a fairly sophisticated knowledge of nutrition.[8]

Glycogen is a carbohydrate that is well known as an instrumental participant in many important cell functions (eg, protection from stress factors, regulation of cell growth and division, spore formation). Carbohydrates comprise approximately 50% to 60% of calories in American diets. Carbohydrate foods provide water-soluble vitamins, minerals, fiber, and calories. Carbohydrate provides approximately 4 calories per gram, similar to protein, but is generally found in less expensive foods such as cereals, breads, vegetables, fruits, grains, rice, potatoes, pasta, and foods made from these products. Many individuals eat foods that are high in simple or refined carbohydrates (eg, donuts, chips). These foods contain high levels of sugar and fat but are high in calories and low in nutrients (ie, empty calories). Complex carbohydrates, which are rich in many nutrients, such as whole grains and insoluble fibers, are a crucial part of a healthy diet.[9]

Fats provide 9 calories per gram, double that of protein and carbohydrates. Limiting, but not omitting, intake of food high in fat is the easiest way to reduce total caloric intake without jeopardizing the nutrient content of the overall diet of individuals who are sedentary. Some fat is essential to a well-balanced diet. Fat ensures that the body has an adequate amount of essential fatty acid and fat-soluble vitamins, which within the Kreb Cycle (a complex series of chemical reactions in all cells involved in the metabolism of nutrients, the utilization of oxygen, and the production of energy [adenosine triphosphate]) mobilize the dormant stores of hormones that are stored in fat cells and is particularly important for the homeostatic mechanism in postmenopausal women. Small amounts of polyunsaturated fats, such as vegetable oils, provide essential fatty acids. Fat-soluble vitamins are available in water-soluble forms and, in the case of vitamin D, from sources other than food (eg, sunlight).[10]

Water needs to be provided in quantities of 1.5 to 2.0 L per day. Inadequate fluid intake can lead to chronic dehydration and electrolyte imbalance.

Physiologic alterations that occur with aging are frequently associated with chronic dehydration. As people become less active, osmoreceptors (cells that influence the release of vasopressin) decrease. Vasopressin, a hormone released from the posterior pituitary gland, increases the absorption of water by the kidneys, thereby preventing excess water loss. Accompanying the reduction of osmoreceptors is a decline in thirst sensitivity. This is often the result of medications but can also be associated with chronic water restriction. Some older adults may voluntarily restrict their fluid intake in a mistaken effort to control problems of incontinence. In fact, by restricting water consumption, the urine becomes overconcentrated, irritates the wall of the bladder, and leads to more of a problem with urinary incontinence. An older individual that consumes 1.5 to 2.0 L of water-based fluids on a daily basis will find that urinary incontinence (along with Kegel exercises) is actually less of a problem. Additionally, providing adequate fluid, along with dietary fiber and exercise, can help prevent constipation and diarrhea, both common chronic complaints of the older, less active individual.[11]

Most water-soluble vitamin requirements do not change with advancing age, with a few notable exceptions. Age-related changes have been noted in vitamin B_6 metabolism, and inadequate intakes have been noted in community-dwelling elderly. Increased requirements have been suggested for older individuals to meet their needs. Older adults may also be at risk for inadequate intake of vitamin B_{12}. Older individuals can maintain serum vitamin B_{12} levels despite low intake, but chronic deficiencies may occur as a result of the presence of atrophic gastritis, a condition associated with advanced age. Atrophic gastritis contributes to a change in gastric pH and a decrease in intrinsic factor production, which is necessary for vitamin B_{12} absorption. Some evidence exists that present requirements for folic acid may be higher than needed for older people, but there appears to be no significant alterations in requirements for vitamins B_1, B_2, C, niacin, biotin, or pantothenic acid (B_5). Fat-soluble vitamins include A, D, K, and E. Requirements for these vitamins are somewhat more complex than those for other vitamins because of the body's physiologic ability to store them. Vitamin A intake needs to be monitored not for potential deficiency but for potential hypervitaminosis. Older persons, who are less efficient at clearing retinyl esters (metabolic byproducts of vitamin A metabolism) from the liver, are more likely to become toxic from high levels of these byproducts, resulting in confusion, dementia, and seizures. Beta carotene, a water-soluble precursor of vitamin A, if taken in large quantities, may not be efficiently cleared from the serum and may cause skin to become orange-hued. Older adults may be at risk for vitamin D deficiency. Vitamin D is known to play an important role in bone metabolism, as it facilitates the absorption of calcium in the intestines, and may be an important factor in immune function, contributing to depressed immune responses often seen in the elderly. Vitamin D deficiency may result from limited intake of dairy products, decreased opportunities for sun exposure, reduction of skin vitamin D precursors, or a diminished ability of kidneys to convert the vitamin to its active form (D_3), which enhances the absorption of calcium.[12]

An adequate intake of vitamin K is generally not a problem because it is produced by bowel bacteria. However, many older people are taking vitamin K antagonists for their anticlotting action or have taken sulfa drugs that kill the bacteria that produce vitamin K in the bowels. Vitamin E is widely available in whole-grain cereals and vegetable oils. Since these are used in many food products and cooking, vitamin E deficiency is generally not regarded as a problem. With a few exceptions, the requirements for minerals and trace metals generally do not change with age. Iron requirements decrease with advancing age due to an increase in tissue iron stores, particularly in women who lose much iron related to menstruation but is not a problem in postmenopausal women. Adequate calcium ingestion is crucial in the older adult. However, the roots of the benefits of calcium intake occur at much earlier stages of life. Increasing calcium intake after osteoporosis has developed, in addition to exercise and potential hormone replacement therapy, may help to stabilize but not increase bone density. Thus, it is important to look at the need for calcium as a lifetime goal. Calcium serves a vital role in every single system of the human body.[13]

Malnutrition and its impact on clinical outcomes may be underestimated in the elderly population. PTAs, as they see a patient on a day-to-day basis, may be the first to recognize signs of malnutrition. It is important to learn the signs of malnutrition. A great deal of information can be gathered from knowing the subtle signs that occur in the skin, hair, eyes, and oral mucosa. For instance, dry, thin, easily plucked hair or "flaky paint" skin is suspect for chronic protein malnutrition. Any fissures around the mouth or glossitis (a swollen tongue) may be indicative of water-soluble vitamin deficiencies. Photophobia (sensitivity to light), Bitot's spots (white spots), in addition to swollen gums and gooseflesh (follicular hyperkeratosis) are indicative of a vitamin A deficiency. These are just a few examples.[14] Table 6-3 provides possible clinical manifestations of nutritional deficiencies that can occur in the aged.

Age-related functional decrements, so long considered inevitable consequences of aging, are now considered to be a function of misuse, disuse, and poor nutrition. Both age-related changes and pathologies have been shown to become symptomatic gradually, which suggests that preventive interventions and management of nutritional balance throughout the lifecycle is clearly an available part of a multidimensional approach to health promotion, disease prevention, and a return to functional levels of activity.[15]

Nutrition screening is one of the first steps that can be taken to address nutrition-related problems among older adults. Rehabilitation professionals should be educated in the possible signs and symptoms of undernutrition or overnutrition and include these observations as a part of a comprehensive evaluation[16] (see Table 6-3). In the absence of regular screening measures in the clinical setting, the presence of malnutrition is frequently overlooked.

COMMON NUTRITIONAL DEFICIENCIES IN THE AGED

Calories/Energy Intake

Unintentional weight loss in older adults is a problem that occurs frequently in community-dwelling and institutionalized individuals. The recommended daily allowance (RDA) for "energy intake" is just enough kilocalories to maintain an energy balance. Four major factors influence energy needs: resting energy expenditure, physical activity, growth, and thermogenesis (heat production secondary to food consumption, exercise, or cold stress). Resting energy expenditure and physical activity both decline with age and decreased activity, therefore, energy needs are lower among the aged or sedentary individual. Linear growth does not occur in the aged organism, although during recovery, healing, and rehabilitation, lean body mass and fat may be laid down requiring energy.[17] Thermogenesis, a relatively minor contributor to energy needs at any age, is not known to differ between aged and younger persons. Resting metabolic rate differs with age chiefly because of lean body mass (metabolically active tissue) and lower levels of activity. Energy output in the form of physical activity declines with age.

Many elderly are ill and with increasing age and illness, interindividual differences in energy requirements and body weight become more pronounced. Limitations on physical activity caused by chronic diseases such as arthritis, hip fractures, emphysema, osteoporosis, congestive heart failure, cerebrovascular accidents, peripheral vascular disease, and other degenerative conditions limit physical activity, and consequently, reduce energy needs in at least

Table 6-3

PHYSICAL MANIFESTATIONS OF MALNUTRITION

NUTRIENT DEFICIENCY	PHYSICAL MANIFESTATION
Protein	Edema; hypoalbuminemia; enlarged liver; diarrhea
Protein/energy	Muscle wasting; sparse, thin, dry, brittle hair; dry, inelastic skin; muscle weakness
Vitamin A	Poor visual accommodation to dark; Bitot's spots (eyes); dryness of the eyes; hair loss; impaired taste; gooseflesh
Vitamin D	Bowed legs, beading of ribs, and other skeletal deformities (rickets)
Vitamin K	Bleeding (poor coagulation of blood)
Thiamin (B$_1$)	Cardiac enlargement; mental confusion; irritability; calf muscle tenderness and foot drop; hypoflexia; hyperesthesia; paresthesia
Riboflavin (B$_2$)	Fissures around mouth; reddened, scaly, greasy skin around the nose and mouth; magenta-colored tongue
Niacin (B$_3$)	Bright red, swollen, painful tongue; pellagrous dermatitis; depression; insomnia; headaches; dizziness; dementia; diarrhea
Pyridoxine (B$_6$)	Neuropathies; glossitis; nasolabial seborrhea
Folic acid	Red, painful, shiny, smooth tongue; skin hyperpigmentation
Vitamin B$_{12}$	Mild dementia; sensory losses in hands and feet; red, smooth, shiny, painful tongue; mild jaundice; optic neuritis; anorexia; diarrhea
Vitamin C	Joint tenderness and swelling; hemorrhages under the skin; spongy gums that bleed easily; poor wound healing; petechiae
Essential fatty acids	Sparse hair growth; dry, flaky skin; depression; psychosis; dementia
Calcium	Poor reflexes; poor cardiovascular accommodation to activity; slow mental processing; depression; dementia
Magnesium	Lethargy and weakness; anorexia and vomiting; tremor; convulsions
Iodine	Goiter
Iron	Pallor; pale, atrophic tongue; spoon-shaped nails; pale conjunctivae
Zinc	Sluggish muscle contraction; poor wound healing; diminished taste and appetite; dermatitis; hair loss; diarrhea

one-tenth of the population over 65 years of age. Among the very old, especially those who are in nursing homes, energy needs are often only slightly above resting basal metabolic levels. While energy needs are lower for some aged, they are extremely high for others. When neuromuscular coordination declines, with reduced mechanical efficiency and increased difficulties in balance control, the energy cost of movement is greatly increased.[18]

Protein/Energy Malnutrition

The current RDA for protein is 0.8 g/kg of high-quality protein per day; this amounts to 56 g for men and 44 g for women.[19] Protein requirements are more likely to be affected by stresses such as disease, which may increase dietary protein requirements by 2 or more times. The reduced contribution of muscle to body protein metabolism in the aged may decrease the ability of the individual to adapt during periods of restricted dietary energy or protein intake, when protein synthesis in vital organs is maintained by mobilization of amino acids from the muscles. The reduction in energy intake is likely to increase protein needs because the efficiency of protein utilization and absorption depends on energy balance.[20]

Chronic protein-energy malnutrition is synonymous with *cachexia* (severe weight loss and muscle atrophy). Cachexia is seen in a number of chronic diseases, and it is always associated with a poor prognosis. Cachexia usually results from low food intake or is secondary to anorexia. In the elderly, common causes of cachexia are cancer, chronic neurological disease with associated paralysis, endstage hepatic or renal disease, and cardiac cachexia resulting from high-dosage digitalis therapy. While cachexia is mainly due to reduced energy and protein intake, additional factors are catabolic effects of disease and excessive losses of nutrients by malabsorption or through protein-losing *enteropathy* (any disease of the intestine). Irrespective of etiology, the development of cachexia has a disastrous consequence in the elderly. As lean muscle mass wastes and the individual becomes frailer and frailer, the ability to produce enough energy for basic ADL is severely restricted. The PTA will play a major role in the provision of feeding programs and ensuring that energy needs are met.[21] It is important that, if the PTA observes that nutritional needs are unmet, these observations be reported to the health care team.

Calcium and Vitamin D

Although there is general agreement that increased dietary calcium consumption and exercise can slow bone loss in the elderly, studies indicate that there is a deficiency in both calcium and exercise in older adults.[22] Several factors negatively influence adequate calcium nutrition in the elderly. Intake of calcium among the aged is low and frequently does not meet the RDA. Absorption of dietary calcium in the gut is poor, and the ability to adapt to a low calcium diet decreases with age.

One significant hormonal event that influences calcium nutrition is menopause in women and andropause in men. Estrogen and testosterone increase calcium absorption and decrease renal losses, so that on the same calcium intake, the estrogen-replete female utilizes dietary calcium better. Postmenopausal estrogen replacement therapy is helpful in preventing negative calcium balance and osteoporosis. Little research has been conclusive on the effects of hormone replacement in men. Growth hormones and hormonal events such as pregnancy also increase absorption and decrease renal losses of calcium. Calcium ingestion and absorption are essential for strong teeth and bones. They help in maintaining the health of the blood, muscle, cardiac, and nervous system functioning. The best sources of calcium are found naturally in milk, dairy products, leafy green vegetables, sardines, tofu, peas, and beans.

The consumption of calcium and vitamin D play an important role in bone health. Reduced supplies of calcium are associated with a reduced bone mass and osteoporosis, whereas a chronic and severe vitamin D deficiency not only contributes to osteoporosis, but leads to *osteomalacia,* a metabolic bone disease characterized by decreased mineralization of bone. Vitamin D insufficiency, the preclinical phase of vitamin D deficiency, is most commonly found in the elderly. There is a significantly increased bone loss during the winter months secondary to the decrease in ultraviolet rays of the sun. This is hypothesized to be a result of the lack of vitamin D necessary for calcium absorption.[23]

Iron

The current RDA for iron is 10 mg/day for individuals 51 years and older. Iron is a mineral for which need declines with age among females; this is a postmenopausal event since iron is no longer lost through menstrual bleeding and childbearing. Counterbalancing decreased iron loss is some evidence that the efficiency of iron absorption may be decreased among the aged. Factors that decrease iron absorption among the aged are frequent use of antacids, calcium supplements, and tea—all of which form complexes with iron in the gut and decrease absorption. Some elderly individuals decrease their intakes of red meat and other animal flesh foods rich in iron because of dental difficulties or limited incomes. Instead they rely on plant foods that are generally lower in bio-available iron. Some older individuals also decrease their intakes of ascorbic acid-rich foods and protein-rich foods, thereby decreasing intakes of ascorbic acid and amino acids, 2 enhancers of iron absorption.[24]

Concerns about iron in the elderly usually focus on its role in blood production. Lack of iron is a causation factor of anemia. Evidence that iron deficiency anemias are a normal part of aging is weak, although the incidence of anemia increases with age. Reductions in hematocrit, which are not associated with dietary iron deficiency, chronic disease, or blood loss, are usually a result of an abnormality in cellular proliferation. Anemias due to other causes are common. In fact, contrary to popular belief, iron deficiency anemia is not the sole or major cause of anemia in the aged; blood losses of iron may be due to alcohol abuse, frequent use of aspirin, infection, neoplasms, and renal disease.[25]

Iron develops the quality of the blood, increases resistance to stress and disease, and is important for proper functioning of the thyroid gland. The best sources of iron are organ meats, lean meat, egg yolks, fish, wheat germ, and leafy green vegetables.

Vitamin B$_{12}$

Different surveys have found either no change or decreased levels of vitamin B$_{12}$ in the elderly. A vitamin B$_{12}$ deficiency is commonly due to lack of gastric intrinsic factor, which causes malabsorption. In pernicious anemia, a disease common in the elderly, the production of gastric intrinsic factor ceases and there is a complete lack of gastric acid production (achlorhydria). Pernicious anemia is an autoimmune disease in which megaloblastic and neurological signs are caused by vitamin B_{12} deficiency. Vitamin B_{12} from the diet cannot be absorbed in the absence of gastric intrinsic factor. The aging process increases the risk of autoimmune disease within the gut. B_{12} deficiency produces both megablastic anemia and neurologic symptoms including mild dementia; sensory losses in the hands and feet; and a painful, red, smooth, and shiny tongue. In addition, a mild jaundice appearance is commonly seen in an individual with a vitamin B_{12} deficiency. In elderly patients with B_{12} deficiency, other associated diseases, such as hypothyroidism, diabetes mellitus, and Addison's disease (adrenal failure), are often found.[26]

Vitamin B_{12} is essential for normal function of all body cells, including brain and nerve cells. The best sources of B_{12} are organ meats, muscle meats, fish, and dairy products.

Folic Acid

Part of the B-complex, folic acid is essential for normal metabolism of growing cells and tissues. Low folic acid levels have been found in depressed institutionalized elderly and elderly in general hospitals as well as among elderly living at home. Folic acid deficiency may stem from many different situations such as inadequate dietary intake due to poor food choices often related to alcoholism, the use of drugs such as anticonvulsants that interfere with the absorption or metabolism of folic acid, the increased use of heat-processed foods with reduced folic acid content, restricted intake associated with poor dentition, gastrointestinal surgery (which reduces folic acid absorption), or impaired folic acid metabolism.

Intakes of 400 µg/day of folic acid are usually sufficient to meet the needs of the older population. Among healthy elderly subjects, low plasma folic acid and tissue folic acid levels are found to be common.[27] In elderly individuals with nutritional folic acid deficiency, folic acid absorption is impaired. This malabsorption of folic acid appears to be related to the deficiency itself and can be reversed by treatment with folic acid. Besides its effect on red blood cells, it has been suggested that folic acid deficiency may produce mental dysfunction in the elderly.[28]

The best natural sources of folic acid include leafy green vegetables, organ meats, and brewer's yeast. Folic acid is also found in most whole grains and beans.

Vitamin C

Vitamin C, or ascorbic acid, is essential for healthy teeth, bones, and red blood cells and is a primary element in the production of synovial fluid in the joints. Ascorbic acid is a potent nonenzymatic protector against free radical damage. Spurred by the proclamations (and longevity) of Linus Pauling, megadoses of vitamin C have been touted as playing a protective role in upper respiratory tract infections and neoplasm.[29]

It has been determined that elderly individuals receiving vitamin C had small but statistically significant increases in body weight and plasma albumin and a reduction in bruising and hemorrhages of the skin. No changes in mood or mobility were observed. The risks of megadoses of vitamin C include rebound scurvy when ascorbic acid is reduced to the RDA, reduced vitamin B_{12} absorption, false-negative fecal occult blood results (leading to delayed diagnosis of colonic cancer), and excessive absorption of dietary iron. It has been concluded that taking too much vitamin C is not worth these risks; however, because vitamin C is not stored, it must be replaced daily.

An association between ascorbic acid and arteriosclerosis has been made. Early vessel changes seen in the arteries of patients with atherosclerosis are similar to those observed in patients with scurvy. Coupled with the finding of low blood ascorbic acid levels in patients with coronary atherosclerosis and acute myocardial infarction, these findings have led to the suggestion that vitamin C may be involved in the pathogenesis of atherosclerosis. Numerous studies have documented lower ascorbic acid levels in plasma, leukocytes, and platelets in older subjects. Not only do ascorbic acid levels decline with age, but the levels of free radicals associated with ascorbate also decline. The decrease in ascorbate radical levels with age may indicate a decline in the free radical defense mechanism with advancing age.[30]

The best natural sources of vitamin C are citrus fruits and juices, tomatoes, green peppers, and strawberries.

Vitamin E

Early studies established that vitamin E levels decline with age. Vitamin E is an antioxidant and helps protect unsaturated fats from abnormal breakdown. It also prolongs the life of red blood cells and functions in maintaining homeostasis in the brain and nervous system.[31] Besides its role as an antioxidant, vitamin E has been suggested to have some effect in the management of intermittent claudication.

Vitamin E appears to play a central role in maintaining the structure and function of the human nervous system. Vitamin E deficiency initiates and perpetuates a progressive neuromuscular degeneration—with irreversible neurologic consequences if treatment is delayed. Vitamin E may also be useful in the treatment of neurological disorders not associated with vitamin E deficiency; its use is being investigated in Parkinson's and Alzheimer's diseases. It appears that vitamin E may help to prevent or retard the degeneration of nerves that occur in Parkinson's disease and delay the onset of cognitive decline in Alzheimer's disease.[32]

The best natural sources of vitamin E are vegetable oils, wheat germ, whole-grain cereals, green vegetables, seeds, and nuts.

Vitamin A

Vitamin A is needed for normal growth, normal vision, and healthy teeth, nails, bones, and glands. Primary functions of vitamin A are its role in dark adaptation, maintaining skin integrity, and blood cell production. A significant decline in light threshold in relation to aging has been demonstrated; however, this did not correlate with serum vitamin A levels and was not improved by vitamin A administration. Follicular hyperkeratosis, a classic sign of vitamin A deficiency, is often seen in elderly subjects but does not appear to be related to a vitamin A deficiency. There is no evidence that plasma vitamin A or the absorption of vitamin A is affected by aging. Vitamin A, however, is the second most commonly used nutritional supplement. In contrast to the rarity of symptoms from vitamin A deficiency in the elderly, vitamin A toxicity is more commonly seen. Symptoms include general malaise, headaches, confusion, liver dysfunction, leukopenia, and hypercalcemia. A severe toxic reaction to too much vitamin A is seizures.[33]

The best natural sources of vitamin A are fish liver oils, dairy products, organ meats, and dark-green and yellow vegetables.

ZINC

Zinc is essential for the general growth and proper development of the reproductive organs. Zinc deficiency in humans can lead to anorexia, impaired immune function, poor wound healing, decreased strength of muscle contraction, and possibly, altered taste acuity. Zinc is also strongly connected to the strength of the immune system.[34] It is estimated that the average daily intake of zinc in elderly persons in the United States ranged from 7 mg to 13 mg with the RDA established at 15 mg. On balance, it appears that serum zinc levels decrease with aging. Similar decreases in hair zinc levels have also been demonstrated with aging. Other studies have found that the zinc concentration in bones and the kidneys also falls after the age of 50.

Zinc has been demonstrated to be necessary for adequate functioning of T cell lymphocytes. Aging is associated with a progressive deterioration in T cell lymphocyte function. The role of zinc in wound healing is now well established. Zinc supplementation has been shown to accelerate healing of leg ulcers in elderly subjects. Zinc deficiency may play a role in the anorexia of aging. Zinc deficiency decreases the responsiveness of the neurotransmitters, which are potent stimulators of food intake as they enhance intake. The effect of zinc supplementation on improving appetite in elderly subjects has been clearly demonstrated. Impotence is extremely common in the elderly, and a strong correlation has been established between hyperzincuria, low serum zinc levels, and impotence in this population.[35]

It appears that zinc levels decline with age, possibly as the result of chronic, long-term marginal zinc intake. This situation can be further aggravated by the hyperzincuria associated with chronic diseases, such as diabetes mellitus, to which the elderly are particularly prone. Zinc deficiency may also play a role in the pathogenesis of dementia based on zinc's essential role in enzyme production necessary for DNA replication, repair, and transcription. Research continues to substantiate lower levels of zinc in the central nervous system (CNS) and brain in patients with Alzheimer's disease.[36]

The best sources of zinc naturally are shellfish, nuts, organ meats, egg yolks, milk, and whole-grain products.

Copper

Copper is needed to utilize iron and for the development of bones, nerves, and connective tissue. Copper serves as a catalyst in the biochemistry of every organ system. In particular, copper plays a role in iron absorption and mobilization, which as previously discussed, is particularly relevant to aging.[37] Copper is a catalyst for lysyloxidase, an enzyme important for the cross-linking of collagen and elastin, and it plays a role in the conversion of dopamine to norepinephrine. Copper deficiency increases serum cholesterol levels, possibly by increasing the rate of cholesterol released from the liver to the circulation. As high dietary zinc accentuates copper deficiency, it is suggested that atherosclerosis is related to the ratio of zinc to copper.[38] Despite the great theoretic interest in the role of copper in the aging process, there is little information concerning copper in the aged population. An increase in serum copper levels is associated with aging. An increase in plasma copper with aging but no change in leukocyte copper levels is also evident.[39] Copper absorption appears similar in aged and young subjects.

The best natural sources of copper are liver, whole-grain cereals, almonds, leafy green vegetables, peas and beans, seafood, kidney, and egg yolks.

Water Intake

Maintaining water balance is essential for health. The environment, pathologies, and the aging process can adversely affect water homeostasis. Dehydration is the most common fluid and electrolyte disturbance in the elderly. The threshold for recognition of thirst is higher in the elderly. Water turnover rate has been shown to be low, and intake may be affected, especially in elders with physical disability.[40] In many instances, cognitive or physical disabilities also reduce the ability to recognize thirst, express thirst, or obtain access to water. In addition, healthy elderly individuals seem to have reduced thirst in response to fluid deprivation. Elderly individuals produced less concentrated urine following fluid deprivation. Since elderly subjects had higher vasopressin levels in response to dehydration, the decreased capacity to concentrate the urine is most likely at the renal level.[41] Fluids as well as solid foods are essential. Approximately 1.5 to 2.0 L of water or other fluids per day is a reasonable goal to strive for in the aged.

An increase in serum sodium concentration is a result of loss of body water in excess of salt loss. Among elderly patients, hypernatremia (dehydration with elevated sodium levels in the serum) is most common in those who are bedbound and not provided with sufficient water to satisfy their thirst or in those whose thirst sensation is diminished by impaired CNS functioning. A net deficit of water is associated with vomiting and diarrhea, diabetes insipidus, and hyperpyrexia (excessive sweating). In general, older patients appear to be predisposed to the development of hypernatremia. Surgery, febrile illnesses, infirmity, and diabetes mellitus account for most of these incidences.[42]

Drug Effects on Nutrition

The frequent use of pharmacologic agents by the elderly increases their vulnerability to malnutrition. Drug-diet interactions occur at all ages but are more common in the elderly because of prescription and over-the-counter drug use on a regular basis. In addition, age-related changes in GI function, liver and renal function, and body composition alter drug and nutrient metabolism. Coexisting disease, undernutrition, and malnutrition may further complicate these interactions.[43]

Drugs may affect nutritional status in the simplest sense by their effects on appetite. More commonly, absorption, metabolism, and excretion of dietary constituents are altered. Dietary factors such as water consumption, amount of food consumed, timing of meals in relation to drug intake, and the constituents consumed may affect absorption and oxidative drug metabolism.

An example of a commonly used drug that increases calcium need is aluminum-containing antacids, which decrease phosphorus absorption, lowering plasma phosphorus and ultimately increasing calcium excretion. Thiazide diuretics, on the other hand, decrease calcium needs by decreasing urinary calcium losses and may have a positive effect on bone mass.[44] Drugs that impact appetite and nutrition will be discussed in greater detail in Chapter 7.

Alcohol

Alcohol is both a drug and a food that provides substantial amounts of energy. It is widely abused by individuals of all ages. Among the aged, its abuse is especially easy since the risks of intoxication from a given dose of alcohol are elevated because lean body mass and total body water decrease with age. The consequence is that the total volume of distribution of alcohol is smaller and peak blood alcohol levels are higher than in younger persons. Greater physiological sensitivity to the effects of alcohol and greater psychological vulnerability to alcohol abuse due to depression, loneliness, and lack of meaningful roles combine to make alcohol abuse risks high in the aged. Alcohol use should be avoided entirely among the aged with known dementia, chronic used psychoactive drugs, a previous history of alcohol abuse, or chronic and extreme depression.[45]

Moderate alcohol use has been associated with some health benefits. Alcohol in moderation is an appetite stimulant, enhancing the taste of food. It increases high-density lipoprotein (HDL) cholesterol levels, thereby lowering atherosclerotic risks. Moderate alcohol intake is also associated with lowered congestive heart failure rates. Since elderly energy intakes are already low, care must be taken to ensure that calories from alcohol do not displace other items in the diet that provide not only energy but protein, vitamins, and minerals.[46]

IDENTIFYING CONDITIONS RESULTING IN FEEDING DISABILITIES

The range of medical diagnoses that might indicate a feeding disability is quite broad. A number of major diagnoses are presented to familiarize the PTA with the potential functional problems of some patients who might be seen in long-term care facilities, assisted living environments, community nutritional programs, and home settings. Although the list presented here is not exhaustive, individual patients within each diagnostic category may present a very different clinical picture and require intervention to attain feeding independence.

Dysphagia

This is a disorder of swallowing that can lead to aspiration and malnutrition. High-risk patients include those with cerebrovascular accidents; altered level of consciousness; head injury; long-term intubation; anoxia; demyelinating disease; brainstem disease; Parkinson's disease; facial/neck recontruction; and respiratory involvement such as pneumonia, chronic obstructive lung disease, or asthma. Warning signs for dysphagia include a decreased level of alertness; drooling; difficulty handling oral secretions; absence of gag, cough, or swallow; moist, wet, gurgly voice quality; or decreased tongue and mouth movements.

Amputations

There are basically 2 kinds of amputation and they are classified by cause. Congenital amputees learn feeding techniques and to adapt to alternative feeding skills as they grow and develop, thus, they usually do not present a feeding concern. Traumatic amputations of an upper extremity, however, lead to "one-handedness" and may result in difficulty with feeding. Amputees who have lost a hand or an arm after they have mastered feeding in the normal developmental sequence will usually need to learn special techniques for one-handed feeding.

Cerebrovascular Accidents

A stroke leading to hemiparesis or hemiplegia will affect functional skills for feeding. Additionally, the individual may have hemianopsia, which is the inability to see in the visual field on the same side as the paralyzed arm. Cognitive abilities may affect the individual's ability to learn particularly when the stroke affects the dominant side of the brain and the individual has receptive, expressive, or global aphasia. The muscles on one side of the mouth may also be paralyzed and the individual will have difficulty holding food in the mouth, chewing, and swallowing.

Arthritis

Arthritic joint changes caused by rheumatoid arthritis or osteoarthritis that affect the upper extremities and potentially the transmandibular joint could also lead to feeding disabilities. Painful joints may limit an individual's ability to manage food containers (eg, opening jars, lifting pots) for food preparation as well as limit his or her functional abilities to feed him- or herself because of weakened grasp, joint deformity, and pain.

Osteoporosis

The individual with severe osteoporosis may develop a severe kyphotic (hunchback) position of the thoracic spine from stress fractures of the vertebrae. This posture compresses all of the internal organs into a smaller space, often making ingestion of any food sources an uncomfortable experience. Postural changes can also make management of food, such as cutting, lifting the upper extremity, and even seeing the food on the plate, very difficult. With severe kyphotic deformity, the patient is required to hyperextend his or her cervical spine in order to keep food in the mouth. Swallowing is extremely difficult and often painful in this extended neck position.

Spinal Cord Injuries

Loss of motor control and sensory input resulting from cervical or thoracic level of quadriplegia or paraplegia can lead to muscle weakness, lack of trunk stability, and in some quadriplegics with higher levels of involvement, difficulty with swallowing. Muscle weakness has obvious implications for feeding problems from a functional perspective. Adaptive feeding equipment is often required to facilitate feeding.

Dementia

In an older population, a loss of cognitive abilities could lead to the inability to accurately and safely interpret their environment. Food items and eating utensils may not be recognized, attention span may be limited, and an inability to distinguish various textures of food may lead to swallowing difficulties and choking. Often, a supervised feeding program is required in this population to ascertain that nutritional needs are met.

Parkinson's Disease

Parkinsonian symptoms, induced by low levels of dopamine and, in many cases, the side effects of psychotropic drugs, cause diminished voluntary movements, slower movement, weaker movement, and uncoordinated and awkward motor function. Nonintentional tremors, rigidity, and difficulty initiating movement may functionally limit the individual's ability to feed him- or herself. Additionally, drooling (the inability to completely close the mouth) and difficult swallowing will impede ingestion of many food items. Often the Parkinson's patient will have decreased tongue and mouth movements, and in many cases, have a hyperactive gag reflex, causing him or her to choke whenever food in present at the back of the tongue.

Muscular Dystrophy

Muscular poor coordination and weakness leading to the inability to accurately control movement is often seen in demyelinating disease such as muscular dystrophy. The muscle groups affected depend on the type of muscular dystrophy; however, in almost all forms, the shoulder girdle is affected and consequently alters the normal feeding process. Positioning is difficult due to muscle weakness, and contractures may limit an individual's functional abilities even further. The patient with muscular dystrophy will also fatigue very rapidly, further compromising his or her ability to complete an entire meal.

Huntington's Chorea

Huntington's chorea also leads to poor coordination; however, the biggest problem is choreoform movements, which lead to involuntary, jerky, and irregular movements of the arm, neck, face, and trunk. Weighted and swivel utensils can assist in aiding these individuals to feed themselves independently. As the disease progresses, all symptoms will increase and often require feeding by caregivers. Swallowing is often a problem in Huntington's chorea, and extra care must be monitored to ensure that the individual does not aspirate on food items.

Chronic Obstructive or Restrictive Lung Disease

A patient with respiratory difficulties will not only have a difficult time catching a breath at rest, but the difficulty in breathing will lead to poor management of solid and liquid food items because of the forced respiratory breathing pattern. Choking becomes a major problem with this diagnostic category. Swallowing may also be a problem.

Visual Problems

An elderly individual may have visual difficulties leading to the inability to see food items or to safely manage eating utensils. This becomes a particularly important problem when the individual is preparing meals in the home environment. The inability to see food labels or knobs on the stove or to distinguish a sharp knife from a table knife often leads to accidents.

Intestinal Problems

The presence of constipation or diarrhea may lead an elderly individual to self-impose food restrictions on him- or herself. Hydration is a problem in both situations.

Tooth Loss and Dentures

Poor dentition or the presence of dentures may also create eating problems. Often dentures are poor fitting and food becomes lodged between the palate of the mouth and the denture plate, making eating uncomfortable. Also, an attempt to eat food without dentures in, or with multiple tooth loss, leads to selection of softer foods, limiting the variety of food items consumed. The presence of dentures also diminishes the gratification of eating by decreasing the sensory input of oral management of food. The inability to fully chew food often leads to choking and swallowing difficulty.

Medications

Although not a specific "diagnosis," many of the drugs that patients are on for numerous conditions cause dehydration, diminish the sense of taste or distort taste (eg, everything tastes "metallic"), and suppress the appetite. Consideration of the types of drugs that patients are taking is an important part of assessing elderly individuals with nutritional problems.

Summary

Although a number of conditions and factors have been presented in this chapter, there are many more that one might encounter in conjunction with a feeding problem. Every patient, regardless of diagnosis or functional ability, must be treated as an individual and individualization of the feeding program must be first and foremost in the health care team member's mind.

With keen observational skills and the development of rapport with each individual patient, the PTA may be among the first to notice a nutritional problem. Timely communication with the PT about these observations is critical to the health and well being of each older adult. Table 6-4 provides a quick nutritional review of systems and describes signs associated with malnutrition for each area of the body and allows assessment and documentation of findings.

Table 6-4

NUTRITIONAL REVIEW OF SYSTEMS

BODY AREA	SIGNS ASSOCIATED WITH MALNUTRITION	FINDINGS
Hair	Lack of natural shine; hair dull and dry; thin and sparse; hair fine, silky, and straight; color changes (flag sign); can be easily plucked	
Face	Skin color loss (depigmentation); skin dark over cheeks and under eyes (malar and supraorbital pigmentation); lumpiness or flakiness of skin of nose and mouth; swollen face; enlarged parotid glands; scaling of skin around nostrils (nasolabial seborrhea)	
Eyes	Eye membranes are pale (pale conjunctivae); redness of membranes (conjunctival injection); Bitot's spots; redness and fissuring of eyelid corners (anguler palpebritis); dryness of eye membranes (conjunctival xerosis); cornea has dull appearance (corneal xerosis); cornea is soft (keratomalacia); scar on cornea; ring of fine blood vessels around corner (circumcorneal injection); xanthelasma	
Lips	Redness and swelling of mouth or lips (cheilosis); especially at corners of mouth (angular fissures and scars)	
Tongue	Swelling; scarlet and raw tongue; magenta (purplish color) tongue; smooth tongue; swollen sores; hyperemic and hypertrophic papillae; atrophic papillae	
Teeth	May be missing or erupting abnormally; gray or black spots (fluorosis); cavities (caries)	
Gums	"Spongy" and bleed easily; recession of gums	
Glands	Thyroid enlargement (front of neck); parotid enlargement (cheeks become swollen)	
Skin	Dryness of skin (xerosis); sandpaper feel of skin (follicular hyperkeratosis); flakiness of skin; skin swollen and dark; red swollen pigmentation of exposed areas (pellagrous dermatosis); excessive lightness or darkness of skin (dyspigmentation); black and blue marks due to skin bleeding (petechiae); lack of fat under skin; xanthoma	
Nails	Nails are spoon-shaped (koilonychia); brittle, ridged nails	
Muscular and skeletal systems	Muscles have "wasted" appearance; bleeding into muscle (musculoskeletal hemorrhages); person cannot get up or walk properly	
INTERNAL SYSTEMS: THIS INFORMATION IS TO BE ABSTRACTED FROM OTHER MEDICAL RECORD SOURCES.		
Cardiovascular	Rapid heart rate (above 100 tachycardia); enlarged heart; abnormal rhythm; elevated blood pressure	
Gastrointestinal	Liver enlargement; enlargement of spleen (usually indicates other associated diseases)	
Nervous	Mental irritability and confusion; burning and tingling of hands and feet (paresthesia); loss of position and vibratory sense; weakness and tenderness of muscles (may result in inability to walk); decrease and loss of ankle and knee reflexes	

NUTRITIONAL INTERVENTION AND PROGRAMS FOR THE ELDERLY

Regardless of the setting of intervention, screening for nutritional problems and special programs that address the nutritional needs of the elderly are recommended. Often the PTA will be the primary member of the "feeding" team in home care agencies, hospital or nursing home-based departments, hospice care, public agencies, or adult day care settings.

When working with an older adult in his or her home, it is often difficult to isolate specific home-making or meal difficulties. An older individual may not be eating because of functional inability to shop or prepare meals, a lack of motivation or interest in eating due to sensory loss or the amount of energy required to prepare and consume a meal, depression or social isolation, or a lack of financial resources for the acquisition of food.

The Team Approach to Nutritional Interventions

The professionals in any care setting for the elderly who are generally involved in patient feeding programs include dietitians, dietetic technicians and assistants, nurses, physicians, physical and occupational therapists and therapist assistants, speech pathologists, psychologists, social workers, and pharmacists. Frequently, dentists are also involved in patient feeding programs when individuals with feeding problems develop severe dental problems. Each member of the team plays a distinct role in managing nutritional programs.

The *dietitian* is responsible for administrative services such as planning meals, supervising food preparation, and delivering the meal to the patient. The dietitian's clinical responsibilities include executing diet orders, making appropriate diet modifications, ensuring that balanced nutrition is provided, and preparing the appropriate diet. The dietitian is chiefly responsible for counseling patients about their nutritional needs, which includes outlining in detail a nutritional plan for each patient. The dietitian possesses the knowledge to accurately access the nutritional needs of patients and become involved in the feeding process. Nutritional aspects of feeding problems are summarized in Table 6-5.

The *nurse* has traditionally been responsible for feeding the patient. Responsibilities include proper positioning of the patient prior to feeding; charting fluid and food intake; and communicating the patient's lack of intake, aversion, or intolerance to food to the dietitian and physician. The nurse is also responsible for integrating and implementing the total patient care plan.

The *occupational therapist* is responsible for assessing oral motor function, instructing the staff and patient on the appropriate body alignment for feeding, determining a patient's ability to self-feed, assessing the patient's need for assistive devices, and working with the patient on chewing and swallowing problems and other functional skills that are prerequisites to feeding independence. Once the occupational therapist has comprehensively evaluated the individual, the certified occupational therapist assistant carries out the feeding program based on the evaluative findings and goals established in the treatment plan, reporting to the occupational therapist routinely regarding progress or difficulties encountered.

The *physical therapist* evaluates deficits in patient mobility and posture and prescribes appropriate feeding activities. The PT is also responsible for evaluating oral motor problems and developing therapeutic interventions to maximize strength, flexibility, endurance, and functional capabilities. Once the PT has comprehensively evaluated the individual, the *physical therapist assistant* carries out the feeding program and therapeutic interventions based on the evaluative findings and goals established in the treatment plan, reporting to the PT routinely regarding progress and/or difficulties encountered.

The *speech pathologist* can provide an extensive assessment of oral motor function and recommend treatment for problems in this area. Depending on experience and background, this professional may be able to provide help in solving behavioral problems and work with problems of bite, tongue thrust, and other oral motor functional problems.

The *social worker* collects social history and demographic data regarding the patient and his or her family and provides the health care team with a summary of the client's financial status and reaction to proposed therapy. If a patient has a financial need that impedes the purchase of appropriate nutritional elements, the social worker may be required to find alternative resources to provide adequate nutrition for the individual, such as "meals-on-wheels." If access to a shopping center is the problem, programs such as "pea-pod," where food can be ordered over the Internet and delivered to the individual's home, are often employed.

The *dentist* can provide assessment of a patient's dental health such as that of the gums and oral structure, as well as particular sensitivity related to the teeth. The dentist will also be the key professional in ascertaining that the patient has appropriately fit dentures or other oral devices.

The *physician* is responsible for identifying feeding as a problem and requests consultation through written orders to the appropriate health care professional: occupational therapist, physical therapist, or speech pathologist.

The *pharmacist* is responsible for evaluating potential drug and nutrient interactions, determining if drugs are suppressing the individual's appetite, or if medications are responsible for dehydration of the patient.

The "feeding team" approach is the most effective model of intervention in geriatric care. The team evaluation not only provides a good communication device but also provides assessment from more than one professional perspective. This places the patient in the center of the team.

Evaluation of Feeding Disabilities

A number of forms containing screening information exist for early identification of feeding problems. In the patient's medical record, for example, information related to feeding and previous nutrition histories can be found in the database and nursing admission form.

Table 6-5

NUTRITIONAL ASPECTS OF FEEDING PROBLEMS

FEEDING PROBLEM	NUTRITIONAL RISK FACTORS—INADEQUATE INTAKE	NUTRITIONAL CONSIDERATIONS
Oral-motor • Chewing • Swallowing • Hyperactive gag • Poor closure	• Puréed foods may be low in calories, protein, vitamins • Loses food from mouth, poor mouth closure • Fatigues easily • Condition accompanied by an inability to self-feed and/or communicate • Frequently on medications that interfere with nutrient absorption and utilization	• Increase calorie density through bread, cereal, carbohydrate supplements • Thickened foods are more easy to swallow than clear liquids • Vitamin-mineral supplement may be needed • Frequent meals in small servings • Adaptive devices
Position • Lack of trunk stability leading to inability to sit up in chair or bed unassisted	• Leads to inadequate intake due to difficult positioning for swallowing • Leads to fatigue	• Position at 45-degree angle with stability to trunk and head • Provide foods easily consumed at highest texture level (chopped, small bite sizes); small frequent meals.
Inability to self-feed	• Inadequate intake caused by frustration, spillage, anger at receiving cold food • Lack of personnel to assist with feeding	• Provision of small servings in finger food size until self-feeding is possible with spoon or fork • Provide adaptive equipment • Thickened foods are easier to self-feed than soups • Provide smaller meals more frequently
Mental confusion	• Inadequate intake or excessive intake due to forgetting that meals were consumed; distractibility during meal	• Provision of between-meal nourishments • Monitor intake and calculate calorie/protein content • Vitamin-mineral supplement • Presenting food with a verbal reminder related to eating

The PTA may often review a form to screen feeding that will include the following:

- Feeding problems—oral-motor, positioning, inability to self-feed, and behavioral
- Nutrition assessment—summary of pertinent findings in the nutrition assessment, that is, clinical signs of malnutrition, biochemical measures, weight/height relationship
- Listing of health care team members included in the patient's feeding program.

(See the appendix at the end of the chapter for an example of useful information that will assist the PTA in carrying out a feeding program.)

Rehabilitation Management of Specific Feeding Problems

The role of the rehabilitation professionals in a feeding program is to coordinate with other disciplines on the "feeding team" and provide a complete evaluation and treatment program specific to the patient's needs.

The occupational therapist evaluates feeding skills as one major component of activities of daily living. Table 6-6 provides an example of a feeding assessment. Feeding assessment and treatment includes the following:

- Oral motor dysfunction
- Upper extremity use
- Eye-hand coordination and/or limb apraxia
- Need for adaptive equipment
- Positioning
- Dietary considerations (ie, food consistency, food preferences)
- Perceptual and cognitive impairments.

The occupational therapist will collaborate with other members of the team as appropriate to develop an effective treatment program and educate the therapist assistant and other disciplines if indicated. This will increase independence in self-feeding abilities and encourage the maximal functional level for individual patients.

The PT will be involved in evaluating and treating the following:

- Head and trunk control
- Cervical range of motion and weakness
- Sitting balance
- Abnormal postural reflex activity interfering with head control and sitting balance
- Gross facial muscle test
- Ability to handle secretions
- Voluntary deep breathing ability
- Breath control and voluntary cough
- Gross motor upper extremity ability
- Wheelchair and bed positioning.

The occupational and physical therapy intervention can further enhance, remediate, and contribute to the patient's feeding program in individual therapy sessions by improving head and trunk control; improving the patient's ability to handle secretions; facilitating sucking and breath control; increasing range of motion of neck, jaw, and extremities; and improving balance, flexibility, strength, endurance, coordination, and eye-hand control (Box 6-1).

Positioning

The position of the patient during feeding proves to be one of the most crucial factors in maintaining adequate protection of the airway. It also allows the individual greater control in manipulation of the food

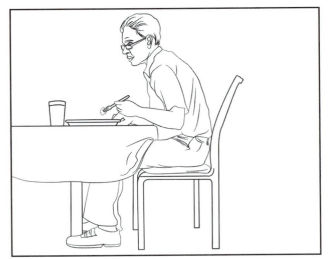

Figure 6-1. Proper positioning for feeding on a chair.

bolus within the mouth. With the trunk in an erect position and slight flexion of the neck, increased tension of the hyoid strap musculature slightly elevates the larynx into its protective position beneath the base of the tongue. More importantly, this position allows gravity to maintain the food source in the mid and anterior mouth, preventing spilling into the pharynx before initiation of the pharyngeal swallow.

If the patient is in a chair, the individual should be in an erect position with the head slightly tilted forward (Figure 6-1). If in bed, the head of the bed should be in the fully upright position such that the patient is erect with the head slightly tilted forward (Figure 6-2). In some instances, the bed may need to be reclined due to postural deformities such as kyphosis of the thoracic spine. Control of the head position can be aided by giving manual assist to the forehead or at the base of the skull.

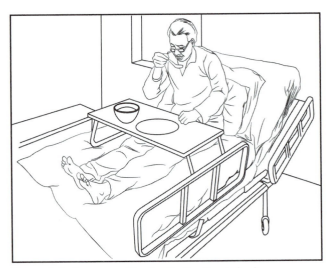

Figure 6-2. Proper positioning for feeding in bed.

Table 6-6

REHABILITATION FEEDING ASSESSMENT

FEEDING ASSESSMENT

Name: _____ Unit/Room: _____

Meal observed: Yes/No Date: _____ Therapist: _____

Sensory Motor Status

Muscle tone: Normal _____ Hypotonic _____ Hypertonic _____

Primitive reflexes: None _____ Startle response _____ Rooting _____ Palmomental _____

Other (describe) _____

Positioning for Feeding

Seating arrangement: Chair at table _____ W/C at table _____ W/C with tray _____

Bean bag _____ Other seating device (describe) _____

Relationship of table/tray to resident (describe) _____

Posture: Upright _____ Reclined (note degree) _____ Lying prone _____

Lying supine _____ Other (describe) _____

Feet supported? Yes _____ No _____

Arm free to reach or assist? Yes _____ No _____

Head control: None _____ Poor _____ Fair _____ Good _____

Trunk control: None _____ Poor _____ Fair _____ Good _____

Feeding Skills/Process

Feeder's position in relation to resident: Front _____ Side _____ Behind _____

Physically supporting _____ N/A – Self-feeder _____

If Fed

Head: Turns toward food _____ Turns away _____ Other (describe) _____
_____

Reaching: Mouth (lifts head) _____ Hands _____ None _____

Assists with feeding: Yes _____ No _____ If yes, describe _____
_____

Bird fed: Beverage _____ Food _____ No _____

Self-Feeding

Eye-hand coordination: None _____ Poor _____ Fair _____ Good _____

Finger feeds: Yes _____ No _____

Equipment used: Spoon _____ Fork _____ Knife _____ Straw _____ Cup _____

Glass _____ Napkin _____

Adaptive equipment used: Yes _____ No _____ (describe) _____
_____

Manages own tray: Yes _____ No _____

Neatness (describe): _____

Monitored for nutritional intake: Yes _____ No _____

Well hydrated: Yes _____ No _____

Box 6-1: **Oral-Motor Exercises for Feeding**

Mandible depression	Request patient to open the jaw and provide resistance by placing hand under the chin and pushing up. This strengthens the hyoid sling musculature as well as strap musculature from sternum-clavicle to thyroid cartilage, hyoid, and mandible. Request patient to make rotary movements with jaw while resisting.
Elevation	When mouth is open, request patient to bite strongly. Provide resistance to closure. Facilitate by providing vibration to masseters prior to resistance and quick stretch of masseters and pterygoids by sharply pushing chin down prior to request to close or bite.
Chewing	Practice with cud or a small firm rubber ball attached to a string. Encourage side-to-side and rotary movements. Facilitate muscles as prescribed above.
Lip compression	Request patient to squeeze lips tightly together. Provide resistance by trying to spread lips apart. Place a tongue blade flat between the lips (not teeth) and push down requesting patient to hold stick tightly. Icing, vibration, and quick stretch of orbicularis oris laterally and opposite the direction of compression to facilitate prior to resistance.
Protrusion	Request patient to push lips outward as in pouting. Provide resistance. Facilitate in the manner prescribed above.
Retraction	Ask patient to smile. Provide resistance by placing the palm over the mouth and resisting retraction with thumb and fingers. Facilitate by icing and vibration to corners of mouth and vibration to cheeks. Provide quick stretch at corners of mouth in direction opposite retraction prior to active or active-resistive movements. Encourage patient to yawn, smile, and frown in exaggerated motions.
Tongue protrusion	Request patient to stick out tongue as far as possible. Provide resistance with a spoon or tongue blade. Facilitate by vibrating genioglossus on either side beneath tongue. Lick a sucker or lick jelly from the lips.
Lateralization	Ask patient to stick out tongue to extreme right and then left. Provide resistance with a tongue blade or spoon. Ask patient to push out the cheek with the tongue on both sides. Provide resistance. Place jelly at corners of mouth, and ask patient to lick.
Tip elevation	Ask patient to push tip of tongue up behind front teeth. Do this with jaw open and closed. With jaw open, request the same movement and provide resistance with tongue blade. Ask patient to run the tip of tongue along the outside of upper teeth. Place jelly on alveolar ridge behind upper teeth, and ask patient to lick. Ask patient to hold a mint in same position with tip of tongue.
Root elevation	Ask patient to say the letter "K." Provide resistance to rise of the base of the tongue with tongue blade or spoon. Ask patient to push against the resistance. Facilitate by vibrating below the chin or provide stretch to glossopharyngeal, palatoglossal, and mylohyoid by sharply pushing base of tongue downward with tongue blade or spoon prior to resistance.
Pharynx-velum	Integrated movements of these structures are elicited by providing stimulation to gag reflex. Touch posterior pharyngeal wall, velum, and palatal arches in the back of the mouth to elicit gag.
Larynx	Provide resistance to elevation of larynx during pharyngeal phase of swallow to strengthen the hyoid sling and thyrohyoid musculature. This should not be done while eating and is otherwise only possible with individuals who have consistent voluntary swallow or initiation is easily stimulated.

Exercise and facilitation of the oral pharyngeal musculature should be carried out twice per day in 20 to 30 minute sessions. When possible, active range of motion and active resistive range of motion techniques should be taught to the patient for independent practice.

Swallowing

In the beginning sessions, the easiest food consistencies should be used (eg, puréed foods, applesauce, pudding). These will require the least intraoral manipulation and allow the patient better control of the food bolus. For persons who are known to have aspiration difficulties or poor swallowing abilities, ice chips should be used. If aspiration occurs, the body is generally able to tolerate small amounts of water. Ice chips also suppress the gag reflex.

Food should be administered using a spoon with small bite-size portions (eg, approximately half of a heaping spoonful). When presenting food, provide "central" facilitation on the tongue to stimulate swallowing and ask the patient to try to push the spoon out of the mouth. This will incorporate the mylohyoid muscle, which is the first to be activated during swallowing. Resist the thrust of the tongue by pushing downward and slightly back while raising the handle of the spoon to "dump" the food onto the tongue. Allow the patient sufficient time to manipulate the bolus. The food bolus will also stimulate increased salivary flow and sensory receptors, which may assist in initiating the swallow. Successful swallowing is the most basic element of oral feeding. Without consistent and reliable performance in this area, the individual is unable to advance to more complex feeding skills.

Chewing

Chewing is not simply the opening and closing of the mandible. The rotary chewing pattern is a complex muscular activity involving coordinated movements of the lips, jaw, cheeks, and tongue. Chewing squeezes juices from foods that combine with increased salivary flow. These liquids pose an additional problem in control. When beginning, use foods that are relatively easy to chew (eg, sliced fruit, cheese). If weakness is more pronounced on one side, the intact or stronger side should be used. Place the food in the mouth on the lower molars, using a fork, tongue blade, or fingers. Ask the patient to chew the food, periodically checking to ensure that food is maintained in an appropriate position and how juices and increased salivary flow are managed. When food has been chewed, shift concentration from "chewing" to "swallowing." Some chewing may continue as the patient attempts to manipulate the food in a position for swallowing (see Box 6-2).

Drinking

Liquids pose the most significant problem for intra-oral manipulation and swallowing. This

---

Box 6-2: Management of Swallowing Disorders

Poor Oral-Motor Control With Good Swallow Reflex

Position: Head up to reduce food falling out of mouth

Chin down when swallowing

Possible recline to 60 degrees

Keep knees flexed

Therapy: Oral-motor exercises

Teach chin up-down for swallow

Difficulty Swallowing Liquids With Poor Swallow Reflex

Position: Sit at 90 degrees with knees flexed

Up in chair for all meals

Tuck chin down to swallow

Turn head to weaker side

Therapy: Give ice chips 15 minutes before meals

Teach chin tuck

Teach double swallow

Turn head to weaker side

Thermal stimulation

Teach clearing of airway

Supraglottic swallow

Oral-motor exercises

Pharyngeal Stage Stasis (Cough After Swallow)

Position: Sit at 90 degrees with knees flexed

Up in chair for all meals

Turn head to weaker side

Therapy: Oral-motor exercises

Ice chips 15 minutes before meals

Teach double swallow

Teach supraglottic swallow

Teach head turning when eating

Difficulty Swallowing With Excess Secretions

Position: Seat patient at 90 degrees with knees flexed

Chin up for spoon, lower chin to chest to swallow

Turn head to weaker side

Therapy: Oral-motor exercises

Teach to swallow frequently

Close mouth when swallowing

consistency is difficult to control and easily runs out of the mouth or into the pharynx and airway. In initial therapy sessions, present small spoonfuls of water in the same manner as described in the section on swallowing. If liquids drool from the mouth when in the recommended position, the head may be returned to a level posture, although extension of the head should be avoided. When attempting to use a glass or cup, begin with a full glass so that the patient does not have to tilt his or her head backward. Place the rim of the glass on the person's lower lip. Avoid pouring liquids into the mouth, instead encourage the patient to take small sips.

Use of a straw requires a considerable amount of function in oral musculature. Shorter straws with larger diameters are somewhat easier as the creation of a pressure differential within the mouth is required to successfully suck fluids. Strength of muscles should be considered and a program of facilitation may be necessary before this is a practical means of maintaining fluid input.

The initial goal of swallowing, chewing, and drinking programs is to assess and establish a functional and adequate means of nutritional support.

ADAPTIVE FEEDING EQUIPMENT

Once feeding has been identified as a problem, the rehabilitation professional has a spectrum of therapeutic modalities available for enhanced intervention. Based upon the evaluation of the patient's status, the plan of action may include diet, physical conditioning and strengthening exercises, swallowing exercises, behavioral modification, use of an assistive device, or the combination of these modalities.

Selection, provision, and training in the use of assistive or adapted feeding devices should only be performed by the registered therapist. Although problems may be common to persons with similar conditions, solutions are unique and need to be tailored to the individual.

The equipment and various solutions to eating presented in this chapter are for the most common symptoms found in a variety of disease conditions. These symptoms and the equipment often prescribed are classified as one-handedness, limitation in joint motion, muscle weakness, poor coordination, and visual problems.

One-Handed Assistive Devices

One-handedness is most common among older persons who have hemiplegia following a cerebrovascular accident. Other neuromuscular conditions may

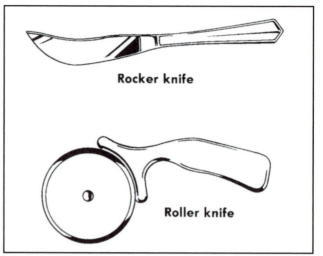

Figure 6-3. Adapted knives.

include amputation or traumatic injury to an upper extremity such as fracture of the wrist, arm, or shoulder or neurological involvement from orthopedic problems in the cervical or thoracic spine. The most difficult eating problem is cutting meat with one hand. Figure 6-3 is an example of a *rocker knife* and a *roller knife*. The rocking motion helps to cut through meat; however, for those who have difficulty mastering the rocking motion, a rolling device may be used (with a sufficient guard over the cutting wheel).

Another problem is buttering bread. Provision of a suctioned board with a low rim around the edge to prevent sliding of the bread may be helpful as shown in Figure 6-4.

Individuals who have suffered a stroke may have hemianopsia, a visual problem that prevents them from seeing objects on one side of their visual field. They cannot see food in dishes placed to their hemianopsic side, so items should be placed in their field of vision. Patients should also be taught to "scan"

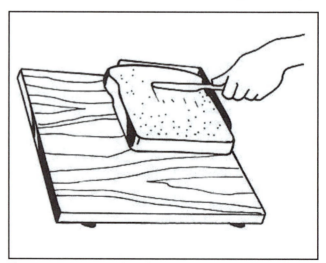

Figure 6-4. Buttering board. Corner keeps bread from sliding.

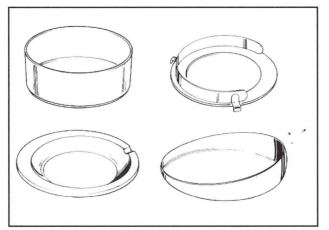

Figure 6-5. Scoop plates.

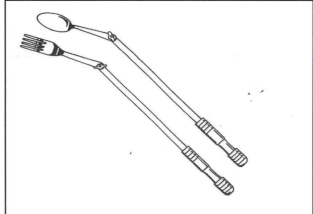

Figure 6-6. Extension utensils.

their plates by turning their head to compensate for the visual field loss.

Another complication may be a degree of poor coordination in the "good" upper extremity. This can affect dexterity (eg, if a patient is right handed and trying to use his or her left extremity for feeding). This problem and related ones can be solved by use of a *scoop dish* or *food guard*. Figure 6-5 demonstrates some possible lipped plates and food guards available on the market.

Assistive Devices for Limitations in Range of Motion

The most prevalent condition interfering with eating that affects range of motion is contractures from severe rheumatoid arthritis. Limitations in shoulders, elbows, wrists, hands, and neck may interfere with movement patterns. Painful movement may also impede motion for eating. The use of *extension utensils* (as shown in Figure 6-6) may assist the individual in compensating for limitations

in range. They are somewhat awkward to use and require practice. The plate should be secured using a nonskid surface such as Dycem or other available rubber surfaces. A scoop dish (as shown in Figure 6-5) is also a helpful adjunct to assisting the person using extension utensils.

Grasp may be a problem with limitations in range or associated disuse weakness, deformities, or painful grasp. The use of *built-up handles* or soft, lightweight materials such as *tubular foam* can be easily adapted to alleviate the problem of holding small, flat silverware. Figure 6-7 shows some examples of prefabricated built-up handles or modification of existing flatware with tubular foam.

When neck range of motion is limited in extension, the individual is unable to tip the head back far enough to drink fluids. *Cut-out plastic glasses* (as shown in Figure 6-8) fit around the nose so that the glass, rather than the neck, can be tipped back to allow liquid to flow into the mouth. Straws are also a convenient means of accommodating for limitations in cervical extension.

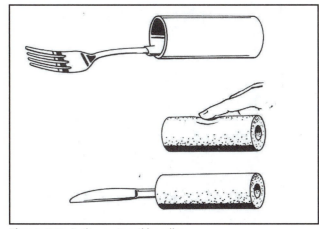

Figure 6-7. Built-up utensil handles.

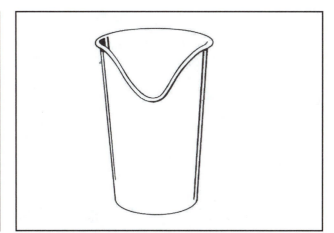

Figure 6-8. Cut-out plastic glass.

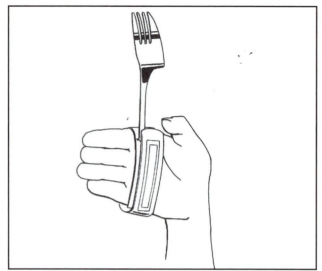

Figure 6-9. Utensil holder.

Assistive Devices for Muscle Weakness

Inability to grasp as a result of extreme muscle weakness prohibits the holding of eating utensils and glasses. Many products are available to address this feeding problem. A *utensil holder* (as seen in Figure 6-9) provides a simple strap with a pocket to

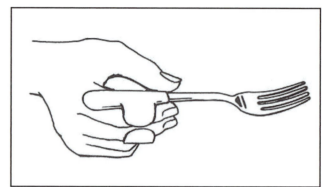

Figure 6-10. Finger ring utensil holder.

hold the eating utensil. The biggest problem with this sort of modification is that the palm must be held in pronation (palm down) or food will spill off of the utensil. *Finger ring* utensils (Figure 6-10) are often a good solution to this problem. The rings are fitted around 2 or more fingers and permit eating in a midposition (thumbs up). Utensils (Figures 6-11A and 6-11B), can be fitted using both *horizontal* and *vertical handles,* allowing an individual to choose the eating position that works best for him or her.

If a slight grasp is present, a *light-weight built-up handle* (see Figure 6-7) allows the person to strengthen the muscles of the hand while using the device. Sometimes a natural tenodesis (closure of the hand with wrist extension) action can be obtained by slightly extending the wrist to initiate grasp. Another method for weak grasp is providing built-up handles on utensils as demonstrated in Figure 6-12. An individual with significant loss of grasp can also weave a flat utensil handle between the fingers to provide natural support and stability of the feeding utensils.

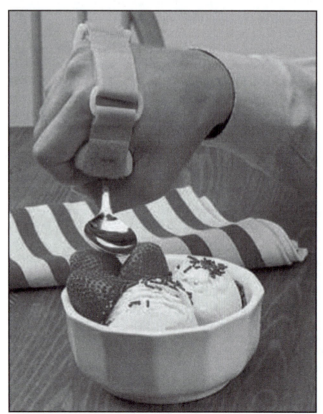

Figure 6-11A. Horizontal utensil handles.

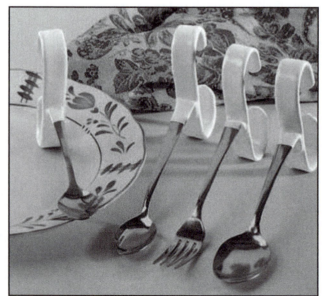

Figure 6-11B. Vertical utensil handles.

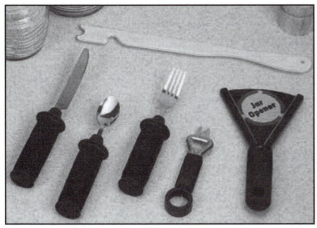

Figure 6-12. Arthritis utensil kitchen kit.

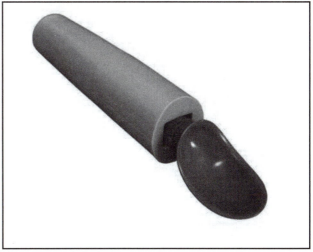

Figure 6-13. Swivel tremor spoons.

Swivel utensils allow the silverware to stay level when there is limited or absent pronation or supination of the forearm (see Figure 6-13).

If an individual is too weak to lift a drinking vessel, the use of *long straws* is helpful. There are straws available that have a large diameter for drinking soups and thicker substances. Accessories such as *support bases* and *straw holders* to secure the cup or glass and position the straw are also helpful. Rotating bases not only secure the vessel but allow the individual to push the straw away from his or her face (see Figure 6-14 for an example). For individuals with moderate weakness, lightweight *2-handled cups* make it possible to lift a drinking vessel with both hands (see Figure 6-15). *Large-handled* or *special-shaped* cups (Figure 6-16) also

provide greater ease of management of glasses and cups when grasp is weak. *Clamp-on handles* (see Figure 6-16) also allow any beverage can, bottle, or glass to be modified.

Assistive Devices for Poor Coordination

In the presence of tremors, spasticity, and uneven jerky movements seen in many neurological disorders, the problem is not strength but the lack of smooth, purposeful movement that results in spills. This is very frustrating for the individual trying to consume a meal. Neuromuscular facilitation techniques need to be employed to gain smoother, more coordinated control of the muscles involved. *Weighted utensils* (Figure 6-17) are often helpful in decreasing extraneous upper extremity movement.

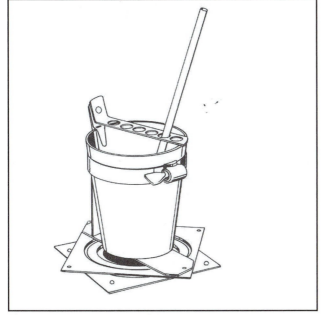

Figure 6-14. Long straw and cup accessories.

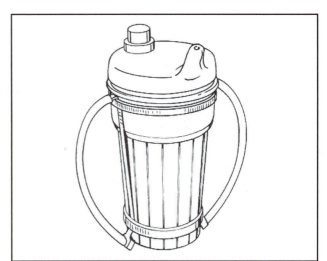

Figure 6-15. Two-handled cup.

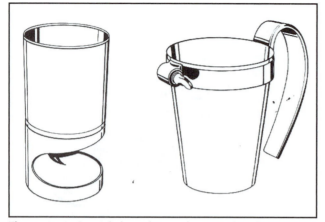

Figure 6-16. Special-shaped cups/clamps on handles.

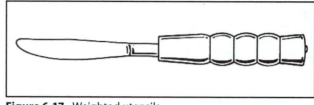

Figure 6-17. Weighted utensils.

Weighting the wrists with cuff weights also helps to diminish shaking and tremors. Scoop dishes, lipped plates, and food guards (see Figure 6-5) are useful adjuncts for the individual with coordination problems. *Suction cup dishes* or *suction cup pads* (Figure 6-18) help to decrease sliding of the plate when motion is difficult to control. It is also advisable that unbreakable dishes be used in the event that a plate is unintentionally relocated from the table to the floor.

With poor coordination, a *covered cup* or glass is helpful in preventing spillage of liquids (Figure 6-19). A *long, soft, flexible plastic straw* is also a great way to accommodate for exaggerated head and neck motion. This aids in preventing injury to the face or mouth as may be the case when a rigid straw is used.

Biting problems often result in the inability to remove food from a utensil without biting it and causing injury to the mouth or broken teeth. A *plastic coated spoon* or a *rubber spoon* (Figure 6-20) can prevent such injury. A regular utensil can be dipped in *Platisol* and baked in an oven to cure the coating, although

this coating is not permanent and eventually will wear down so it needs to be monitored for breakdown.

Problems in chewing or swallowing due to poor coordination are best dealt with through a comprehensive program of neuromuscular re-education as described in the previous section of this chapter. Some of the goals include controlling drooling, developing a better sucking reflex, and developing better swallowing and chewing patterns. Often, persons with these problems can be fed soft foods or liquids by squirting them into the back of the mouth with condiment dispensers (Figure 6-21). The presence of food in the back of the mouth facilitates swallowing. The use of ice chips also will decrease the gag reflex and prevent choking by diminishing the intensity of this reflex.

Assistive Devices With Visual Problems

Individuals who are blind can be trained to use the clockwise method of locating food. Food guards or scoop dishes (see Figure 6-5) are helpful in preventing food from being pushed off the plate.

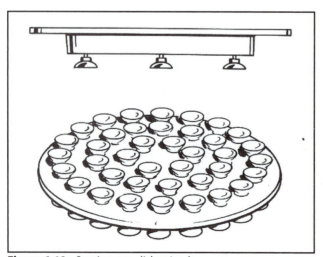

Figure 6-18. Suction cup dishes/pads.

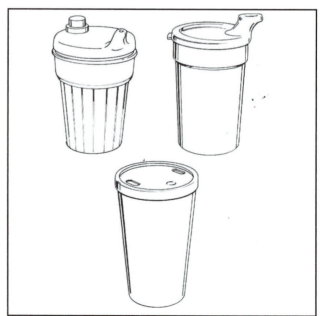

Figure 6-19. Covered cups.

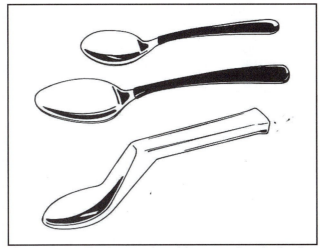

Figure 6-20. Plastic-coated, rubber-coated soft feeding spoons.

Independence in eating is a basic human drive that can be facilitated in elderly persons with physical disabilities by appropriate evaluation and treatment. If restoration of the disability is only partial, independence in eating still can be accomplished by accurately selecting specific assistive devices that enhance the utilization of remaining functional capabilities. Most conditions involving one-handedness, limitation in range of motion, weakness, poor coordination, or a combination of these have a device or group of devices that can provide a functional solution to the particular problem.

CONCLUSION

As America ages, the older population becomes increasingly diverse. Variation in the type and severity of diseases and conditions that present for care

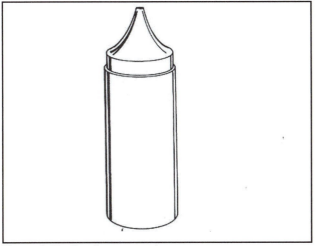

Figure 6-21. Condiment container.

intensifies. Diagnosis and treatment become considerably more complex. A thoughtful approach to the interplay among factors contributing to each individual's state of health and the careful balancing of the provision of health care options is needed to ensure the delivery of appropriate, cost-effective health care for all.

Malnutrition is a frequent and serious problem in the elderly. Malnutrition contributes significantly to morbidity and mortality in the elderly. The routine provision of nutrition screening and intervention will enhance disease management and outcome, and positively impact each older person's health and quality of life. Implementation of the minimum recommendations regarding nutritional screening and intervention will help to ensure consistency in the level and quality of nutritional care provided by multiple disciplines across the continuum of settings through which older persons access care. Adequate nutrition is considered central to the maintenance of good health, the slowing of degenerative changes, and support of the capacities elders need to live active, satisfying lives. A partnership between nutritionists and rehabilitation therapists is a crucial step toward enhancing health, rather than treating the disease after functional manifestations have appeared. What is now known about nutrition, aging, and rehabilitation needs to be advanced to the forefront. Health promotion and disease prevention can delay, or potentially eliminate, chronic disorders and the so-called "inevitable" aging process.

PEARLS

- The age-related changes in the GI system, such as decreased saliva, a decline in the sense of taste and smell, and a decrease in esophageal mobility and intestinal motility will have the most effect on nutrition in the elderly.

- General deconditioning from inactivity and bed rest is a primary factor affecting nutritional intake and directly impacts functional capabilities.

- Many chronic conditions, such as Alzheimer's disease, cerebrovascular accident, and diabetes mellitus, lead to nutritional difficulties.

- Most significant GI changes that accompany advancing age lead to decreased metabolism, resulting in a decrease in energy requirement.

- A decrease in energy required to meet metabolic demands at rest is a reflection of the attempt to maintain a homeostatic body weight and compensate for energy expenditure from physical activity.

- The component that most affects energy needs is muscle protein.

- Nutrients that make up a well-balanced diet include protein, carbohydrates, fat, water, water-soluble vitamins, fat-soluble vitamins, and minerals.

- There are subtle signs of malnutrition that occur in the skin, eyes, and oral mucosa.

  o Dry, thin, and easily plucked hair or flaky skin is suspect for chronic protein malnutrition.

  o Fissures around the mouth or tongue may be indicative of water-soluble vitamin deficiencies.

  o Sensitivity to light, white spots or swelling of the gums, and gooseflesh are indicative of vitamin A deficiency.

- Limitations on physical activity caused by chronic conditions reduce energy needs.

- Frequent use of medications by the elderly increases their vulnerability to malnutrition.

- Drugs may affect nutritional status by affecting appetite, making eating much less gratifying for an older individual.

- Dysphagia may be one of the most important conditions leading to feeding disabilities.

- A swallowing disorder can lead to aspiration and malnutrition.

- One-handedness, limitations in joint range, muscle weakness, poor coordination, and visual problems can lead to difficulties with eating.

- Many adaptive or assistive feeding devices will allow an elderly individual to be more independent in feeding him- or herself.

REFERENCES

1. Novak D. Nutrition in early life: how important is it? *Clin Perinatol.* 2002;29:203-223.

2. White House Conference on Aging. Nutrition and Aging. *Health Care Food Nutr Focus.* 2006;23:1,3-5.

3. Bates CJ, Benton D, Biesalski HK, et al. Nutrition and aging: a consensus statement. *J Nutri Health Aging.* 2002;6:103-116.

4. Krassie J, Toberts DC. The independent older Australian: implications for food and nutrition recommendations. *J Nutr Health Aging.* 2001;5:11-16.

5. O'Neill PS, Wellman NS, Himburg SP, Johnson P, Elfenbien P. Aging in community nutrition, diet therapy, and nutrition and aging textbooks. *Gerontol Geriatr Educ.* 2005;25:65-83.

6. Bales CW, Ritchie CS. Sarcopenia, weight loss, and nutritional frailty in the elderly. *Annu Rev Nutr.* 2002;22:309-323.

7. Kuczmarski MF, Weddle DO. Position paper of the American Dietetic Association: nutrition across the spectrum of aging. *J Am Diet Assoc.* 2005;105:616-633.

8. Evans WJ. Protein nutrition, exercise and aging. *J Am Coll Nutr.* 2004;23(suppl 6):601S-609S.

9. Samokhvalov V, Ignatiov V, Kondrashova M. Reserve carbohydrates maintain the viability of Saccharomyces cerevisiae cells during chronological aging. *Mech Ageing Dev.* 2004;125:229-235.

10. Archer VE. Does dietary sugar and fat influence longevity? *Med Hyptheses.* 2003;60:924-929.

11. Ahluwalia N. Aging, nutrition and immune function. *J Nutr Health Aging.* 2004;8:2-6.

12. Drewnowski A, Warren-Mears VA. Does aging change nutrition requirements? *J Nutr Health Aging.* 2001;5:70-74.

13. Drewnowski A, Shultz JM. Impact of aging on eating behaviors, food choices, nutrition, and health status. *J Nutr Health Aging.* 2001;5:75-79.

14. Guigoz Y Lauque S, Vellas BJ. Identifying the elderly at risk for malnutrition: the mini nutritional assessment. *Clin Geriatr Med.* 2002;18:737-757.

15. Chen CC, Schilling LS, Lyder CH. A concept analysis of malnutrition in the elderly. *J Adv Nurs.* 2001;36:131-142.

16. Stratton RJ, King CL, Stroud MA, Jackson AA, Elia M. Malnutrition universal screening tool predicts mortality and length of hospital stay in acutely ill elderly. *Br J Nutr.* 2006;95:325-330.

17. Wallace JI, Schwartz RS. Epidemiology of weight loss in humans with special reference to wasting in the elderly. *Int J Cardiol.* 2002;85:15-21.

18. Ledikwe JH, Blanck HM, Kettel Khan L, et al. Dietary energy density is associated with energy intake and weight status in US adults. *Am J Clin Nutr.* 2006;83:1362-1368.

19. Krieger JW, Sitren HS, Daniels MJ, Langkamp-Henken B. Effects of variation in protein and carbohydrate intake on body mass and composition during energy restriction: a meta-regression. *Am J Clin Nutr.* 2006;83:260-274.

20. de Graaf C. Effects of snacks on energy intake: an evolutionary perspective. *Appetite.* 2006;47:18-23.

21. Von Haehling S, Genth-Zoth S, Anker SD, Volk HD. Cachexia: a therapeutic approach. *Int J Cardiol.* 2002;85:173-183.

22. Devine A, Dhaliwal SS, Dick IM, Bollerslev J, Prince RL. Physical activity and calcium consumption in the elderly. *Asia Pac J Clin Nutr.* 2004;13(suppl):S133.

23. Gennari C. Calcium and vitamin D nutrition and bone disease of the elderly. *Public Health Nutr.* 2001;4:547-559.

24. Fleming DJ, Jacques PF, Tucker KL, et al. Iron status of the free-living, elderly Framingham Heart Study cohort: an iron-deplete population with a high prevalence of elevated iron stores. *Am J Clin Nutr.* 2001;73:638-646.

25. Joosten E, Van Loon R, Billen J, Blanckaert N, Fabri R, Pelemans W. Serum transferring receptor in the evaluation of the iron status in elderly hospitalized patients with anemia. *Am J Hematol.* 2002;69:1-6.

26. Meertens L, Solano L. Vitamin B_{12}, folic acid and mental function in the elderly. *Invest Clin.* 2005;46:53-63.

27. Clarke R, Grimley Evans J, Schneede J, et al. Vitamin B_{12} and folate deficiency in later life. *Age Ageing.* 2004;33:34-41.

28. Malouf M, Grimley EJ, Areosa SA. Folic acid with or without vitamin B_{12} cognition and dementia. *Cochrane Database Syst Rev.* 2003;CD004514.

29. Moller P, Viscovich M, Lykkesfeldt J, Loft S, Jensen A, Poulsen HE. Vitamin C supplement decreases oxidative DNA damage in mononuclear blood cells of smokers. *Eur J Nutr.* 2004;43:267-274.

30. Bader N, Bosy-Westphal A, Koch A, Mueller MJ. Influence of vitamin C and E supplementation on oxidative stress induced by hyperbaric oxygen in healthy men. *Ann Nurt Metab.* 2006;50:173-176.

31. Navarro A, Gomez C, Sanchez-Pino MJ, et al. Vitamin E at high doses improves survival, neurological performance, and brain mitochondrial function in aging male mice. *Am J Physiol Regul Integr Comp Physiol.* 2005;289:R1392-R1399.

32. Landmark K. Could intake of vitamins C and E inhibit development of Alzheimer dementia? *Tidsskr Nor Laegeforen.* 2006;126:159-161.

33. Aguilera A, Bajo MA, del Peso G, et al. True deficiency of antioxidant vitamins E and A in dialysis patients. Relationship with clinical patterns of atherosclerosis. *Adv Perit Dial.* 2002;18:206-211.

34. Bogden JD. Influence of zinc on immunity in the elderly. *J Nutr Health Aging.* 2004;8:48-54.

35. Mocchegiani E, Costarelli L, Giacconi R, et al. Zinc homeostasis in aging: two elusive faces of the same "metal." *Rejuvenation Res.* 2006;9:351-354.

36. Flinn JM, Hunter D, Linkous DH, et al. Enhanced zinc consumption causes memory deficits and increased brain levels of zinc. *Physiol Behav.* 2005;83:793-803.

37. Musci G Persichini T, Casadei M, et al. Nitrosative/oxidative modifications and ageing. *Mech Ageing Dev.* 2006;127:544-551.

38. Harless W, Crowell E, Abraham J. Anemia and neutropenia associated with copper deficiency of unclear etiology. *Am J Hematol.* 2006;81:546-549.

39. Squitti R, Barbati G, Rossi L, et al. Excess of nonceruloplasmin serum copper in AD correlates with MMSE,CSF(beta)-amyloid, and h-tau. *Neurology.* 2006;67:76-82.

40. Leiper JB, Seonaid Primrose C, Primrose WR, Phillimore J, Maughan RJ. A comparison of water turnover in older people in community and institutional settings. *J Nutr Health Aging.* 2005;9:189-193.

41. Natsume O. A clinical investigation of nocturnal polyuria in patients with nocturia: a diurnal variation in arginine vasopressin secretion and its relevance to mean blood pressure. *J Urol.* 2006;176:660-664.

42. Stookey JD, Pieper CF, Cohen HJ. Is the prevalence of dehydration among community-dwelling older adults really low? Informing current debate over the fluid recommendation for adults aged 70+ years. *Public Health Nutr.* 2005;8:1275-1285.

43. Bailey DN, Briggs JR. The effect of parenteral nutrition fluids on the binding of therapeutic drugs to human serum in vitro. *Ther Drug Monit.* 2004;26:31-34.

44. Shineha R. Current topics of nutrition–new goods and drugs. *Nippon Rinsho.* 2001;59(suppl):943-944.

45. Finfgeld-Connett DL. Self-management of alcohol problems among aging adults. *J Gerontol Nurs.* 2005;31:51-58.

46. Krause N. Race, religion, and abstinence from alcohol in late life. *J Aging Health.* 2003;15:508-533.

APPENDIX

Observations of Feeding Ability

A. Sucking

- Does patient choke when sucking? _____
- Can patient suck through a straw? _____
- Is there adequate lip closure?_____
- Does food or liquid drool from the mouth during the sucking process?_____

B. Swallowing

- Is swallowing done automatically and involuntarily?_____
- Can patient swallow when asked?_____
- Does patient drool?_____
- Does the mouth remain "gaped" open when patient is relaxed? _____
- What foods can patient swallow most easily?_____
- What foods are difficult to swallow? _____
- Is there any difference in ability to swallow liquids, semisolid foods, or solid foods?_____
- Is there any difference between thin and thick liquid?_____

C. Biting
- Does patient bite the spoon?_____
- Can patient bite voluntarily?_____
- Can patient open mouth voluntarily after biting?_____
- Does patient pull food off the spoon with his or her lips?_____

D. Chewing
- Does patient chew automatically?_____
- Is there tongue thrust during chewing?_____
- Does patient suck rather than chew?_____
- Is there a deficiency of tongue movement in chewing?_____
- Can patient transfer food from one side of the mouth to the other side? _____
- Is there rotary movement in the tongue and jaw during chewing? _____
- Does food get stuck in the palatal arch?_____
- What foods can patient chew? _____
- Can patient chew gum?_____
- Condition of teeth:_____

E. Related Behaviors
- Can patient bring hands or fingers to mouth?_____
- Can patient using feeding utensils?_____
- Can patient cut meat?_____
- Can patient butter bread?_____
- Can patient open wrappers?_____
- Does patient drink from a cup?_____
- Can patient hold a cup/glass/carton?_____
- Is the face and/or oral region sensitive to touch?_____
- Does patient make any abnormal facial expressions when feeding? _____
- Can patient sit upright during feeding?_____ How long?_____
- Does patient have visual problems?_____
- Does patient have hearing problems?_____
- Can patient locomote self to dining room?_____
  - Ambulatory?_____ Distance?_____
  - Wheelchair locomotion?_____
- Can patient communicate?_____ How?_____
- Is patient confused/disoriented?_____
- Does patient use adaptive equipment (ie, shoulder support slings, wrist support splints, built-up handle utensils)?
  Specify: _____

Section II

Care of the Geriatric Patient

Drugs and Function in the Elderly

Older people require special consideration where medications are concerned. Advanced age brings changes that may alter how an older individual reacts to medicines. An impaired digestive system may interfere with drug absorption. Declines in liver and kidney function may decrease the ability to metabolize and remove drugs, which can lead to toxic drug levels. As a person ages, the ability to maintain a steady state (or homeostasis) decreases. In addition, an older person may have a higher sensitivity to medications, leading to adverse reactions even in normal drug doses. If aging causes a decline in understanding, memory, vision, or coordination, patients may not use drugs safely and effectively. Adverse reactions to drugs occur 3 times more frequently in the older population. An unwanted drug response can change an independent older person into a confused nonfunctional patient. For these reasons, it is important for the PTA to understand and consider the individual's health and tolerances to drugs and to be aware of possible side effects that the older adult might experience.

This chapter looks at the difference in drug usage and effects in the elderly. Polypharmacy, multipharmacy, and general information related to drug prescription in older people are provided, including behavioral issues that are often masked by prescription medications. Dosages and prescription management are discussed and problems specific to drug usage in the elderly are presented. The problems inherent in mixing drugs with alcohol and multiple over-the-counter medication, herbs, and vitamins are also discussed as they relate to functional abilities, cognitive performance, and adverse effects.[1] This chapter is intended to provide a user-friendly format for the PTA to refer to on a day-to-day basis, providing easy-to-read tables listing adverse effects of drugs and drugs commonly used in the elderly for various conditions and specific system effects. Each table gives the intended effects of each drug class, indication for use, functional ramifications, and side effects of medications used in the pharmaceutical management of elderly patients.

STATISTICS RELATED TO DRUG USE IN THE ELDERLY

Providing safe and effective drug therapy is one of the greatest challenges in the elderly. The elderly use more drugs than any other age group and have many chronic disorders that affect drug response. Acute or chronic disorders can further deplete the already diminished physiologic reserves of the elder, increasing his or her risk of adverse drug effects.

Aging alters *pharmacodynamics,* or how drugs affect the body and the individual's response to a drug at a given concentration.[2] An older individual may have a different physiologic and biomechanical response due to an alteration of drug action related to aging changes.[3] Additionally, *pharmacokinetics,* or how the body handles absorption, distribution, metabolism, and excretion, may affect the choice,

Bottomley J. *Geriatric Rehabilitation: A Textbook for the Physical Therapist Assistant* (pp 151-232).
© 2010 SLACK Incorporated

dosage, and frequency of drugs prescribed.[4] For the elderly, drug therapy may be further complicated because of cost and accessibility of the drugs. For example, elderly individuals will often decrease the recommended dosage in order to save money if they are on a limited budget.

People over the age of 65 use more drugs than any other age group in the US population. The prevalence of prescription drug use among ambulatory, community-dwelling adults increases substantially with advancing age. Among people over the age of 65, 90% use more than one drug per week, more than 40% use 5 or more drugs per week, and 12% use 10 or more drugs per week.[5] Over 75% of older adults receive a prescription for one or more drugs with each visit to a physician, and the medication is often the only treatment prescribed.[6] The elderly also purchase more over-the-counter drugs and herbal and vitamin compounds than any other age group in the United States.[7] Drug use is greatest among the frail elderly, hospitalized patients, and nursing home residents. A nursing home resident is typically given 7 to 8 different drugs on a daily basis.[8]

When prescribed and used appropriately, most drugs can benefit the elderly. Drugs are critical for the prevention and treatment of acute and chronic disorders. Many drugs directly modulate disease; others control symptoms that reduce quality of life. Nonetheless, the elderly are at substantial risk of having adverse drug reactions. Among ambulatory people over the age of 65, adverse events occur at a rate of about 50 events per 1000 persons per year. Nearly 30% of these events result from drug errors, predominantly in drug prescribing and monitoring, as well as lack of patient adherence.[9]

POLYPHARMACY

Although pharmacotherapy for the elderly can treat diseases and improve well-being, its benefits can be compromised by drug-related problems.[10] Unfortunately, the cure can become the disease. Patients who are cared for by several physicians may end up on several drugs prescribed separately by more than one doctor for the same condition or different disorders. Without appropriate communication between the patient, pharmacy, and prescribing physicians, adverse reactions are much more likely to occur. This frequent practice of visiting multiple physicians can lead to serious drug-drug interactions. The patient should routinely talk to each health care provider about all the drugs—both prescription and nonprescription—he or she is taking. It is also important that PTAs review the medications that each patient is on and be aware of potential side

effects and adverse reactions.[11] It is within the role of the PTA as patient advocate to encourage the patient or caregiver to create a list of all medications, including exact dosages. This list should be reviewed at each doctor's appointment and updated accordingly. The PTA should ask the patient or caregiver about any drug changes following each visit to the physician.

Although the terms *multipharmacy* and *polypharmacy* are often used interchangeably, the terms actually mean different things. Polypharmacy is the use of multiple drugs for the same condition (eg, taking more than one beta blocker or anti-inflammatory) whereas multipharmacy is the use of multiple drugs to treat multipathology and conditions associated with aging. In the elderly, it is not unusual to have a medically complex older person being treated for several conditions. The use of many drugs increases the risk of drug interactions as well as adverse reactions to the drugs and may affect patient compliance with physical therapy interventions.[12]

As previously discussed, advancing age brings changes that can alter how a person reacts to a prescribed medication; how drugs work in the body; the time required for drugs to be absorbed, distributed, and remain effective in the body; as well as how they are eliminated. Through the study of pharmacokinetics, we understand more about the interactions that determine specific drug effects as well as the individual diversity of different drug responses. Depending on several factors, including body weight, health, activity level, nutrition, and age, we all respond to drugs differently.[13]

AGING AND DRUG EFFECTS IN THE ELDERLY

The elderly are particularly more sensitive to the actions of many drugs. With age come changes in the digestive system that may alter the absorption of drugs. Liver function can make it harder for the body to break down (metabolize) and eliminate certain drugs. The aging changes in the circulatory and nervous systems may affect responsiveness to many drugs (see Chapter 3); changes in mental functioning may impact the ability of an older person to comply with directions for usage so that taking medicines according to instructions is more difficult.

With age, the changes in the nervous system show increased susceptibility to many commonly used drugs. Some drugs, such as the opioid analgesics, benzodiazepines, anti-psychotics, and anti-Parkinsonian drugs, must be used with caution as the older adult may be more reactive to the drug. Similarly, organs other than the liver may also be more susceptible to drugs, such as anti-hypertensives and nonsteroidal anti-inflammatory drugs (NSAIDs), which are discussed in greater detail later in this chapter.[14]

The most important effect of aging is the reduction in renal clearance, where excretion of the drug is slower, increasing liability to the effects of *nephrotoxic* (destructive or toxic to kidney cells) drugs. Acute illness exacerbates renal clearance, especially if accompanied by dehydration. Metabolism of the drug by the liver can also be reduced in the elderly, exacerbating the problems of clearing the drug from the system.

In elderly patients, drugs are used in many cases as a substitute for effective social or behavioral measures (ie, to control behavior). The complications of multiple drug use pose a serious threat from adverse reactions (eg, dizziness, confusion, or changes in muscle function, which is often the reason for falls). While unnecessary medication use should be avoided, elderly patients should not be denied effective treatments, such as those for the prevention of stroke in atrial fibrillation, insulin for diabetes, or drugs needed to treat the loss of bone mass in osteoporosis.[15]

The ability of an older adult to swallow a pill should also be considered. The form of medicine should be appropriate for effectiveness. For example, more fluid may be required to wash a tablet down, the tablet may need crushing, or the drug may need to be delivered in a liquid form. The ability to open containers also needs to be considered. Different containers exist to aid dispensing and concordance with medications (eg, dosage boxes, blister packs, screw-topped bottles). These often need to be requested specifically at the local pharmacy, but the patient or caregiver may not be aware that these options exist. Careful observation or noting comments by the patient regarding difficulty opening meds may present the opportunity for the PTA to discuss container options.

In the very old, manifestations of normal aging may be taken as signs of disease and lead to inappropriate prescribing. Self-medication with over-the-counter drugs, leftover tablets from a previous illness, or medicines from a relative or friend may also create a negative drug interaction, leading to safety issues and falls.

The net result of pharmacokinetic and pharmacodynamic changes is that the tissue concentration of a drug commonly increases by over 50% and debilitated patients may show an even larger change.[16] Adverse reactions can be vague and nonspecific such as confusion, constipation, hypotension, and falls. For all these reasons, it is vital that an older person's medication is reviewed regularly and maintained on the lowest dosage of a drug as possible to gain the desired effect. It will be crucial for the PTA to be a close observer of potential side effects of a patient's drugs. Since PTAs may be the clinician seeing the patient on a consistent basis, they may be the first to identify negative side effects to a new drug; the interaction of drugs; or the potential mixing of over-the-counter drugs, vitamins and herbs, and alcohol.[17]

Dosages and Monitoring Side Effects

Because physical changes make older people more sensitive to drugs, the elderly generally require lower doses to achieve the desired effects and to avoid toxic overdoses. Unfortunately, the side effects of drugs and the misuse and abuse of drugs are distinctly more serious problems in the elderly. Adverse reactions to medication occur frequently in older people and it is often more difficult for the elderly to eliminate their effects. It has been estimated that as many as 1 in 4 drugs administered to the elderly in skilled nursing facilities may be ineffective or unneeded. Compounding the problem, many elderly people use nonprescription drugs without the knowledge of their physician[18] and many misuse drugs by taking less than the prescribed dosage in a misguided attempt to reduce costs.

Particular drug problems occur more frequently in the elderly compared to younger individuals, and some drugs widely used by elderly people may present special concerns.[19] One example is that of diuretic drugs, which are commonly used because they reduce the amount of water in the body, an effect that ultimately reduces the workload of the heart and arteries. These "water pills" increase the flow of urine and are used to treat hypertension, heart failure, and other ailments common to older people; yet, they also cause a loss of potassium and other minerals from the body. A potassium deficiency will produce symptoms that range from weakness, listlessness, and a loss of appetite to an irregular heartbeat. A potassium deficiency can be resolved by reducing the dosage, changing the diuretic, or taking a potassium supplement. Many foods contain potassium, but it is difficult to increase the amount of dietary potassium by eating certain foods. Generally, problems of potassium depletion will require taking a potassium supplement to prevent or resolve the problem if the same diuretic is continued.[20]

Many older people receive antihypertension medications that may make them feel depressed, drowsy, or suddenly faint, especially when they try to stand up. The elderly are more likely to experience adverse effects from sedatives and tranquilizers. Barbiturates are particularly risky because they can cause severe mental confusion or even psychosis if taken to excess.

For example, benzodiazepine tranquilizers, taken in ease the nervousness and stress of everyday life, may also cause drowsiness, shakiness, and confusion in older people. If it is necessary for an older person to take a tranquilizer, the drug needs to be carefully prescribed and a dosage established that is lower than what is normally indicated for a younger person. It is vital that the older person, once prescribed a tranquilizer, be closely monitored for ill effects.

Digitalis medicines, prescribed to improve the strength and efficiency of the heart, also can be a serious problem for elderly individuals. Older people sometimes develop symptoms of toxicity from these drugs, including excessive fatigue, loss of appetite, vision problems, and psychological disturbances. These symptoms occur in the elderly because they are commonly given digitalis for longer periods and they do not eliminate the drug as readily as younger persons. Older persons sometimes will receive lower doses of digitalis medications because the medicine can accumulate to toxic levels over time.[21]

Mixing Drugs and Alcohol

In an effort to alleviate some of the age-related problems of loneliness and boredom that many elderly people face, some older people use drugs, such as alcohol, prescription drugs, and illegal (street) drugs. A National Institute of Drug Abuse[22] survey indicated that two-thirds of all persons over the age of 65 use prescription drugs and, except for cardiovascular medications, the most commonly used drugs were sedatives and tranquilizers. More than half of all the persons using tranquilizers and sedatives said they could not perform their daily activities without these drugs. In many cases, the abuse or misuse of a drug is purely unintentional; for example, when an individual attends a social event and mixes alcohol with his or her daily medications, he or she runs the risk of drug-alcohol interaction. The use of many drugs along with alcohol can cause harmful interactions.[23] Another example is the use of antidepressant medications, which when combined with alcohol, could cause dizziness, loss of consciousness, and falls. Many drugs will carry a label that indicates that the drug should not be mixed with alcohol. Even drugs such as over-the-counter cold and allergy medications are potentially negatively affected by alcohol consumption.

Misuse of Drugs in the Elderly

Perhaps the most common form of drug misuse in the elderly is multiple drug use. This involves taking too many drugs or inappropriately taking drugs that interact with each other. Elderly persons often have numerous symptoms or illnesses. Sometimes there is a tendency for each new symptom to result in a visit to the physician and a new prescription, all too frequently without sufficient regard to the schedule of medicine already being taken. This pattern can lead to a patient taking a surprising number of medicines, some of which may interact harmfully with each other.[24]

Often the older person expects a medicine for every new symptom. Sometimes a symptom can be resolved by reducing the dose of another medicine, reorganizing the schedule of medicine, or using a less harmful approach altogether, such as the use of ice to reduce pain and inflammation. With multiple drug use, it is hardly surprising that, in many instances, a person can get confused and take too little or too much of one or more drugs or experience unwanted side effects from drug interactions. Older people often need assistance in following drug therapies, especially if they have multiple diseases that require the correct use of several medicines each day. When the drugs are not taken as prescribed, they may be ineffective, and the mixing of certain medications may cause negative drug interactions, which are far more likely and more severe.[25]

CLASSES OF DRUGS

More elderly patients affected by severe and chronic diseases are treated in primary care and drugs are more likely to be prescribed than any other form of treatment. Throughout the tables in this chapter, drugs will be presented as various drug classes. Medicines in the same class often share important characteristics in their chemistry, how they work in the body, and even the problems or side effects they may cause. Any or all drugs in a given class can be expected to behave in a similar way. Each drug class is presented and lists the generic names in its class. Following each generic name, widely recognized brand names are provided in parentheses. Although a complete listing of all available drugs is not possible, these classes represent the elderly's most frequently used drug groups and brand names. Table 7-1 provides a listing of some of the most commonly prescribed medications.

Certain drugs are prescribed more frequently than others.[26] Table 7-2 provides an overview of the most commonly prescribed drug classes used by Medicare patients, and Table 7-3 provides the classes and defines each drug category most frequently used by older adults. These tables will assist the PTA in determining which drug groups are better at treating certain conditions in the elderly.

Table 7-1

CLASSES OF COMMONLY PRESCRIBED MEDICATIONS

DRUG CLASS	PURPOSE OF DRUGS	GENERIC (TRADE NAME EXAMPLES)	
ACE inhibitors *(angiotensin-converting enzyme)*	Used to reduce hypertension by blocking the angiotension enzyme; these drugs help to relax the arterial walls and reduce work of the heart	• Benazepril *(Lotensin)* • Enalapril *(Vasotec)* • Lisinopril *(Prinivil, Zestril)* • Perindopril *(Aceon)* • Ramipril *(Altace)* • Trandolapril *(Mavik)*	• Captopril *(Capoten)* • Fosinopril *(Monopril)* • Moexipril *(Univasc)* • Quinapril *(Accupril)* • Spirapril *(Renormax)*
Adrenocortical steroids *(cortisone-like drugs)*	Glucocorticoids involved in glucose metabolisms and the body's ability to deal with stress; decrease inflammation and suppress immune system response Mineralocorticoids maintain fluid and electrolyte balance	• Amcinonide *(Cyclocort)* • Budesonide *(Pulmincort)* • Dexamethasone *(Decadron)* • Flunisolide *(AeroBid, Nasarel)* • Glucocorticoids *(Cortisol, Corticosterone)* • Halcinonide *(Halog)* • Methylprednisolone *(Medrol)* • Prednisone *(Deltasone)*	• Betamethasone *(Celestone)* • Cortisone *(Cortone)* • Fludrocortisone *(Florinef)* • Fluorometholone *(FML)* • Hydrocortisone *(Cortef)* • Mineralocorticoids *(Aldosterone)* • Paramethasone *(Haldrone)* • Rimexolone *(Vexol)*
Aminoglycosides	Anti-infectives; anti-bacterial agents	• Amikacin *(Amikin)* • Kanamycin *(Kantrex)* • Netilmicin *(Netromycin)* • Streptomycin	• Gentamicin *(Garamycin)* • Neomycin • Paromomycin *(Humatin)* • Tobramycin *(Tobrex)*
Analgesics	Decrease mild to moderate pain; anti-inflammatory; decrease elevated body temperature; decrease blood clotting	• Acetaminophen *(Tylenol)* • Lidocaine cream *(Emla)* • Propoxyphene *(Darvon)* • Nonsteroidal anti-inflammatory drugs	• Aspirin • Morphine • Tramadol *(Ultram)*
Anti-Alzheimer's drugs	Drugs used to lighten affect, slow the progression of the disease, and delay onset; improve alertness; slow memory loss	• Donepezil *(Aricept)* • Ginkgo biloba • Rivastigmine *(Exelon)* • Vitamin E	• Galantamine • Metrifonate *(Bilarcil)* • Tacrine *(Cognex)*
Anti-anginal drugs	Dilate arteries to provide blood and oxygen to heart muscle; decrease pain produced by tissue ischemia; decrease chest pain	• Bepridil *(Vascor)* • Nicardipine *(Cardene)* • Nifedipine *(Adalat, Procardia)* • Nitrates	• Diltiazem *(Cardizem)* • Beta blockers • Verapamil *(Calan, Isoptin)*

(Continued)

Table 7-1 continued

CLASSES OF COMMONLY PRESCRIBED MEDICATIONS

DRUG CLASS	PURPOSE OF DRUGS	GENERIC (TRADE NAME EXAMPLES)	
Anti-anxiety drugs	Reduce anxiousness	• Benzodiazepines • Chlormezanone *(Trancopal)* • Hydroxyzine *(Atarax, Vistaril)* • Meprobamate *(Equanil)*	• Buspirone *(Buspar)* • Lorazepam *(Ativan)* • Paroxetine *(Paxil)*
Anti-arrhythmic drugs	Regulate heart rhythm	• Acebutolol *(Sectral)* • Amiodarone *(Cardarone)* • Digitoxin *(Crystodigin)* • Disopyramide *(Norpace)* • Flecainide *(Tambocor)* • Lidocaine *(Xylocaine)* • Procainamide *(Procan)* • Propranolol *(Inderal)* • Tocainide *(Tonocard)* • Verapamil *(Calan, Isoptin)*	• Adenosine *(Adenocard)* • Atenolol *(Tenormin)* • Digoxin *(Lanoxin)* • Dofetilide *(Tikosyn)* • Ibutilide *(Corvert)* • Mexiletine *(Mexitil)* • Propafenone *(Rythmol)* • Quinidine *(Quinaglute, Quinidex, Quinora)* • Sotalol *(Betapace)*
Anti-arthritic drugs	Reduce inflammation and pain associated with arthritis	• Aspirin • Chloroquine *(Aralen)* • Etanercept *(Enbrel)* • Leflunomide *(Arava)* • Penicillamine *(Cuprimine)* • NSAIDs	• Azathioprine *(Imuran)* • COX-II inhibitor family • Infliximab *(Remicade)* • Adrenocorticosteroids
Disease-modifying anti-rheumatics (DMARDs)	Reduce or slow the progression of arthritic changes	• Etanercept *(Enbrel)* • Methotrexate *(Rheumatrex)*	• Leflunomide *(Arava)*
Anti-asthmatic drugs *also called bronchodilators*	Reduce inflammation and spasm in bronchial tubes; can act as anti-leukotrienes	• Beclomethasone *(Beclovent, Vanceril)* • Flunisolide *(AeroBid)* • Triamcinolone *(Azmacort)* • Montelukast *(Singulair)* • Zileuton *(Zyflo)* • Albuterol *(Proventil, Ventolin)* • Bitolterol *(Tornalate)*	• Fluticasone *(Flovent)* • Ipratropium *(Atrovent)* • Ephedrine *(Efed II)* • Zafirlukast *(Accolate)* • Aminophylline *(Phyllocontin)* • Dyphylline *(Lufyllin)* • Epinephrine *(Adrenaline, Bronkaid, Primatene Mist)*

(Continued)

Table 7-1 continued

CLASSES OF COMMONLY PRESCRIBED MEDICATIONS

DRUG CLASS	PURPOSE OF DRUGS	GENERIC (TRADE NAME EXAMPLES)	
Anti-asthmatic drugs *(continued)*	Reduce inflammation and spasm in bronchial tubes; can act as anti-leukotrienes	• Isoetharine *(Bronkosol)* • Metaproterenol *(Alupent)* • Pirbuterol *(Maxair)* • Terbutaline *(Brethaire)*	• Isoproterenol *(Isuprel)* • Oxtriphylline *(Choledyl)* • Salmeterol *(Serevent)* • Theophylline *(Bronkodyl)*
ANTIBIOTICS/ANTI-INFECTIVES			
Cephalosporins	Anti-infective family of drugs (any generic name: Cefa-) that destroys bacteria and reduces its replication by producing protective cell walls	• Cefaclor *(Ceclor)* • Cefadroxil *(Duricef, Ultracef)* • Cefamandole *(Mandol)* • Cefazolin *(Ancef, Kefzol)*	• Cefatrizine *(Cefaperos)* • Cefdinir *(Omnicef)* • Moxalactam *(Moxam)* • Loracarbef *(Cefobid)*
Macrolide antibiotics	Anti-infective drugs that prevents organism growth by interfering with the formation of essential proteins	• Azithromycin *(Zithromax)* • Dirithromycin *(Dynabac)* • Erythromycin *(E-Mycin, Ilosone, Erythrocin, E.E.S)*	• Clarithromycin *(Biaxin)* • Troleandomycin *(TAO)*
Penicillins	Anti-infective family of drugs that destroys infecting bacteria	• Amoxicillin (Amoxil, Larotid) • Ampicillin *(Omnipen, Amoxicillin/Clavulanate, Polycillin, Principen, Tocillin)* • Ampicillin/Sulbactam *(Unasyn)* • Bacampicillin *(Spectrobid)* • Carbenicillin *(Geocillin, Pyopen)* • Dicloxacillin *(Dynapen, Pathocil)*	• Cloxacillin *(Cloxapen, Tegopen)* • Mezlocillin *(Mezlin)* • Oxacillin *(Prostaphlin)* • Penicillin V *(Pen Vee K)* • Ticarcillin *(Ticar)* • Methicillin *(Staphcillin)* • Nafcillin *(Nafcil, Unipen)* • Penicillin G *(Pentids)* • Piperacillin *(Pipracil)* • Ticarcillin/Clavulanate *(Timentin)*
Tetracyclines	Anti-infective family of drugs that prevents the growth and multiplication of organisms by interfering with formation of essential proteins	• Demeclocycline *(Declomycin)* • Methacycline *(Rondomycin)* • Oxytetracyline *(Terramycin)*	• Doxycycline *(Doryx)* • Minocycline *(Minocin)* • Tetracycline *(Sumycin, Achromycin V, Panmycin)*

(Continued)

Table 7-1 continued

CLASSES OF COMMONLY PRESCRIBED MEDICATIONS

DRUG CLASS	PURPOSE OF DRUGS	GENERIC (TRADE NAME EXAMPLES)	
Other anti-infective drug classes Amebicides Anti-fungal Anti-leprosy Anti-malarial Anti-tuberculosis Anti-viral Oxazolidinones			
Fluoroquinolones	Block the bacterial enzyme required for DNA synthesis and cell reproduction; arrest bacterial growth (in low dosage) and kill bacteria in larger doses	• Ciprofloxacin *(Cipro)* • Gatifloxacin *(Tequin)* • Levofloxacin *(Levaquin)* • Moxifloxacin *(Avelox)* • Ofloxacin *(Floxin)* • Trovafloxacin *(Trovan)*	• Fleroxacin *(Quinodis)* • Grepafloxacin *(Raxar)* • Lomefloxacin *(Maxaquin)* • Norfloxacin *(Noroxin)* • Sparfloxacin *(Zagam)*
Miscellaneous anti-infective drugs	Reduce infection by bacteria	• Atovaquone *(Mepron)* • Chloramphenicol *(Chloromycetin)* • Clindamycin *(Cleocin)* • Furazolidone *(Furoxone)* • Lincomycin *(Lincocin)* • Nalidixic Acid *(NegGram)* • Vancomycin *(Vancocin)*	• Colistin *(Coly-Mycin S)* • Linezolid *(Zyvox)* • Pentamidine *(Pentam 300)* • Nitrofurantoin *(Furadantin, Macrodantin)* • Novobiocin *(Albamycin)* • Trimethoprim *(Proloprim, Trimpex)*
Anti-cancer drugs	Chemotherapy drugs that block the genetic activity of cancerous cells, impairing reproduction; anti-neoplastics	• Chlorambucil *(Leukeran)* • Flutamide *(Eulexin)* • Liposomal Doxorubicin *(Evacet)* • Mercaptopurine *(Purinethol)*	• Cyclophosphamide *(Cytoxan)* • Hydroxyurea *(Hydrea)* • Tamoxifen *(Nolvadex)* • Methotrexate *(Rheumatrex)*
Anti-cholinergic drugs	Blocks the passage of impulses through the parasympathetic nerves (parasympatholytic)	• Atropine • Hyoscyamine • Anti-depressant drugs • Anti-Parkinsonism drugs • Muscle relaxants *(some)*	• Belladonna • Scopolamine • Anti-histimines *(some)* • Anti-spasmodics *(some)*
Anti-coagulant drugs	Prevent clotting of blood	• Anisindione *(Miradon)* • Warfarin *(Coumadin)*	• Discumarol
Blood flow agents	Enhance circulation in peripheral vascular diseases	• Cilostazol *(Pletal)* • Pentoxifylline *(Trental)*	• Ginkgo biloba *(various)*

(Continued)

Table 7-1 continued

CLASSES OF COMMONLY PRESCRIBED MEDICATIONS

DRUG CLASS	PURPOSE OF DRUGS	GENERIC (TRADE NAME EXAMPLES)	
Anti-convulsant drugs	Reduce and prevent epileptic seizures	• Acetazolamide *(Diamox)* • Carbamazepine *(Tegretol)* • Clorazepate *(Tranxene)* • Ethosuximide *(Zarontin)* • Felbamate *(Felbatol)* • Lamotrigine *(Lamictal)* • Paramethadione *(Paradione)* • Phenacemide *(Phenurone)* • Phensuximide *(Milontin)* • Primidone *(Mysoline)* • Trimethadione *(Tridione)*	• Clonazepam *(Klonopin)* • Diazepam *(Valium)* • Ethotoin *(Peganone)* • Gabapentin *(Neurontin)* • Levetiracetam *(Keppra)* • Mephenytoin *(Mesantoin)* • Methsuximide *(Celontin)* • Oxcarbazepine *(Trileptal)* • Phenobarbital *(Luminal)* • Phenytoin *(Dilantin)* • Topiramate *(Topamax)* • Valproic Acid *(Depakene)*
ANTI-DEPRESSANT DRUGS			
Bicyclic anti-depressants	Reduce the symptoms of depression	• Fluoxetine *(Prozac)*	• Venlafaxine *(Effexor)*
Tetracyclic anti-depressants	Reduce the symptoms of depression	• Maprotiline *(Ludiomil)*	• Mirtazapine *(Remeron)*
Tricyclic anti-depressants	Reduce the symptoms of depression	• Amitriptyline *(Elavil, Endep)* • Clomipramine *(Anafranil)* • Desipramine *(Norpramin)* • Doxepin *(Adapin, Sinequan)*	• Amoxapine *(Asendin)* • Imipramine *(Tofranil)* • Protriptyline *(Vivactil)* • Nortriptyline *(Aventyl, Pamelor)* • Trimipramine *(Surmontil)*
Other anti-depressants	Reduce the symptoms of depression	• Bupropion *(Wellbutrin)* • Hypericum *(St. John's wort)* • Paroxetine *(Paxil)* • Trazodone *(Desyrel)*	• Fluvoxamine *(Luvox)* • Nefazodone *(Serzone)* • Sertraline *(Zoloft)* • Monoamine oxidase (MAO) inhibitors
ANTI-DIABETIC DRUGS			
Oral alpha-glucoside inhibitors	Assist in balancing glucose and insulin levels	• Acarbose *(Precose)*	• Miglitol *(Glyset)*
Oral biguanides	Assist in balancing glucose and insulin levels	• Metformin *(Glucophage)*	
Oral meglitinides	Assist in balancing glucose and insulin levels	• Repaglinide *(Prandin)*	

(Continued)

Table 7-1 continued

CLASSES OF COMMONLY PRESCRIBED MEDICATIONS

DRUG CLASS	PURPOSE OF DRUGS	GENERIC (TRADE NAME EXAMPLES)	
Oral sulfonylureas	Assist in balancing glucose and insulin levels	• Acetohexamide (Dymelor) • Chlorpropamide (Diabinese) • Glipizide (Glucotrol) • Glyburide (DiaBeta, Micronase)	• Glimepiride (Amaryl) • Tolazamide (Ronase, Tolinase • Tolbutamide (Orinase)
Oral thiazolidinediones	Assist in balancing glucose and insulin levels	• Pioglitazone (Actos)	• Rosiglitazone (Avandia)
Injectable anti-diabetic drugs	Assist in balancing glucose and insulin levels	• Insulin	
Oral spray	Assist in balancing glucose and insulin levels	• Insulin (Oralgen)	
Anti-diarrhea drugs	Assistn in solidifying bowel, movements decrease runny stool and abdominal cramping	• Loperaminde (Imodium)	
Anti-emetric drugs	Reduce nausea; anti-motionsickness drugs; often used to treat vestibular problems	• Chlorpormazine (Thorazine) • Dimenhydrinate (Dramamine) • Diphenhydramine (Benadryl) • Hydroxyzine (Atarax, Vistaril) • Meclizine (Antivert, Bonine)	• Cyclizine (Marezine) • Granisetron (Kytril) • Ondansetron (Zofran) • Prochlorperazine (Compazine) • Promethazine (Phenergan) • Scopolamine (Transderm Scop) • Trimethobenzamide (Tigan)
Anti-fungal drugs	Reduce growth of fungus	• Amphotericin B (Fungizone) • Fluconazole (Diflucan) • Griseofulvin (Fulvicin, Grisactin) • Ketoconazole (Nizoral) • Miconazole (Monistat) • Nystatin (Mycostatin)	• Butenafine (Mentax) • Flucytosine (Ancobon) • Itraconazole (Sporanox) • Lipid Amphotericin B (Abelcet) • Terbinafine (Lamisil) • Tioconazole (Vagistat-1)

(Continued)

Table 7-1 continued

CLASSES OF COMMONLY PRESCRIBED MEDICATIONS

DRUG CLASS	PURPOSE OF DRUGS	GENERIC (TRADE NAME EXAMPLES)	
Anti-glaucoma drugs	Reduce the symptoms of glaucoma and slow structural damage to the eye	• Acetazolamide *(Diamox)* • Brimonidine *(Alphagan)* • Dipivefrin *(Propine)* • Dorzolamide *(Cosopt, Trusopt)* • Latanoprost *(Xalatan)* • Metipranolol *(Optipranolol)*	• Betaxolol *(Betoptic)* • Brinzolamide *(Azopt)* • Epinephrine *(Glaucon)* • Levobunolol *(Betagan)* • Pilocarpine *(Pilocar)* • Timolol *(Betimol, Timoptic, Timoptic-XE)*
Anti-gout drugs	Decrease inflammation and discomfort of joints affected by gout	• Allopurinol *(Zyloprim)* • Diclofenac *(Cataflam, Voltaren)* • Ibuprofen *(Advil, Motrin, Nuprin)* • Indomethacin *(Indocin)* • Ketoprofen *(Orudis)* • Mefenamic Acid *(Ponstel)* • Sulfinpyrazone *(Anturane)*	• Colchicine • Fenoprofen *(Nalfon)* • Piroxicam *(Feldene)* • Sulindac *(Clinoril)* • Naproxen *(Anaprox, Naprosyn)* • Oxaprozin *(Daypro)* • Probenecid *(Benemid)*
Anti-histamine drugs	Block histamine, stopping symptoms such as swelling and itching of the eyes Nonsedating or minimally sedating	• Azatadine *(Optimine)* • Brompheniramine *(Dimetane)* • Chlorpheniramine *(Chlor-Trimeton, Sudahist, Teldrin)* • Cyclizine *(Marezine)* • Cyproheptadine *(Periactin)* • Diphenhydramine *(Benadryl)* • Hydroxyzine *(Atarax)* • Meclizine *(Antivert, Bonine)* • Pheniramine *(part of Triaminic)* • Pyrilamine *(part of Triaminic)*	• Azelastine *(Astelin)* • Carbinoxamine *(Clistin)* • Cetirizine *(Zyrtec)* • Clemastine *(Tavist)* • Doxylamine *(Unisom)* • Loratadine *(Claritin)* • Orphenadrine *(Norflex)* • Fexofenadine *(Allegra)* • Promethazine *(Phenergan)* • Tripelennamine *(Pyribenzamine, PBZ)* • Triprolidine *(Actifed)*

(Continued)

Table 7-1 continued

CLASSES OF COMMONLY PRESCRIBED MEDICATIONS

DRUG CLASS	PURPOSE OF DRUGS	GENERIC (TRADE NAME EXAMPLES)	
Anti-hypertensive drugs *Also see other classes:* *ACE inhibitors* *Beta blockers* *Calcium channel blockers* *Diuretics*	Decrease systemic blood pressure	• Amlodipine/Benazepril *(Lotrel)* • Bisoprolol/ Hydrochlorothiazide *(Ziac)* • Clonidine *(Catapres)* • Enalapril/Felodipine *(Lexxel)* • Guanethidine *(Ismelin)* • Hydralazine *(Apresoline)* • Hydrochlorothiazide Benazepril *(Lotensin)*	• Carvedilol *(Coreg)* • Doxazosin *(Cardura)* • Guanabenz *(Wytensin)* • Guanfacine *(Tenex)* • Minoxidil *(Loniten)* • Reserpine *(Serpasil)* • Methyldopa *(Aldomet)* • Prazosin *(Minipress)* • Terazosin *(Hytrin)*
Anti-osteoporotic drugs	Increase and/or stabilize bone mineral mass	• Alendronate *(Fosamax)* • Calcitonin *(Miacalcin)* • Estrogen *(various brands)* • Risedronate *(Actonel)*	• Anti-estrogens *(SERMs)* • Calcium *(various)* • Raloxifene *(Evista)* • Tiludronate *(Skelid)*
Anti-Parkinsonism drugs	Manage the signs and symptoms associated with Parkinson's disease	• Amantadine *(Symmetrel)* • Bromocriptine *(Parlodel)* • Diphenhydramine *(Benadryl)* • Levodopa *(Dopar, Prolopa)* • Levodopa/Benserazide *(Prolopa)* • Levodopa/Carbidopa *(Sinemet, Sinemat CR)*	• Benztropine *(Cogentin)* • Ropinirole *(Requip)* • Tolcapone *(Tasmar)* • Vitamin E *(various)* • Pergolide *(Permax)* • Selegiline *(Eldepryl)* • Trihexyphenidyl *(Artane)*
Catechol o-methyl tranferase (COMT)	Anti-Parkinsonism drug	• Tolcapone *(Tasmar)*	
Anti-platelet drugs	Platelet aggregation inhibitor, prevent clots from forming	• Aspirin • Clopidogrel *(Plavix)* • Sulfinpyrazone *(Anturane)* • Tirofiban *(Aggrastat)*	• Aspirin/Dipyridamole • Dipyridamole *(Persantine)* • Ticlopidine *(Ticlid)*
Anti-psoriatic drug	Decrease the symptoms associated with psoriosis; decrease itchy and crusty skin patches	• Acitretin *(Soriatane)* • Methotrexate	• Etretinate

(Continued)

Table 7-1 continued

CLASSES OF COMMONLY PRESCRIBED MEDICATIONS

DRUG CLASS	PURPOSE OF DRUGS	GENERIC (TRADE NAME EXAMPLES)	
Anti-psychotic drugs	Major and minor tranquilizers; neuroleptic effect	• Chlorprothixene *(Taractan)* • Haloperidol *(Haldol)* • Molindone *(Moban)* • Pimozide *(Orap)* • Risperidone *(Risperdal)*	• Clozapine *(Clozaril)* • Loxapine *(Loxitane)* • Olanzapine *(Zyprexa)* • Quetiapine *(Seroquel)* • Thiothixene *(Navene)*
Phenothizines	Anti-psychotic drug family derivatives	• Acetophenazine *(Tindal)* • Chlorpromazine *(Thorazine)* • Fluphenazine *(Permitil, Prolixin)* • Mesoridazine *(Serentil)* • Triflupromazine *(Vesprin)*	• Promazine *(Sparine)* • Trifluoperazine *(Stelazine)* • Perphenazine *(Trilafon)* • Prochlorperazine *(Compazine)* • Thioridazine *(Mellaril)*
Thienobenzodiazepines	Anti-psychotic drug family derivatives	• Olanzapine *(Zyprexa)*	
Anti-pryretic drugs	Reduce fever	• Acetaminophen *(see NSAIDs; COX-II inhibitors)*	• Aspirin
Anti-spasmodic drugs (synthetic)	Reduce spasms	• Anisotropine *(Valpin)* • Glycopyrrolate *(Robinul)* • Isopropamide *(Darbid)* • Methantheline *(Banthine)* • Methscopolamine *(Pamine)*	• Clidinium *(Quarzan)* • Hexocyclium *(Tral)* • Mepenzolate *(Cantil)* • Propantheline *(Pro Banthine)* • Tridihexethyl *(Pathilon)*
ANTI-TUSSIVE DRUGS			
Cough suppressants	Suppress coughs	• Dextromethorphan *(Hold DM, Suppress, Benylin)* • Hydromorphone *(Dilaudid)*	• Codeine *(various brands)* • Hydrocodone *(Hycodan)* • Benzonatate *(Tessalon)* • Promethazine *(Phenergan)*
ANTI-ULCER DRUGS			
Antacids	Reduce acid content in the stomach	• Various brands	
Antibiotics	Reduce infection in the gastrointestinal tract	• Amoxicillin • Metronidazole • Tetracycline • Misoprostol	• Clarithromycin • See Histamine H_2 blockers and proton pump inhibitors *(Continued)*

Table 7-1 continued

CLASSES OF COMMONLY PRESCRIBED MEDICATIONS

DRUG CLASS	PURPOSE OF DRUGS	GENERIC (TRADE NAME EXAMPLES)	
Miscellaneous anti-ulcer drugs		• Amoxicillin/Clarithromycin/ Lansoprazole *(Prevac)* • Bismuth Subsalicylate *(Pepto-Bismol)*	• Sucralfate *(Carafate)* • Misoprostol *(Cytotec)* • Ranitidine bismuth citrate *(Tritec)*
Anti-viral drugs	Counteract the effects of infection (anti-infective)	• Abacavir *(Ziagen)* • Amantadine *(Symmetrel)* • Cidofovir *(Vistide)* • Efavirenz *(Sustiva)* • Foscarnet *(Foscavir)* • Indinavir *(Crixivan)* • Nelfinavir *(Viracept)* • Oseltamivir *(Tamiflu)* • Ribavirin *(Virazole)* • Stavudine *(Zerit)* • Vidarabine *(Vira A)* • Zanamivir *(Relenza)*	• Acyclovir *(Zovirax)* • Amprenavir *(Agenerase)* • Didanosine *(Videx)* • Famciclovir *(Famvir)* • Ganciclovir *(Cytovene)* • Lamivudine *(Epivir)* • Nevirapine *(Viramune)* • Penciclovir *(Denavir)* • Saquinavir *(Invirase)* • Valacyclovir *(Valtrex)* • Zalcitabine *(Hivid)* • Zidovudine *(Retrovir)*
Barbiturates	A group of CNS depressants with potent sedative-hypnotic properties that promote sleep	• Amobarbital *(Amytal)* • Butabarbital *(Butisol)* • Metharbital *(Gemonil)* • Phenobarital *(Luminal, Solfoton)*	• Aprobarbital *(Alurate)* • Mephobarbital *(Mebaral)* • Pentobarbital *(Nembutal)* • Secobarbital *(Seconal)* • Talbutal *(Lotusate)*
Benzodiazepines	Share common abilities with barbituates; promote relaxation and sleep but have a different chemical structure	• Alprazolam *(Xanax)* • Chlordiazepoxide *(Librium)* • Diazepam *(Valium, Vazepam)* • Flurazepam *(Dalmane)* • Ketazolam *(Loftran)* • Nitrazepam *(Mogadon)* • Prazepam *(Centrax)* • Temazepam *(Restoril)*	• Bromazepam *(Lectopam)* • Clonazepam *(Klonopin)* • Clorazepate *(Tranxene)* • Estazolam *(Prosom)* • Halazepam *(Paxipam)* • Lorazepam *(Ativan)* • Oxazepam *(Serax)* • Quazepam *(Doral)* • Triazolam *(Halcion)*

(Continued)

Table 7-1 continued

CLASSES OF COMMONLY PRESCRIBED MEDICATIONS

DRUG CLASS	PURPOSE OF DRUGS	GENERIC (TRADE NAME EXAMPLES)	
Beta blockers	Block beta-adrenergic, which blocks sympathetic nervous system effects, slowing the heart rate and force by expanding vessel walls and lowering blood pressure	• Acebutolol *(Sectral)* • Betaxolol *(Kerlone)* • Bisoprolol Hydrochlorothiazide *(Ziac)* • Carteolol *(Cartrol)* • Labetalol *(Normodyne, Trandate)* • Metoprolol *(Lopressor)*	• Atenolol *(Tenormin)* • Bisoprolol *(Zebeta)* • Carvedilol *(Coreg)* • Nadolol *(Corgard)* • Pindolol *(Visken)* • Timolol *(Blocadren)* • Penbutolol *(Levatol)* • Propranolol *(Inderal)*
Bisphosphonates	Stabilize bone mass; used in treating osteoporosis, osteopenia, and Paget's disease	• Alendronate *(Fosamax)* • Tiludronate *(Skelid)*	• Risedronate *(Actonel)*
Calcium blockers	Calcium channel-blocking drugs; block the normal passage of calcium through cell walls and inhibit artery narrowing	• Amlodipine *(Norvasc)* • Diltiazem *(Cardizem, Tiazac)* • Isradipine *(DynaCirc)* • Nifedipine *(Adalat CC, Procardia XL)* • Verapamil *(Calan, Isoptin, Verelan)*	• Bepridil *(Vascor)* • Felodipine *(Plendil)* • Nicardipine *(Cardene)* • Nisoldipine *(Sular)* • Nimodipine *(Nimotop)*
Cholesterol-reducing drugs	Enhance the breakdown of cholesterol	• Atorvastatin *(Lipitor)* • Cholestyramine *(Questran, Prevalite)* • Clofibrate *(Atromid-S)* • Dextrothyroxine *(Choloxin)* • Fluvastatin *(Lescol)* • Lovastatin *(Mevacor)* • Pravastatin *(Pravachol)*	• Cerivastatin *(Baycol)* • Colestipol *(Colestid)* • Fenofibrate *(Tricor)* • Gemfibrozil *(Lopid)* • Niacin *(Nicobid, Slo-Niacin)* • Simvastatin *(Zocor)*
COX-II inhibitors	Anti-inflammatory drugs	• Celecoxib *(Celebrex)*	• Rofecoxib *(Viox)*
Decongestants	Reduce congestion in the upper respiratory tract, eyes, ears, nose, and throat	• Ephedrine *(Efedron, Ephedrol)* • Naphazoline *(Naphcon, Vasocon)*	• Oxymetazoline *(Afrin, Duration)* • Phenylephrine *(Neo-Synephrine)*

(Continued)

Table 7-1 continued

CLASSES OF COMMONLY PRESCRIBED MEDICATIONS

DRUG CLASS	PURPOSE OF DRUGS	GENERIC (TRADE NAME EXAMPLES)	
Decongestants *(continued)*		• Phenylpropanolamine *(Propadrine, Propagest)* • Pseudoephedrine *(Afrinol, Sudafed, others)*	• Tetrahydrozoline *(Tyzine, Visine, others)* • Xylometazoline *(Otrivin)*
Digitalis preparations	Increase the force of the heart's contractions, helping to improve circulation	• Deslanoside *(Cedilanid-D)* • Digoxin *(Lanoxicaps, Lanoxin)*	• Digitoxin *(Crystodigin)*
Diuretics	Help eliminate excess salt and water from the kidneys by making patient urinate more often; reduce swelling caused by fluid buildup in the tissues	• Acetazolamide *(Diamox)* • Bumetanide *(Bumex)* • Erthacrynic Acid *(Edecrin)* • Indapamide *(Lozol)* • Metolazone *(Diulo, Zaroxolyn)*	• Amiloride *(Midamor)* • Chlorthalidone *(Hygroton)* • Furosemide *(Lasix)* • Triamterene *(Dyrenium)* • Spironolactone *(Aldactone)*
Thiazide diuretics		• Bendroflumethiazide *(Naturetin)* • Benzthiazide *(Aquatag, Exna, Marazide)* • Chlorothiazide *(Diuril)* • Hydrochlorothiazide *(Esidrix, HydroDiuril, Oretic)*	• Cyclothiazide *(Anhydron)* • Hydroflumethiazide *(Diucardin, Saluron)* • Methyclothiazide *(Enduron, Aquatensen)* • Polythiazide *(Renese)* • Trichlormethiazide *(Metahydrin, Naqua)*
Ergot derivatives		• Bromocriptine *(Parlodel)* • Methysergide *(Sansert)*	• Ergotamine *(Bellergal)* • Pergolide *(Permax)*
5-alpha-reductase inhibitors		• Finasteride *(Proscar)*	
Hematopoietic agents		• Filgrastim *(Neupogen)*	
HMG-CoA reductase inhibitors		• Atorvastatin *(Lipitor)* • Fluvastatin *(Lescol)* • Pravastatin *(Pravachol)*	• Cerivastatin *(Baycol)* • Lovastatin *(Mevacor)* • Simvastatin *(Zocor)*

(Continued)

Table 7-1 continued

CLASSES OF COMMONLY PRESCRIBED MEDICATIONS

DRUG CLASS	PURPOSE OF DRUGS	GENERIC (TRADE NAME EXAMPLES)	
HORMONES			
Androgens	Male sex hormones; treat periandropausal symptoms	• Fluoxymesterone *(Halotestin)* • Methyltestosterone *(Android, Metandren, Oreton)*	• Testosterone *(Androderm, Andriol, Testoderm, Testone)*
Estrogens	Female sex hormones	• Chlorotrianisene *(Tace)* • Diethylstilbestrol *(DES, Stilphostrol)* • Estradiol *(Estrace, Estraderm)* • Plant-derived synthetic conjugated estrogens *(Cenestin)*	• Estrogens, conjugated *(Premarin)* • Estropipate *(Ogen)* • Quinestrol *(Estrovis)* • Estrone *(Theelin)* • Ethinyl estradiol *(Estinyl)*
Progestins	Female sex hormones	• Hydroxyprogesterone *(Duralutin, Gesterol, others)* • Medroxyprogesterone *(Curretab, Prempro, Premphase)*	• Norethindrone *(Micronor, Norlutate, Norlutin)* • Progesterone *(Gesterol 50, Progestaject)*
Thyroid hormones	Increase levels of the hormone thyroxine	• Levothyroxine *(Synthroid)* • Nafarelin *(Synarel)*	• Liothyronine *(Cytomel)*
H$_2$ blockers	Histamine (H$_2$) blocking drugs	• Cimetidine *(Tagamet)* • Famotidine *(Pepcid)*	• Nizatidine *(Axid)* • Ranitidine *(Zantac)*
Hypnotic drugs	Sedatives and sleep inducers See also Barbiturates	• Acetylcarbromal *(Paxarel)* • Estazolam *(ProSom)* • Ethinamate *(Valmid)* • Glutethimide *(Doriden)* • Paraldehyde *(Paral)* • Quazepam *(Doral)* • Triazolam *(Halicion)* • Zolpidem *(Ambien)*	• Chloral Hydrate *(Noctec)* • Ethchlorvynol *(Placidyl)* • Flurazepam *(Dalmane)* • Methyprylon *(Nodular)* • Propiomazine *(Largon)* • Temazepam *(Restoril)* • Zaleplon *(Sonata)*

(Continued)

Table 7-1 continued

CLASSES OF COMMONLY PRESCRIBED MEDICATIONS

DRUG CLASS	PURPOSE OF DRUGS	GENERIC (TRADE NAME EXAMPLES)	
Immunosuppresants	Suppress the immune system response	• Azathioprine (Imuran) • Cyclophosphamide (Cytoxan) • Hydroxychloroquine (Plaquenil) • Sirolimus (Rapamune)	• Chlorambucil (Leukeran) • Cyclosporine (Sandimmune) • Leflunomide (Arava) • Tacrolimus (Prograf)
Monoamine oxidase inhibitor drugs (MAO inhibitors)	Anti-depressant drugs	• Isocarboxazid (Marplan) • Tranylcypromine (Parnate)	• Phenelzine (Nardil)
Muscarinic receptor antagonists	Anti-incontinence drugs	• Tolterodine (Detrol)	
Muscle relaxants	Produce skeletal muscle relaxation	• Baclofen (Lioresal) • Chlorphenesin Carbamate (Maolate) • Chlorzoxazone (Paraflex, Parafon Forte) • Cyclobenzaprine (Flexeril) • Diazepam (Valium) • Meprobamate (Equanil, Miltown)	• Carisoprodol (Rela, Soma) • Dantrolene (Dantrium) • Metaxalone (Skelaxin) • Orphenadrine (Norflex) • Methocarbamol (Robaxin)
Neuramidase inhibitors	Anti-viral, anti-influenza drugs	• Oseltamivir (Tamiflu)	• Zanamivir (Relenza)
Nitrates	Cause the vessels to dialate, reducing angina	• Amyl Nitrate (Amyl Nitrate Vaporole, others) • Erythrityl Tetranitrate (Cardilate) • Isosorbide Dinitrate (Isordil, Sorbitrate, others)	• Isosorbide Mononitrate (Ismo, Imdur) • Nitroglycerin (Nitrostat, Nitrolingual, Nitrogard, Nitrong, etc) • Pentaerythritol Tetranitrate (Duotrate, Peritrate)
Non-inflammatory steroidal drugs (NSAIDs)	Reduce pain and inflammation	• Ketorolac (Toradol) • Nabumetone (Relafen) • Tolmetin (Tolectin, Tolectin DS)	• Meloxicam (Mobic) • Sulindac (Clinoril)

(Continued)

Table 7-1 continued

CLASSES OF COMMONLY PRESCRIBED MEDICATIONS

DRUG CLASS	PURPOSE OF DRUGS	GENERIC (TRADE NAME EXAMPLES)	
Acetic acids	Mild analgesic, reducing pain and inflammation; reduce the substance that causes pain and inflammation (prostaglandin)	• Bromfenac sodium *(Duract)* • Diclofenac potassium *(Cataflam)* • Diclofenac sodium *(Voltaren)*	• Etodolac *(Lodine)* • Indomethacin *(Indochron E-R, Indocin, Indocin SR)*
Fenamates	Mild analgesic, reducing pain and inflammation; reduce the substance that causes pain and inflammation (prostaglandin)	• Meclofenamate *(Meclomen)*	• Mefenamic Acid *(Ponstel)*
Oxicams	Mild analgesic, reducing pain and inflammation; reduce the substance that causes pain and inflammation (prostaglandin)	• Piroxicam *(Feldene)*	
Propionic acids	Mild analgesic, reducing pain and inflammation; reduce the substance that causes pain and inflammation (prostaglandin)	• Diflunisal *(Dolobid)* • Flurbiprofen *(Ansaid)* • Ketoprofen *(Orudis, Oruvail)* • Oxyphenbutazone *(Oxalid)* • Oxaprozin *(Daypro)* • Suprofen *(Profenal)*	• Fenoprofen *(Nalfon)* • Ibuprofen • Naproxen *(Naprosyn)* • Naproxen Sodium *(Aleve, Anaprox, Anaprox DS)*
Opioid drugs	Narcotic analgesic pain medications	• Alfentanil *(Alfenta)* • Fentanyl *(Actiq, Sublimaze, Duragesic)* • Hydrocodone *(Hycodan)* • Levorphanol *(Levo-Dromoran)* • Methadone *(Dolophine)* • Morphine *(Astramorph, Duramorph, MS Contin, Roxanol)*	• Codeine • Hydromorphone *(Dilaudid)* • Meperidine *(Demerol)* • Oxycodone *(OxyContin)* • Propoxyphene *(Darvon)* • Oxymorphone *(Numorphan)* • Sufentanil *(Sufenta)*
Pain syndrome modifiers	Break the pain cycle by inhibiting nerve conduction	• Carbamazepine *(Tegretol)* • Phenytoin *(Dilantin)* • Samarium-EDTMP *(Quadramet)*	• Gabapentin *(Neurontin)* • Strontium-89 *(Metastron)*
Potassium replacement products	Replace potassium in the body	• K-Dur	• Potassium chloride *(various brands)*

(Continued)

Table 7-1 continued

CLASSES OF COMMONLY PRESCRIBED MEDICATIONS

DRUG CLASS	PURPOSE OF DRUGS	GENERIC (TRADE NAME EXAMPLES)	
Protease inhibitors	Anti-AIDS and anti-viral drugs; supress HIV reproduction by inhibiting the enzyme protease	• Amprenavir *(VX-1478, Agenerase)* • Indinavir *(Crixivan)*	• Nelfinavir *(Viracept)* • Ritonavir *(Norvir)* • Saquinavir *(Fortovase, Invirase)*
Radiopharmaceuticals	Radioactive drugs	• Samarium-EDTMP *(Quadramet)*	• Strontium-89 *(Metastron)*
Salicylates	Analgesic; mild anti-platelet and anti-pyretic (anti-fever)	• Aspirin *(variety of products)* • Choline salicylate *(Arthropan)* • Magnesium salicylate *(Doan's, Magan, Mobidin)*	• Sodium salicylate • Sodium thiosalicylate *(Rexolate, Tusal)* • Salsalate *(Amigesic, Disalcid, Salsitab)*
Sedatives/sleep inducers	*(see Hypnotic drugs)*		
Selective serotonin reuptake inhibitors (SSRIs)	Anti-depressent drugs that restore normal levels of the neurotransmitter serotonin by inhibiting reuptake	• Citalopram *(Celexa)* • Fluvoxamine *(Luvox)* • Paroxetine *(Paxil)* • Trazodone *(Desyrel)*	• Fluoxetine *(Prozac)* • Nefazodone *(Serzone)* • Sertraline *(Zoloft)* • Venlafaxine *(Effexor)*
Selective estrogen receptor modulators (SERMs)	Enhance remineralization of bone and prevent bone loss associated with menopause; anti-osteoporosic group of drugs; increase bone density and reduce low-density lipids	• Raloxifene *(Evista)*	• Tamoxifen *(Nolvadex)*
Vaccines	Immune system modulators; anti-viral drugs made of purified virus that has been inactivated; stimulate the immune system to make antibodies	• Influenza vaccine *(Fluogen, Flu-Shield, Fluzone, FluMist)* • Lyme disease vaccine *(LYMErix)*	• Pneumococcal vaccine *(Prevnar)* • Varicella virus vaccine *(Varivax)*

(Continued)

Table 7-1 continued

CLASSES OF COMMONLY PRESCRIBED MEDICATIONS

DRUG CLASS	PURPOSE OF DRUGS	GENERIC (TRADE NAME EXAMPLES)	
Vasodilators	Dilate the peripheral vascular systems	• Cyclandelate (Cyclospasmol) • Ethaverine (Ethaquin, Isovex)	• Nylidrin (Arlidin) • Isoxsuprine (Vasodilan) • Papaverine (Cerespan, Pavabid)
Xanthines	Bronchodilators	• Aminophylline (Phyllocontin, Truphylline) • Dyphylline (Dilor, Lufyllin)	• Oxtriphylline (Choledyl) • Theophylline (Bronkodyl, Slo-Phyllin, Theolair, etc)

Sometimes elderly individuals receive prescriptions for drugs by their physician, who may not be trained in geriatric-specific pharmacology, that are inappropriate, and in some cases too dangerous to be used in the elderly.[27] It is important that the PT be on the watch for inappropriately prescribed medications and that the PTA be attentive to subtle changes in behavior or physical status of a patient who has started a new drug. Many medications that are safe in most patients pose serious risks in older patients, including functional decline, delirium, falls, and poorer outcomes. Some specific drugs prescribed within the classes listed in Table 7-1 are considered high-risk drugs[28] for the elderly. These drugs create concerns relative to the safe use due to the potential for significant negative side effects. Table 7-4 provides a list of drugs that are potentially harmful and describes the negative effects that should be watched for by the PT and PTA.

PRESCRIPTION DRUG FAMILIES DELINEATED BY SYSTEM AND CONDITIONS

This section presents user-friendly tables listing the various drugs prescribed by condition or diagnosis; brief descriptions are provided related to each section and pathology, and some tables will apply to more than one condition. For instance, Table 7-5 provides a listing of drugs used for pain management, which is used in many circumstances. Geriatric patients are a unique subset with multiple comorbidities that usually have significant functional implications. Geriatric patients have impaired homeostasis and wide interindividual

variability (see Chapters 1 and 3). Comprehensive assessment captures the complexity of the problems that characterize many older patients and can be used to guide management, including prescribing drugs. Prescribing medications for geriatric patients requires an understanding of the efficacy of the medication in frail older people, assessing the risk of adverse drug events, weighing the risk-to-benefit ratio, providing an appropriate dose that does not result in multiple negative side effects, and carefully monitoring the patient's response. This requires an understanding of changes in pharmacokinetics and pharmacodynamics and attention to medication management issues.

Given that most disease occurs in older people and that older people are the major recipients of drug interventions, it it crucial that the PTA understand the effects and side effects of frequently prescribed drugs intended to manage various conditions in geriatric patients.[29,30]

Pain Management

Chronic pain in the elderly is a significant and common problem. An estimated 18% of older Americans take analgesic medications on a regular basis; 63% of individuals surveyed had been prescribed pain medications in the past 6 months.[31] Management of patients with chronic pain is complicated by the multiple medications typically prescribed for the elderly. Increased sensitivities to medications and an increased rate of side effects also occur in older adults. In particular, NSAIDs are associated with a much higher incidence of gastrointestinal bleeding in people older than 60 years of age compared with younger individuals (4% versus 1%, respectively).[32]

To reduce the number of pain medications that elderly patients are taken by, the American Geriatrics

Table 7-2

CLASSES OF PRESCRIPTION DRUGS MOST COMMONLY USED BY MEDICARE PATIENTS

CARDIOVASCULAR DRUGS

Anti-anginal

Anti-arrhythmic

Anti-hypertensive agents

Sympatholytics

Beta blockers

Vasodilators

ACE inhibitors

Antilipemic agents

Cardiac glycosides

DIURETICS

Thiazide

Potassium sparing

Loop

TRANQUILIZERS

Minor

Major

ANTI-COAGULANTS

Coumadin

Heparin

BENZODIAZEPINES

Temazepam

Triazolam

Flurazepam

ANALGESICS

Nonnarcotic

Acetaminophen

Aspirin

Narcotic

DIABETIC PRODUCTS

Insulin preparations

Oral hypglycemics

ANTACIDS

Sodium bicarbonate

Aluminum hydroxide

Aluminum and magnesium hydroxide

Magaldrate

CATHARTICS

Castor oil

Psyllium

ANTIBIOTICS

Erythromycin

Amoxicillin

ANTI-INFLAMMATORIES

NSAIDs

Aspirin

Ibuprofen

Naproxen

COX-II inhibitors

Andrenal corticosteroids

ANTI-SPASMODICS

Dicyclominehydrochloride

THYROIDALS

Thyroidal hormones

Antithyroid agents

VITAMINS AND HERBS

All over-the-counter preparations

Society Panel on Chronic Pain in Older Persons has made a number of reasonable suggestions.[31] First, there should be a comprehensive approach to each patient. Treatable physical causes and psychiatric disorders that could be making treatment success more difficult need to be examined. Next, *nociceptive pain syndromes* (arthropathies, myofascial, nonarticular inflammation, ischemic disorders, and visceral pain) need to be separated from *neuropathic pain syndromes* (postherpetic neuralgia, trigeminal neuralgia, diabetic neuropathy, poststroke pain, postamputation pain, myopathic or radiculopathic pain, etc). It is possible that these 2 categories may cross over and that there are pain syndromes, such as chronic recurrent headaches, vasculopathic pain, or somatization disorders, that do not fit into a particular category. Categorizing patients into these 2 main groups can make choosing treatment medications more rational.

In general, the nociceptive pain syndromes respond better to analgesics; the neuropathic pain syndromes respond less well. Neuropathic pain responds better to some of the adjuvant pain therapies such as tricyclic anti-depressants and anti-seizure medications.

Patient Example

An 82-year-old female presents with severe, constant pain secondary to spinal stenosis, having undergone 5 resections of a lipoma in the lumbosacral region. She is afraid to use opioids because of a history of rectal stricture and constipation. She had

Table 7-3

CLASSES AND DEFINITIONS OF USE OF PRESCRIPTION DRUGS COMMONLY USED BY THE ELDERLY

CLASS	DEFINITIONS
Anti-acid	Reduces acid in the upper GI tract
Analgesic	Relieves pain; decreases sensitivity to pain without causing loss of consciousness
Antibiotic	Chemical substance produced by microorganisms that has the capacity to destroy or inhibit the growth of bacteria or other microorganisms; used in infectious diseases
Anti-coagulant	Reduces or suppresses the clotting of the blood
Anti-depressant	Reduces or prevents depression by stimulating the mood of a depressed person
Anti-histamine	Counteracts the action of histamine, a naturally occurring substance that causes capillaries to dilate; reduces sensitivity to allergens
Anti-hypertensive	Reduces blood pressure
Anti-inflammatory	Counteracts or suppresses inflammation
Anti-Parkinsonian	Reduces the movement and CNS effects of Parkinson's disease
Anti-psychotic	Reduces manic-depression, psychosis, or extreme agitation; also called neuroleptic drugs
Anti-spasmodic	Reduces spasms in any system
Barbiturate	Depresses the CNS and causes a sedative-hypnotic effect
Benzodiazephine	Sedative-hypnotic drugs that promotes relaxation and sleep by suppressing the CNS
Cardiovascular drug	Treats cardiac and/or vascular disorders such as clotting disorders, arrhythmias, fluid retention, or hypertension
Cathartic	Quickens or increases the evacuation from the bowels and produces emptying of the bowel; also called GI anti-spasmodic medication or laxatives
Diabetic product	Regulates blood sugar by reducing the level of glucose in the blood or increasing availability of insulin to balance a sugar/insulin imbalance
Diuretic	Reduces fluid retention and reduces the fluid load on the cardiovascular system
Hypoglycemic	Helps the system increase the level of glucose in the blood
Muscle relaxant	Facilitates muscle relaxation due to spasm after injury
Sedative-hypnotic	Tranquilizing drugs (including barbiturates and benzodiazepines) that promote relaxation and sleep; depresses the CNS and causes a sedative-hypnotic effect

an anaphylactic reaction to penicillin 40 years ago and an urticarial reaction (skin rash, hives, raised itchy bumps on skin) to aspirin a few years later. She subsequently used etodolac (Lodine) without reaction but also without obtaining pain relief. She responded to intramuscular ketorolac but not to the oral form of treatment. Is it reasonable to try Viox for pain relief? Are there any other oral medications that might be of benefit?

For this patient, the gerontologist tried Viox (rofecoxib) on a regularly scheduled regime to replace the etodolac (Lodine). Rofecoxib is believed to be safer in the elderly; however, long-term use of doses above 25 mg per day has not been tested. Celecoxib (Celebrex) appears to be safe in much higher doses (400 mg twice a day) than typically used for osteoarthritis (200 mg per day). However, celecoxib has only been tested in and approved for patients with familial adenomatous polyposis. The efficacy of this higher dose for the treatment of chronic pain or osteoarthritis has not been established. Because this patient seems to have a neuropathic pain syndrome component (spinal stenosis), her physician tried a low-dose tricyclic at bedtime and added an anti-seizure medication—gabapentin

Table 7-4

HIGH-RISK DRUGS WITH NEGATIVE SIDE EFFECTS IN THE ELDERLY

CLASS	CONCERNS IN PRESCRIBING IN THE ELDERLY
Anti-acid	Decreases the breakdown of food in the upper GI tract by reducing available stomach acids that lead to immotility and malnourishment. Depletes the system of trace nutrients as well as calcium.
Analgesic	This NSAID has an extreme adverse effect on the CNS, and long-term use is usually avoided in the elderly. Immediate and long-term use avoided in elderly due to asymptomatic GI disorders. Some analgesics are ineffective when taken orally and should be avoided in the elderly. NSAIDs are available without prescription. Serious adverse effects include peptic ulceration and upper GI bleeding; risk is increased when dose is increased. NSAIDs can also increase the risk of cardiovascular events and cause fluid retention.
COX-II inhibitor	Causes less GI irritation and platelet inhibition than other NSAIDs, although still a risk of GI bleeding if taking other drugs, such as anti-coagulants or low-dose aspirin. Also increased risk of bleeding with pre-existing GI problems. Renal clearance of serum creatinine is a problem and can lead to heart failure, renal impairment, cirrhosis, and fluid volume depletion.
Non-COX-selective	Long-term use can cause GI bleeding, renal failure, hypertension, and heart failure.
Opiods	An opioid analgesic has more adverse effects such as confusion and hallucinations.
Antibiotic	Over-use results in a suppression of the immune system response to infection in the elderly
Anti-coagulant	May cause easy bruising and problems with bleeding in the elderly. Increased sensitivity to anti-coagulant with age.
Anti-depressant	Strong anti-cholinergic (blocks conduction through parasympathetic nerves) and sedating effects in the elderly. Some anti-depressants have a long half-life and may cause excessive stimulation of the CNS, such as sleep disturbances and increased agitation.
Anti-histamine	Over-the-counter and prescription anti-histamines have cholinergic properties. Anti-histamines are commonly included in other drugs, such as cough and cold preparations. Cough and cold medications without antihistamines are available and provide safer alternatives for the elderly.
Anti-hypertensive	Can cause systemic and orthostatic hypotension (drop in blood pressure with position change). Lower starting doses may be necessary to reduce the risk of adverse effects.
Anti-inflammatory	Long-term use results in GI bleeding and ulceration.
Anti-Parkinsonian	Clearance is reduced in the elderly, making them more susceptible to orthostatic hypotention and confusion.
Anti-psychotic	Increased risk of adverse effects in the CNS and extrapyramidal system. Can reduce paranoia but worsen confusion. Increased risk of tardive dyskinesia (which is often irreversible). Can have side effects including sedation, orthostatic hypotension, anti-cholinergic effects, and motor restlessness. Drug-induced parkinsonism can develop.
Anti-spasmodic	GI antispasmodics are highly anti-cholinergic and usually produce substantial toxicity in the elderly. Recommended that these drugs be avoided in the elderly.
Barbiturate	Can cause severe depression of the CNS and have a sedative-hypnotic effect with a long half-life.
Cardiovascular drug	Orthostatic hypotension and CNS effects are more frequent in the elderly. Can cause slowing of the heart rate and depression, constipation, impotence, sedation, and problems with renal clearance (especially in the diuretics) and should only be used in very low doses. Anti-arrhythmic drugs may induce heart failure in the elderly. Other problems include dry mouth, urinary frequency, incontinence, hypertension, and fluid imbalances.

(Continued)

Table 7-4 continued

HIGH-RISK DRUGS WITH NEGATIVE SIDE EFFECTS IN THE ELDERLY

CLASS	CONCERNS IN PRESCRIBING IN THE ELDERLY
Diuretic	Clearance decreases serum creatinine levels and causes electrolyte imbalances and reduction of left ventricular ejection fraction. Risk of hypokalemia and hyperglycemia. Dehydration, dizziness, and fatigue are also significant side effects.
Hypoglycemic	Prolonged half-life in the elderly and can cause prolonged, serious hypoglycemia.
Laxative (stimulant)	Stimulant laxatives may exacerbate bowel dysfunction such as diarrhea, cramping, and gas.
Muscle relaxant	Most muscle relaxants and anti-spasmodics are poorly tolerated by the elderly, resulting in anti-cholinergic effects, sedation, and overall weakness and fatigue.
Sedative-hypnotic	Sensitivity to benzodiazepines is increased in the elderly and should be used in the lowest doses possible. Nonpharmaceutical approaches to treating insomnia should be sought (eg, environmental modifications such as noise and color; limited caffeine intake, limited daytime napping, modified bedtime). Long-term use can lead to drowsiness, impaired memory, and impaired balance, which leads to falls and fractures.

(Neurontin).[33] The pharmacist suggested reconsidering the use of long-term narcotics. If combined with a regular bowel regimen (remember that the elderly can be more sensitive to drugs than younger people), judicial use of either a short-acting or long-acting agent may prove useful. Finally, the physician recommended nonpharmacologic and alternative therapies. Education programs, cognitive-behavioral programs, exercise programs, physical therapy, acupuncture, transcutaneous nerve stimulation (TENS), massage therapy, and other approaches can be helpful. These therapies also carry the advantage of having few reported adverse side effects.

Table 7-5 presents some of the most commonly prescribed pain medications used in the elderly. It provides generic and trade names, the method of action of the drug, and potential side effects.

MUSCULOSKELETAL SYSTEMS

Myopathy and Myositis

Polymyositis and myopathies respond to high doses of immunosuppressant drugs in most cases. The most common medication used is the *corticosteroid prednisone*. Prednisone therapy usually leads to improvement within 2 or 3 months, at which point the dose can be tapered to a lower level to avoid the significant side effects associated with high doses of prednisone. Unresponsive patients are often given a replace-ment or supplementary immunosuppressant, such as *azathioprine (AZA)*, *cyclosporine*, or *methotrexate*. *Intravenous immunoglobulin* treatments may help some people who are unresponsive to other immunosuppressants. Pain can usually be controlled with an over-the-counter analgesic such as *aspirin*, *ibuprofen*, or *naproxen*. Avoiding weight gain helps prevent over-taxing weakened muscles and stressing the joints. Individuals with myopathies may also experience difficulty swallowing and should be referred to a speech therapist if this poses a problem. Standard drug therapy of adult polymyositis, dermatomyositis, and inclusion body myositis includes high-dose corticosteroids and cytotoxic drugs (methotrexate, AZA, and cyclophosphamide).[34]

Osteoporosis

Bone disorder drugs treat diseases that weaken the bones, such as osteoporosis (brittle bone disease), in women past menopause as well as older men. They also are prescribed for *Paget's disease*, a painful condition that weakens and deforms bones, and they are used to control calcium levels in the blood. Bone is living tissue. Like other tissue, bone is constantly being broken down and replaced with new material. Normally, there is a balance between the breakdown of old bone and its replacement with new bone, but when something goes wrong with the process, bone disorders may result.[35] See Tables 7-6 and 7-7 for drug dosages, precautions, side effects, and interactions with other drugs and nutrients used in the treatment of bone disorders such as osteoporosis and Paget's disease.[36,37]

Table 7-5

COMMONLY USED PAIN MEDICATIONS IN THE ELDERLY

DRUG	TRADE NAME	METHOD OF ACTION	SIDE EFFECTS
INDOLE ACETIC ACIDS			
Tolmetin	*Tolectin*	Inhibits the biosynthesis of prostaglandin, which can cause pain and inflammation	Dizziness, drowsiness, depression, rash, pruritus, headache, nervousness, chest pain, hypertension, tinnitis, edema, nausea, vomiting, asthenia, heartburn
Sulindac	*Clinoril*	As above	Drowsiness, dizziness, headache, nausea, vomiting, pruritus, rash, diarrhea
Indomethacin	*Indocin*	As above	Drowsiness, dizziness, somnolence, depression, fatigue, nausea, tinnitus, headache, diarrhea, vomiting
FENAMIC ACIDS			
Meclofenamic acid	*Meclomen*	As above	Dizziness, tinnitus, edema, headache, nausea, vomiting, diarrhea, rash
Mefenamic acid	*Ponstel*	As above	Diarrhea, nausea, vomiting, abdominal, pain, anorexia, pyrosis, drowsiness, dizziness, rash, nervousness, headache, blurred vision, insomnia
PROPIONIC ACIDS			
Ibuprofen	*Motrin*	As above	Cramps, constipation, pruritus, tinnitus, dizziness, anxiety, headache, nausea, vomiting, aseptic, meningitis
Fenoprofen	*Nalfon*	As above	GI symptoms, occult blood in stool, somnolence, dizziness, rash, tremor, pruritus, headache, nervousness, dyspnea, fatigue, insomnia, decreased hearing
Naproxen	*Naprosyn*	As above	Blurred vision, edema, anorexia, shortness of breath, indigestion, tinnitus, constipation, nausea, drowsiness, dizziness, headache
Naproxen sodium	*Anaprox*	As above	Shortness of breath, indigestion, tinnitus, edema, itching, dizziness, drowsiness, headache, nausea, vomiting
Ketoprofen	*Orudis*	As above	Headache, dizziness, drowsiness, constipation, nausea, vomiting, tinnitus, visual disturbances, urinary tract infection
PYRAZOLES			
Phenylbutazone	*Butazolidin*	As above	Aplastic anemia, edema, water retention, GI distress, nausea, dyspepsia, rash
PHENYLACETIC ACIDS			
Diclofenac sodium	*Voltaren*	As above	Peptic ulceration, GI bleeding, abdominal cramps, headache, fluid retention, diarrhea, indigestion, constipation, dizziness, tinnitus, rash, pruritus

(Continued)

Table 7-5 continued

COMMONLY USED PAIN MEDICATIONS IN THE ELDERLY

DRUG	TRADE NAME	METHOD OF ACTION	SIDE EFFECTS
OXICAMS			
Piroxicam	*Feldene*	As above	Stomatitis, anorexia, GI distress, nausea, constipation, flatulence, diarrhea, dizziness, somnolence, headache, malaise, tinnitis, anemia, leukopenia, edema
SALICYLATE			
Diflunisal	*Dolobid*	As above	Abdominal cramps, diarrhea, rash, fatigue, somnolence, insomnia, dizziness, nausea, vomiting, dyspepsia, tinnitus
Salsalate	*Disalcid*	As above	Tinnitus, abdominal pain, abnormal liver function, anaphylactic shock, angio-edema, vertigo, rash, bronchohepatitis, hypotension, nephritis
Aspirin	*Bufferin*	As above	Stomach pain, heartburn, nausea, vomiting, increased rate of GI distress
COX-II-SELECTIVE NSAIDs			
COX-II inhibitors	*Celecoxib*	Selectively inhibits COX-II sites, resulting in the bio-synthesis of prostaglandin	Liver dysfunction, increased liver enzymes, decline in kidney function in those with kidney disease, fluid accumulation that mimics congestive heart disease, blood clots, vessel constriction
Oral steriods	*Medrol*	Short-term anti-inflammatory	Weight gain, stomach ulcers, osteoporosis, collapse of joints, increased blood sugar, exacerbation of infection
TUMOR NECROSING FACTOR INHIBITOR			
	Rituxam Abatacept	Blocks the protein that causes inflammation and promotes joint distruction	Aching joints, chills, cough, fever, headache, hives, itching, nausea, shakes, sneezing, swelling, throat irritation or tightness, upper respiratory tract infection
Opioid analgesics	*Morphine (see Table 7-1)*	Used for neuropathic pain; to treat acute pain	Addictive, nausea, drowsiness, constipation, respiratory depression
Non-narcotic opiods	*Fiorocet Fiorinal Imitrex Tramadol Prialt*	Acute pain management; used for severe intractable chronic pain	Rebound headaches, abdominal cramps, bloating, dizziness, drowsiness

In osteoporosis, the inside of the bones becomes porous and thin. Over time, this condition weakens the bones and makes them more likely to break. Osteoporosis is 4 times more common in women than in men. This is because women have less bone mass than men, tend to live longer and take in less calcium, and need the female hormone estrogen to keep their bones strong. If men live long enough, they are also at risk of getting osteoporosis later in life.

Once total bone mass has peaked—around age 35—all adults start to lose it. In women, the rate of bone loss increases during menopause when estrogen levels fall. Bone loss may also occur if both ovaries are removed by surgery. Ovaries make estrogen. *Hormone replacement therapy* is one approach to preventing osteoporosis; however, not all people can use it. Bone disorder drugs are a good alternative for people who already have osteoporosis or who are at risk of developing

Table 7-6

DRUGS COMMONLY USED FOR BONE DISORDERS

ALENDRONATE

Dosage for osteoporosis

The usual dose is 10 mg once a day. Treatment usually continues over many years.

Dosage for Paget's disease

The usual dose is 40 mg once a day for 6 months.

This medicine works only when it is taken with a full glass of water first thing in the morning, at least 30 minutes before eating or drinking anything or taking any other medicine. Do not lie down for at least 30 minutes after taking it because the drug can irritate the esophagus, the tube that delivers food from the mouth to the stomach.

Precautions

People with low levels of calcium in their blood should not take this medicine. It also is not recommended for women on hormone replacement therapy or for anyone with kidney problems. Digestive or swallowing problems could also create a risk for side effects.

Side effects

Common side effects include constipation, diarrhea, indigestion, nausea, pain in the abdomen, and pain in the muscles and bones. These problems usually go away as the body adjusts to the medicine and do not usually interfer with normal activities.

Interactions

Taking aspirin with alendronate may increase the chance of upset stomach, especially if the dose of alendronate is more than 10 mg per day. If an analgesic is necessary, switch to another drug, such as acetaminophen (Tylenol) or use buffered aspirin. Ask a physician or pharmacist for the correct medication to use.

Some calcium supplements, antacids, and other medicines keep the body from absorbing alendronate. To prevent this problem, do not take any other medicine within 30 minutes of taking alendronate.

CALCITONIN

Nasal spray

The usual dose is one spray into the nose once a day, alternating nostrils.

Injectable

The recommended dosage depends on the condition for which the medicine is prescribed and may be different for different people.

Precautions

Calcitonin nasal spray may cause irritation or small sores in the nose. The injectable form has caused serious allergic reactions in a few people. The nasal spray is not known to cause such reactions, but the possibility exists.

Side effects

The most common side effects of calcitonin nasal spray are nose problems such as dryness, redness, itching, sores, bleeding, and general discomfort. These problems should go away as the body adjusts to the medicine, but if they do not or if they are very uncomfortable, check with a physician. Other side effects that should be brought to a physician's attention include headache, back pain, and joint pain.

Injectable calcitonin may cause minor side effects such as nausea or vomiting; diarrhea; stomach pain; loss of appetite; flushing of the face, ears, hands, or feet; and discomfort or redness at the place on the body where it is injected. Medical attention is not necessary unless these problems persist or cause unusual discomfort. Anyone who has a skin rash or hives after taking injectable calcitonin should check with a physician as soon as possible.

(Continued)

Table 7-6 continued

DRUGS COMMONLY USED FOR BONE DISORDERS

Interactions
Calcitonin may keep certain other drugs for Paget's disease, such as etidronate (Didronel), from working as they should.

RALOXIFENE
Dosage
The usual dose is 60 mg tablet once daily.
Precautions
A rare, but serious side effect of raloxifene is an increased risk of blood clots that form in the veins and may break away and travel to the lungs. This is about as likely in women who take raloxifene as it is in women who take estrogen. Individuals with a history of blood clots in their veins should not take raloxifene. Women who have had breast cancer or cancer of the uterus may not be able to safely use raloxifene.
Side effects
Common side effects include hot flashes, leg cramps, nausea, and vomiting. Women who have these problems while taking raloxifene should check with their physicians.
Interactions
Raloxifene may affect blood clotting. Patients who are taking other drugs that affect blood clotting, such as warfarin (Coumadin), should be monitored closely for bruising or bleeding.

it. Risk factors include lack of regular exercise, early menopause, being underweight, and a strong family history of osteoporosis.[38]

Bone disorder drugs are available only with a physician's prescription and come in tablet, nasal spray, and injectable forms. Commonly used bone disorder drugs are *alendronate (Fosamax), calcitonin (Miacalcin, Calcimar),* and *raloxifene (Evista).* Raloxifene belongs to a group of drugs known as *selective estrogen receptor modulators* (SERMs), which act like estrogen in some parts of the body but not in others. This makes the drugs less likely to cause some of the harmful effects that estrogen may cause. Unlike estrogen, raloxifene does not increase the risk of breast cancer. In fact, research suggests that raloxifene may even reduce that risk.

General Precautions for Bone Disorder Drugs

To keep bones strong, the body needs calcium and vitamin D. Dairy products and fish such as salmon, sardines, and tuna are good sources of both calcium and vitamin D. People who are taking bone disorder drugs for osteoporosis and who do not get enough of these nutrients in their diets should check with their physicians about taking supplements. Other important bone-saving steps are avoiding smoking and alcohol and getting enough of the kind of exercise that puts weight on the bones (such as walking or lifting weights).

Rheumatoid Arthritis

First-string medications prescribed for rheumatoid arthritis include pain relievers, anti-inflammatory agents, and disease-modifying anti-rheumatic drugs (DMARDs).[39] DMARDs are used to slow the progress of the disease. Traditionally, doctors first prescribed pain relievers to people with RA and administered more powerful drugs later only after the disease becomes worse. Recently, many doctors have changed their approach, prescribing more powerful drugs earlier to halt disease progression and reduce or prevent joint damage.[40] Table 7-8 provides a listing of medications used in the treatment of RA and other degenerative joint diseases.

CARDIOVASCULAR SYSTEM

Atherosclerosis and Ischemic Heart Disease

Most of the drugs prescribed for atherosclerosis seek to lower cholesterol levels. Many popular lipid-lowering drugs can reduce low-density lipoprotein (LDL) cholesterol by an average of 25% to 30% when combined with a low-fat, low-cholesterol diet. Lipid-lowering drugs include *bile acid resins, "statins"* (drugs that effect HMG-CoA reductase, an enzyme that controls the processing of cholesterol), *niacin*, and *fibric acid* derivatives such as *gemfibrozil (Lobid)*. Aspirin helps prevent thrombosis, and a variety of other medications can be used to treat the effects of atherosclerosis[41,42] (see Table 7-9A).

Table 7-10 provides a brief listing of drugs used to treat hyperlipidemia[43] and potential side effects of these cholesterol-reducing drugs.

Angina Pectoralis

Angina[44] is chest pain or discomfort that occurs when the heart muscle does not get enough blood and/or oxygen, creating an ischemic state. It may feel like pressure or a squeezing pain in the chest. Some individuals mistake angina for indigestion. Pain may also radiate to the shoulders, arms, neck, jaw, or back. Angina is a symptom of CAD, the most common symptom of heart disease. CAD happens when a sticky substance called *plaque* builds up in the arteries that supply blood to the heart, reducing blood flow.

Table 7-7

DRUGS COMMONLY USED FOR OSTEOARTHRITIS AND DEGENERATIVE JOINT DISEASE[38,39]

Medications for osteoarthritis include anti-inflammatory drugs to reduce swelling, drugs to reduce pain, and drugs that help the functioning of the joints.

NSAIDs These drugs, which include aspirin, ibuprofen, and naproxen, reduce pain and inflammation and may be used for both short- and long-term pain relief.

COX-II inhibitors A newer generation of NSAIDs called COX-II inhibitors, or "super aspirins," are as effective as the older NSAIDs. These compounds do not cause as much of the GI irritation of the older anti-inflammatory drugs, but there have been concerns that they raise the risk of heart problems.

A note about NSAIDs and COX-II inhibitors

NSAIDs, such as ibuprofen and naproxen, relieve inflammation as well as pain. One disadvantage, however, is that they have been known to cause an assortment of side effects, including irritation and bleeding in the stomach and a decrease in kidney function.

Concerns have been raised regarding naproxen. The Food and Drug Administration (FDA) is working with the National Institutes of Health to review the available scientific information on naproxen following the decision of the National Institute on Aging to stop a clinical trial studying NSAIDs in people at risk of developing Alzheimer's disease. Early information from the study showed some evidence of a higher risk of heart problems when compared to a dummy pill.[37]

The FDA advises patients who take over-the-counter naproxen products to carefully follow the instructions on the label. The recommended doses for naproxen is 220 mg twice daily and should not be taken for longer than 10 days without physician approval. NSAIDs also should be used with caution by anyone who drinks alcohol.

The safety of COX-II inhibitors has also been called into question. Vioxx was pulled by its manufacturer, Merck, in 2004 because a study on how it can work against colon cancer showed a small increased risk of cardiovascular problems. In 2005, the FDA asked Pfizer to stop selling Bextra (valdecoxib) because of an increased risk for heart problems and a higher risk for a rare, serious skin reaction.

Celebrex, another COX-II inhibitor, may also increase the risk of heart attack at high doses or with long-term use. Like Vioxx, Celebrex was being studied to see if it helped prevent colon cancer in certain people. Results of that study showed the rate of heart attack was 2.5 times higher in those taking 400 mg of Celebrex and more than 3 times higher in people taking the 800 mg dose than in those taking a dummy pill. The study was stopped immediately. However, another study did not show an increase in heart attacks. More research is being done, so the use of this medication should be discussed with a doctor.[37]

Corticosteroids These drugs reduce inflammation and can be very effective in treating arthritis, although they also may have significant side effects. Patients may receive injections of corticosteroids directly into the affected joint. Frequent injections may damage the joint cartilage. Note: Patients treated chronically with high-dose corticosteroids become increasingly weak because of a superimposed corticosteroid myopathy.[39]

Table 7-8

DRUGS COMMONLY USED FOR TREATMENT OF RHEUMATOID ARTHRITIS

NSAIDs Primarily decrease joint inflammation but do not slow or alter the progression of RA.

DMARDs This class of drugs has been found to slow or halt the progession of RA by interfering with the immune system response that leads to joint erosion. *Gold therapy* compounds containing elemental gold were among the first drugs identified as DMARDs.

Steroids (methylprednisolone and prednisone) These steroids are available as pills or for injection into a joint. Symptoms will start to decrease within 24 hours after getting the first dose of the drug. Extremely effective in reducing inflammation but are associated with serious adverse side effects. Some serious side effects, especially at high doses, include a breakdown of support tissues, such as muscle, tendon, and bone. Osteoporosis is a particularly important problem, and bone status and posture should be monitored by the clinician. Steroids are used for severe flare-ups and when NSAIDs and DMARDs do not work.

Biologic response modifiers These drugs selectively block parts of the immune system called cytokines, which play a role in inflammation.

Anti-malarial drugs Found to be effective in treating RA by halting or slowing the progression by increasing the pH within the cells. This is believed to disrupt the ability of these cells to process antigenic proteins. Decrease in T-cell stimulation results in a decrease in the immune system response.

Tumor necrosis factor inhibitors (etanercept, infliximab, and adalimumab) These medications work well for people who do not have much luck with DMARDs. The doctor may give them along with some DMARDs, particularly methotrexate. Etanercept requires injections 2 times per week. Infliximab is injected into a vein during a 2-hour procedure. Adalimumab requires injections every 2 weeks.

Interleukin-1 inhibitor (nakrina) This medication requires daily injections. These block cytokines, a substance that causes degeneration of joints. Interleukin-1 is a factor that induces fever, controls lymphocytes, and increases the number of bone marrow cells.[41]

There are 3 types of angina: stable, unstable, and variant. Unstable angina is the most dangerous. It does not follow a pattern and can happen without physical exertion. It does not go away with rest or medicine and is a sign that a heart attack is imminent.[45]

There are many treatment options including rest, medications (*nitroglycerin, beta blockers, calcium channel blockers*), percutaneous transluminal coronary angioplasty (PTCA), or a coronary artery bypass graph (CABG). When patients continue to have angina despite maximally tolerated combinations of drug intervention, cardiac catheterization with coronary arteriography is typically indicated. Depending on the location and severity of the disease in the coronary arteries, patients can be referred for balloon angioplasty, PTCA, or CABG to increase coronary artery blood flow. Surgery is always the last resort.

Drugs are one of the first treatment approaches to treating chest pain. Resting, sublingual (placed under the tongue) nitroglycerin tablets, and nitroglycerin sprays all relieve angina by reducing the heart muscle's demand for oxygen. Nitroglycerin also relieves spasm of the coronary arteries and can redistribute coronary artery blood flow to areas that need it most. Short-acting nitroglycerin can be repeated at 5-minute intervals. When 3 doses of nitroglycerin fail to relieve the angina, further medical attention is recommended. Short-acting nitroglycerin can also be used prior to exertion to prevent angina. If an individual is having chest pain, it is advised that the patient bring nitroglycerin with him or her to therapy sessions. It is also important that the distinction between stable and unstable angina be made. Someone with stable angina is able to manage the pain by utilizing preventive nitroglycerin as described above. However, an individual who has recently been diagnosed with angina, or has experienced exacerbations in symptoms, may be unstable and suffering an acute episode that may be a life-threatening emergency. Careful monitoring is cruicial.

Longer-acting nitroglycerin preparations, such as *Isordil tablets, Nitro-Dur transdermal systems* (patch form), and *Nitrol ointment* are useful in preventing and reducing the frequency and intensity of episodes in patients with chronic angina. The use of nitroglycerin preparations can be limited by headaches and

Table 7-9

TYPES OF MEDICATIONS COMMONLY USED FOR ATHEROSCLEROSIS AND ISCHEMIC HEART DISEASE

Cholesterol-lowering medications When diet and exercise fail to lower levels of cholesterol and other blood fats, medication may be needed. Some examples of cholesterol-lowering medications are *lovastatin, colestipol, fluvastatin, pravastatin, atorvastatin, cholestyramine, fenofibrate, gemfibrozil, rosuvastatin,* and *niacin.*

Blood pressure-lowering medications High blood pressure causes the heart to enlarge. Untreated, it increases the risk of stroke, heart attack, and kidney and heart failure. Many different types of medication are used to treat high blood pressure.

Nitrates *Nitroglycerin* is one type of nitrate medication that is often prescribed to treat coronary artery disease. Nitrates dilate the arteries that supply the heart with blood. In doing so, they increase the flow of blood and oxygen to the heart. Nitrates also reduce the workload of the heart by decreasing the amount of blood returning to the heart for pumping to the rest of the body.

Beta blockers *Atenolol, carvedilol,* and *metoprolol* are 3 commonly prescribed beta blocker medications. Beta blockers slow the heart rate and decrease the force needed to contract the heart muscle. In doing so, beta blockers reduce the workload of the heart.

Calcium channel blockers *Nifedipine, verapamil, amlodipine,* and *diltiazem* are examples of commonly prescribed calcium channel blockers. These medications open up the coronary arteries and may also decrease the heart muscle's needs for blood and oxygen.

Aspirin Aspirin has the ability to stop blood clots from forming within the coronary arteries. It reduces the risk of heart attack in people who have coronary heart disease. Studies have shown that a daily baby aspirin is just as effective as an adult aspirin.

light-headedness due to an excess lowering of blood pressure. The side effects of drugs commonly used to treat chest pain are listed in Table 7-11.

Beta blockers also relieve angina by inhibiting the effect of adrenaline on the heart. Inhibiting adrenaline decreases the heart rate, lowers the blood pressure, and reduces the pumping force of the heart muscle, all of which reduce the heart muscle's demand for oxygen. Examples of beta blockers include *propranolol (Inderal), metoprolol (Lopressor),* and *atenolol (Tenormin).* Side effects include worsening of asthma, excess lowering of the heart rate and blood pressure, depression, fatigue, impotence, increased cholesterol levels, and shortness of breath due to diminished heart muscle function (congestive heart failure).

Calcium channel blockers relieve angina by lowering blood pressure and reducing the pumping force of the heart muscle, thereby reducing muscle oxygen demand. Calcium channel blockers also relieve coronary artery spasm. Calcium channel blockers include *nifedipine (Procardia), verapamil (Calan),* and *diltiazem (Cardizem).* Verapamil and diltiazem also lower the heart rate. Side effects include swelling of the legs, excess lowering of the heart rate and blood pressure, and depressing heart muscle function, thereby causing an increased shortness of breath.

A recent study found that patients with high blood pressure taking short-acting calcium blockers (*Procardia, Cardizem,* and *Calan*) had a higher rate of heart attacks.[46] This has not been shown for the longer-acting preparations (*Procardia-XL, Cardizem-CD,* and *Calan-SR*) and has not been confirmed by other long-term studies. Until other studies are available, no conclusive statements can be made about the safety of these agents. Many of the commonly prescribed anti-anginal drugs have several negative adverse effects that may have an impact on functional mobility, safety, and falls. Table 7-11 provides a listing of anti-anginal agents, their method of action, and their side effects.[46]

Cardiomyopathy/Congestive Heart Disease[47]

One or more of the following types of medicines may be prescribed for congestive cardiomyopathy[47]:

- Digitalis
- Diuretics
- Vasodilators
- Beta blockers

Table 7-10

DRUGS COMMONLY USED TO TREAT HYPERLIPIDEMIA (REDUCE CHOLESTEROL LEVELS) AND THEIR SIDE EFFECTS

DRUG	METHOD OF ACTION	SIDE EFFECTS
Cholestyramine	Decreases plasma LDL cholesterol levels	Nausea, diarrhea
Clofibrate gemfibrozil	Lowers plasma triglycerides by decreasing LDL and IDL levels	Nausea, diarrhea, fatigue, weakness, myalgia, myositis, arrhythmias, blood dyscrasias (abnormal blood condition [eg, Hodgkin's]), angioneurotic syndrome (necrosis of the walls of the blood vessels)
Lovastatin Pravastatin	Decreases plasma LDL cholesterol levels; may decrease triglycerides and increase HDL levels	Nausea, diarrhea, fatigue, weakness, myalgia, myositis
Niacin	Lowers plasma triglycerides by decreasing VLDL levels	Nausea, diarrhea, cutaneous vasodilation, sensation of warmth when administered
Pravachol	Decreases plasma LDL cholesterol levels; may decrease triglycerides and increase HDL levels	Nausea, diarrhea, fatigue, weakness, myalgia, myositis
Probucol	Decreases LDL and HDL cholesterol; inhibits deposition of fat into the arterial wall	Nausea, diarrhea, parasthesias, arrhythmias, blood dyscrasias, angioneurotic syndrome
Simvastatin (Zocor)	Decreases plasma LDL cholesterol levels; may decrease triglycerides and increase HDL levels	Nausea, diarrhea, fatigue, weakness, myalgia, myositis

Note: HDL indicates high density lipoproteins; LDL, low density lipoproteins; IDL, intermediate density lipoproteins; VLDL, very low density lipoproteins.

- Angiotensin converting enzyme (ACE) inhibitors
- Angiotensin receptor blockers

Digitalis helps the heart muscle to have stronger pumping action. *Diuretics* help eliminate excess salt and water from the kidneys by making patients urinate more often, which helps reduce the swelling caused by fluid buildup in the tissues. *Vasodilators*, *beta blockers*, and *ACE inhibitors* lower blood pressure and expand the blood vessels so blood can move more easily through them. This action makes it easier for the heart to pump blood through the vessels.

Patients may also be given *anti-coagulant medications* to prevent clots from forming due to pooling of blood in the heart chambers. Medicines called *anti-arrhythmic drugs* prevent abnormal heart rhythms (arrhythmias) and may be given, but some of these drugs can also reduce the force of heart contractions. Automatic implantable cardioverter defibrillators (AICDs) can treat life-threatening arrhythmias, which are relatively common in severe cardiomyopathy.[48]

Medications for Congestive Heart Failure

Although there is no known cure, heart failure can be treated successfully. Treatment consists of lifestyle changes and drug therapy to improve patients' quality of life.[49] Lifestyle changes include quitting smoking, losing excess weight, drinking less alcohol, and eating healthy low-saturated fat and low-salt foods. Regular, modest exercise (once cleared by the physician) is also helpful for many patients. Yet, even with lifestyle changes, most heart failure patients must take medication. Some drugs used to treat congestive heart failure are presented in Table 7-12.

Conductive System Diseases

Drug therapy can manage many arrhythmias, but finding the right drug and dose requires care and can take some time. Common drugs for suppressing arrhythmias include *beta blockers*, *calcium channel blockers*, *quinidine*, *digitalis preparations*, and *procainamide*. Because of their potential serious side effects, stronger, desensitizing drugs are used only to treat life-threatening arrhythmias. All of the drugs used to treat arrhythmias have possible side effects, ranging from mild complications with beta blockers and calcium channel blockers to more serious effects of desensitizing drugs that can, paradoxically, cause arrhythmias or make them worse. Response to drugs is usually measured by EKG, Holter monitor, or electrophysiologic study.[50]

Table 7-11

ANTI-ANGINAL AGENTS—DRUGS THAT DECREASE CHEST PAIN AND SIDE EFFECTS OF THE DRUGS IN THE ELDERLY

DRUGS	METHOD OF ACTION	SIDE EFFECTS
Nitroglycerin	Relaxes smooth muscle in arterial and venous beds; direct dilatation of coronary conductive vessels	Transient headache, nausea, vomiting, dizziness, flush on face and neck, rapid pulse, skin rash (with patch), tachycardia, hypotension, weakness, and poor endurance
Calcium channel blockers	Blocks active and inactive calcium channels; prevents the influx of calcium	Hypotension, dizziness, headache, peripheral edema, fatigue, constipation, nausea, edema, rash, AV block, weakness, drowsiness, complaints of paresthesia
	Nonselective block of β-adrenergic receptors	
	Selectively dilates coronary arteries, resulting in increased oxygen supply to heart muscle; inhibits clotting	Dizziness, weakness, syncope flushing, nausea, vomiting, skin rash, GI distress, headache, postural hypotension

Most of the drugs used for treatment have potential side effects and should be carefully monitored by a doctor. The goal of treatment is to control the rate and rhythm of the heart and to prevent the formation of blood clots. If the arrhythmia is caused by heart disease, the heart disease will also be treated. The American Heart Association recommends aggressive treatment.

In atrial fibrillation, a digitalis drug, most commonly digoxin, is usually prescribed to control the heart rate. Digitalis drugs slow the heart's electrical impulses, helping to restore the normal rate and rhythm. These drugs also increase the ability of the heart's muscular layer to contract and pump properly. Beta blockers and calcium channel blockers can also be used for this purpose. Beta blockers slow the speed of electrical impulses through the heart. Some calcium channel blockers dampen the heart's response to erratic electrical impulses. Table 7-13 provides a list of drugs that are often prescribed in the attempt to manage the heart's rhythm. Amiodarone is fairly efffective for atrial flutter. This drug is often able to maintain the heart's proper rhythm and can also help control the heart rate when the flutter occurs.

The risk of heart attack, stroke, or peripheral vascular thrombosis is increased with any arrhythmia. To prevent blood clots, aspirin or warfarin (Coumadin) is administered. Warfarin, however, has potential side effects of bleeding, especially in older patients.

Hypertension

There are many different classes of medications used to lower blood pressure[51]; those most commonly used are listed in Table 7-14. The use of drugs to treat high blood pressure often has significant side effects and may lead to increased dizziness, lack of energy, and falls.[52] The most common adverse reactions to antihypertensive drugs are provided in Table 7-15.

Peripheral Vascular Disease

Peripheral vascular disease (PVD)[53] includes a group of diseases in which blood vessels become restricted or blocked. Typically, the patient has PVD from atherosclerosis, a disease in which fatty plaques form in the inside walls of blood vessels. Other processes, such as blood clots, further restrict blood flow in the blood vessels. Drug interventions for PVD are the same as those described that are related to atherosclerosis. Additionally, claudication (pain or a tired feeling in the legs) is often a problem that restricts ambulation. Table 7-16 is a summary of drugs used to reduce blood clots and plaque buildup; these drugs are used for atherosclerosis, ischemic heart disease, and PVD.

Table 7-12

DRUGS COMMONLY USED FOR THE TREATMENT OF CONGESTIVE HEART FAILURE

Beta blockers Reduce the heart rate and the output of blood by counteracting a hormone called noradrenalin. (Beta blockers are not recommended for people with severe heart failure.)

Diuretics Help patients with fluid retention and/or high blood pressure to reduce the amount of fluid in the body. Possible side effects include the loss of too much potassium, weakness, muscle cramps, joint pains, and impotence.

Digitalis Increases the force of the heart's contractions, helping to improve circulation. Possible side effects include nausea, vomiting, loss of appetite, diarrhea, confusion, and new heartbeat irregularities.

ACE inhibitors and angiotensin II receptor blockers (ARBs) May improve survival among heart failure patients and may slow or prevent the loss of heart pumping activity, according to recent studies. Originally developed as a treatment for high blood pressure, ACE inhibitors help heart failure patients by, among other things, decreasing the pressure inside blood vessels. As a result, the heart does not have to work as hard to pump blood through the vessels. About 1 in 4 patients develop a chronic dry cough. Other possible side effects include skin rashes, fluid retention, excess blood potassium, kidney problems, and an impaired sense of taste.

Nitrate and/or hydralazine May be prescribed to patients who cannot take ACE inhibitors or ARBs. These medications help relax tension in blood vessels and improve blood flow. Possible side effects include headaches, rapid heartbeat, and joint pain.

Cardiac Output

The primary function of the heart is to provide an efficient blood pump in order to generate and sustain an arterial blood pressure necessary to provide adequate perfusion of organs. The heart achieves this by contracting its muscular walls around a closed chamber to generate sufficient pressure to propel blood from the cardiac chamber (eg, left ventricle), through the aortic valve, and into the aorta. Each time the heart beats, a volume of blood is ejected. The amount of blood put out by the left ventricle of the heart in one contraction is called the *stroke volume*; when this is multiplied by the number of beats per minute, or the heart rate, it is termed the *cardiac output*. In other words, cardiac output is the amount of blood that is pumped by the heart per unit time, measured in liters per minute (L/min). A normal adult's heart can easily pump 5 quarts (4.7 L) of blood a minute. Cardiac output, therefore, is the amount of blood the heart pumps through the circulatory system in 1 minute. Many of the conditions of the cardiovascular system discussed result in poor cardiac output. For instance, plaque buildup or artherosclerosis in the vessel walls decrease the amount of blood delivered to the peripheral vascular system, the brain, and all of the body's organs.[54] Arrhythmias reduce the strength and efficiency of the heart and reduce cardiac output. Several drugs are prescribed to enhance cardiac output. Table 7-17 provides a list of drugs commonly used to affect cardiac output and improve the circulation to all body parts by improving the strength of heart contractions.[55]

PULMONARY SYSTEM

Pneumonia

If the disease is found early, most people can be treated at home with *antibiotics*, but elderly people or those who are immunocompromised are routinely hospitalized because their risk of death is higher. In healthy people, antibiotics can cure bacterial pneumonia and improve recovery from other organisms such as mycoplasma.[56] Viral pneumonia usually clears up on its own. Drugs that are prescribed depend on the type of organism causing the infection. Because bacteria are complete life forms, they perform many chemical processes to stay alive. They must manufacture their structural elements, digest and assimilate nutrients, replicate themselves as they multiply, and protect themselves from hostile elements in their environment. Antibiotics hinder these processes. Some can kill bacteria by interrupting a vital process. Others merely slow them down or stop them from multiplying until the body's immune system can kill them.[57]

Chronic Obstructive Pulmonary Disease

The purpose of drug prescription with COPD[58] is to open the airways, clear the bronchial tubes of secretions, reduce inflammation of the

Table 7-13

DRUGS USED TO STABILIZE HEART RHYTHM—ANTI-ARRHYTHMIC DRUGS

DRUG	METHOD OF ACTION	SIDE EFFECTS
Quinidine	Depresses pacemaker rate, conduction, and excitability	Nausea, vomiting, abdominal pain, diarrhea, headache, tinnitus, disturbed vision, and worsening arrhythmia
Procainamide hydrochloride	Supresses automaticity, decreases conduction velocity, prolongs effective refractory period	Hypotension, worsening ventricular arrhythmia, systemic lupus erythema, arthritic symptoms and arthralgia, fever, rash
Lidocaine	Suppressor of abnormal cardiac activity, acting exclusively on sodium channels	Paresthesias, tremor, convulsions, drowsiness, light-headedness
Propranolol	Nonselective blockage of β-adrenergic receptors	Dizziness, fatigue, lightheadedness, nausea, vomiting, bronchospasm, bradycardia, peripheral vascular insufficiency
Verapamil	Coronary vasodilator, blocks both activated and inactivated calcium channels	Hypotension, peripheral edema, bradycardia, dizziness, headache, fatigue, constipation, nausea
Amiodarone	Effective blocker of inactivated sodium channels, blocks α- and β-adreno receptors	Halo in peripheral vision fields, yellowing of cornea, photodermatitis, grayish/blue skin discoloration
Disopyramide	Depresses pacemaker rate, conduction and excitability	Dry mouth, urinary retention, constipation, blurred vision, dry nose, and eyes, bloating, malaise, fatigue, weakness, low endurance
Quinidine polygalacturonate	Slows conduction time, prolongs refractory period, depresses excitability of the heart muscle	Disturbed vision, headache, diarrhea, nausea, vomiting, abdominal pain, confusion, vertigo, fever, delirium, syncope, apprehension
Quinidine gluconate	Prolongation of refractory period, decrease in excitability of ectopic heart muscle activity and irritability	Disturbed vision, headache, diarrhea, nausea, vomiting, abdominal pain, confusion, vertigo, fever, delirium, syncope, apprehension
Isoproterenol	Increases cardiac output; increases venous return to heart	Sweating, mild tremors, nervousness, tachycardia with palpitations, lowers peripheral vascular resistance

bronchial tree, and fight infections.[59] Table 7-18 provides a review of drugs commonly used to decrease the effects and symptoms of COPD.

Asthma and Resistive Pulmonary Diseases

Drugs used in the treatment of asthma and resistive pulmonary diseases have a great deal of overlap with those used in the treatment of COPD.[61] Table 7-19 shows drugs that are prescribed in these pulmonary conditions to decrease the inflammation of the airways, prevent inflammation of the airways, and decrease the spasms that often occur with resistive pulmonary conditions.

NEUROMUSCULAR SYSTEM

Cerebrovascular Accidents

Drugs prescribed for cerebrovascular accidents[63,64] are aimed at preventing stroke from occurring. Following a stroke, medications are available, if used in a timely fashion, to break up clots causing acute ischemia or arterial blockage. Medications used to prevent and treat stroke are listed in Table 7-20.

Confusion and Delirium

There are a large number of possible causes of delirium. Metabolic disorders are the single most

Table 7-14

DRUGS COMMONLY USED TO TREAT HYPERTENSION[52]

Diuretics Sometimes called "water pills," diuretics work by eliminating excess water and salt from the body. Diuretics are usually the first medications used when treating high blood pressure or they are used in combination with other drugs. They are inexpensive and highly effective.
Beta blockers These drugs reduce the heart rate and the output of blood by counteracting hormones called adrenaline and noradrenaline.
ACE inhibitors These drugs interfere with the production of angiotensin II, which causes arteries to constrict and increases salt retention.
ARBs ARBs block the angiotensin receptor found in many tissues, primarily in vascular smooth muscle. ARBs are rarely associated with dry cough, a common side effect in patients on ACE inhibitors.
Calcium channel blockers These drugs work by relaxing the blood vessels and reducing the heart rate. Patients taking calcium channel blockers should not eat grapefruit or drink grapefruit juice because these can interfere with the calcium channel blocker and increase the risk of side effects.
Vasodilators These drugs cause the vessel walls to dilate, relaxing their walls and lowering blood pressure.
CNS agents These drugs prevent the brain from sending impulses that stimulate blood vessels to constrict. Constriction raises blood pressure.

Table 7-15

SIDE EFFECTS OF ANTI-HYPERTENSIVE DRUGS

DRUG	METHOD OF ACTION	SIDE EFFECTS
Vasodilator	Relaxation of the peripheral vessel decreases system pressure	Dizziness; can lower blood pressure too much, resulting in reflex tachycardia, postural hypotension, weakness, nausea, fluid retention, and headaches; can lead to falls
ACE inhibitor	Reduces blood pressure by inhibiting the enzyme that converts angiotensin I to angiotension II	Possible allergic reaction resulting in skin rash, GI discomfort, dizziness, chest pain, persistent dry cough, increased risk of falls
Calcium channel blocker	Block calcium's entry into vascular smooth muscle cells (originally developed to treat chest pain and arrhythmias—also found to be effective in treating hypertension)	Excessive vasodilation, swelling in feet and ankles, orthostatic hypotension, increased risk of falls

common cause, accounting for 20% to 40% of all cases. This type of delirium, termed *metabolic encephalopathy*, may result from organ failure, including liver or kidney failure. Other metabolic causes include diabetes mellitus, hyperthyroidism and hypothyroidism, vitamin deficiencies, and imbalances of fluids and electrolytes in the blood. Severe dehydration can also cause delirium.[65]

Drug intoxication (*intoxication confusional state*) is responsible for up to 20% of delirium cases, either from side effects, overdose, or deliberate ingestion of a mind-altering substance. Medicinal drugs with delirium as a possible side effect or result of overdose include the following:[66]

- Sedatives, including barbiturates, benzodiazepines, and ethanol (drinking alcohol)
- Anticholinergics, including atropine, scopolamine, chlorpromazine (an anti-psychotic), and diphenhydramine (an anti-histamine)
- Anti-depressant drugs
- Anti-convulsant drugs

Table 7-16

DRUGS PRESCRIBED TO REDUCE BLOOD CLOTS AND PLAQUE FORMATION IN THE VASCULAR SYSTEM: ANTI-COAGULANT, ANTI-THROMBOTIC, AND THROMBOLYTIC DRUGS COMMONLY PRESCRIBED

DRUG	METHOD OF ACTION	WHEN PRESCRIBED
ANTI-COAGULANT Heparin	Inhibits synthesis and function of clotting factors	Used primarily to prevent and treat venous thromboembolism
ORAL ANTI-COAGULANT Anisindione Dicumarol Warfarin Coumadin Panwarfin	Inhibits synthesis and function of clotting factors	Used primarily to prevent and treat venous thromboembolism
ANTI-THROMBOTIC Aspirin Dipyridamole Sulfinpyrazone	Inhibits platelet aggregation and platelet-induced clotting	Use primarily to prevent arterial, thrombus formation
THROMBOLYTIC Anistreplase Streptokinase Urokinase	Facilitates clot dissolution	Used to reopen occluded vessels in arterial and venous thrombosis

- NSAIDs, including ibuprofen and acetaminophen
- Corticosteroids, including prednisone
- Anti-cancer drugs, including methotrexate and procarbazine
- Lithium
- Cimetidine
- Antibiotics
- L-dopa.

Dementias

Up to 15% of the aging population suffer from the symptoms of dementia: memory loss, disorientation, and confusion. Dementia can be a side effect of medicines; it may also be related to high blood pressure or conditions like Huntington's disease (a genetic disorder), Parkinson's disease (involuntary tremors), or Creutzfeldt-Jakob disease (a viral infection). Treatment of these diseases can, to a small extent, reverse the dementia. However, some 60% of those with symptoms of dementia have Alzheimer's disease, a slow, progressive mental deterioration that, so far, cannot be cured.

Alzheimer's disease is a particularly tragic disorder. It can affect people as early as in their 40s, but is more common among the elderly. Among the first signs of Alzheimer's include loss of short-term or recent memory (eg, forgetting to shut off a light or the stove, or to pick up the kids from school). As the disease gets worse, the person tends to become lost more easily and begins to forget how to do simple tasks like adding up numbers or reading the newspaper. Later on, all mental functions deteriorate, although the rest of the body is usually spared.[67]

Treatment today consists largely of keeping the patient nourished, reducing agitation through tranquilizers, and helping the family cope through support groups. There is one medication—Cognex—that can alleviate the symptoms of Alzheimer's in some. It is not a cure and does not work for many people, but it is definitely worth trying.

Table 7-17

DRUGS PRESCRIBED TO IMPROVE CARDIAC OUTPUT

DRUG	METHOD OF ACTION	SIDE EFFECTS
Cardiotonic glycoside	Increases cardiac output, improves contractility, decreases heart rate, controls dysrhythmias Increases influx of calcium ions into myocardial cells by altering the electric properties of cell membrane (sodium-potassium pump) Decreases conduction velocity through A-V node	Nausea, vomiting, anorexia, diarrhea, nervousness, headache, hypokalemia, visual disturbances, dysrhythmias (usually conduction disturbances) Prolonged pulse interval on EKG indicates toxicity
Calcium channel blocker	Increases CO by decreasing heart rate and increasing ventricular filling time Blocks influx of calcium ions, decreases smooth muscle contractions, and relaxes coronary arteries In some cases, may lower CO by decreasing contractility of cardiac muscle	Headache, hypotension, flushing, pedal edema, constipation, vertigo, dysesthesia, atrioventricular block
Beta blocker	Cardioselective blockers inhibit beta-1 receptors in the heart, relieving hypertension angina and dysrhythmias Nonselective blockers inhibit beta-1 and beta-2 receptors Both types may decrease CO by decreasing ventricular contractility Bradycardia in patients with compromised ventricular function	Lightheadedness, depression, mild paresthesia, hypotension, respiratory distress, heart failure, dysrhythmias, decreased peripheral circulation Increased respiratory distress with COPD or asthma
Vasopressor	Stimulates beta-receptors in the heart Increases CO by increasing strength of muscle contraction (improving stroke volume) or increasing heart rate	Nausea, vomiting, tachycardia, dysrhythmias, palpitation MAO inhibitors may increase effects
Coronary vasodilator	Relaxes smooth muscle of coronary arteries, increases blood supply, and relaxes smooth muscle in vascular system May improve cardiac output	Headache, flushing, nausea, vomiting, vertigo, hypotension Glaucoma patients at risk for increase in intraocular pressure
Peripheral vasodilator	Relaxes smooth muscle in peripheral vascular system, blood pressure; also decreases preload and pulmonary capillary pressure May improve cardiac output by decreasing afterload and allowing more efficient ventricular function	Nausea; vomiting; abdominal discomfort; reduced lightheadedness, headache, anxiety, muscle, twitching, skin rash, tachycardia, palpitations, angina Can raise the blood glucose level in individuals with diabetes
Diuretic	Inhibits renal absorption of sodium in combating chronic congestive heart failure Relieves concomitant edema Can increase or decrease CO by affecting preload rhythm of heart volumes	Fatigue, anorexia, diarrhea, skin rash, vertigo, tinnitus, loss of electrolytes, hypokalemia, weakness, muscle cramps Severe potassium loss affecting quality and contractions Severe dehydration

There is no medication available that can cure Alzheimer's disease or stop its progression. While researchers continue to try to find a cure, medication is available that provides some relief of symptoms.[68]

Acetyl cholinesterase inhibitors are used to improve cognitive functioning in the early stage of Alzheimer's disease. These drugs increase the availability of the neurotransmitter, acetylcholine, which is often reduced in patients with Alzheimer's disease. Three medications in this class have been approved by the FDA for the treatment of mild to moderate symptoms of dementia in patients with Alzheimer's disease. They are *Aricept (donepezil), Exelon (rivastigmine),* and *Reminyl (galantamine)*.

One newer medication that works on a different neurotransmitter system in the brain has been approved by the FDA for the treatment of moderate to severe symptoms of dementia in patients with Alzheimer's disease. *Namenda (memantine)* is thought to regulate glutamate through its action on the N-methyl-D-aspartate (NMDA) receptors in the brain.

Parkinson's Disease

Table 7-21 provides the drugs currently being used to treat Parkinson's disease. All medications may have side effects, which can include mental confusion, hallucinations, and dyskinesia (abnormal movements).

PERIPHERAL NERVOUS SYSTEM: NEUROSENSORY SYSTEM

Herpes Zoster

The antiviral drugs *acyclovir, valacyclovir,* and *famciclovir* can be used to treat herpes zoster (shingles) and possibly shorten the course of the illness. Their use results in more rapid healing of the blisters when drug therapy is started within 72 hours of the onset of the rash. In fact, the earlier the drugs are administered, the better because early cases can sometimes be stopped. If taken later, these drugs are less effective but may still lessen the pain. Antiviral drug treatment does not

---

Table 7-18

DRUGS COMMONLY USED FOR CHRONIC OBSTRUCTIVE PULMONARY DISEASE[60]

Bronchodilators Help open narrowed airways. Short-acting bronchodilators, both beta-agonists and anti-cholinergics, are the backbone of therapy for COPD. Long-acting bronchodilators are used for moderate to severe COPD.

The most common side effect of taking beta-agonists is muscle tremor. This side effect often goes away after taking the medication for several weeks. High doses of beta-agonists can cause adverse effects such as a change in blood pressure, increase in heart rate, restlessness, apprehension, and headaches.

Anti-cholinergic drugs block the chemical produced by bodies that normally cause the airways to contract. They also decrease mucous secretions or phlegm.

Corticosteroids or steroids can be given orally or intravenously during acute symptoms of COPD to help reduce any inflammation and bronchospasm. The use of inhaled corticosteroids remains one of the most controversial issues in COPD pharmacology. Data from studies show a modest reduction in the frequency of COPD exacerbations with inhaled corticosteroids.

Antibiotics Fight infection and are frequently given at the first sign of a respiratory infection.

Expectorants help loosen and expel mucous secretions from the airways.

Oxygen is only helpful when there is a low level of oxygen in the blood. Being short of breath does not necessarily mean that you are not getting enough oxygen. Tests can be done to check blood oxygen levels. Low oxygen levels over months or years can put a strain on the heart, leading to heart problems. Oxygen is given to prevent heart strain. It is considered a drug and can have side effects.

A **flu vaccine** is generally recommended for people with COPD. Chronic inflammation of the airways and poor airway clearance increases the susceptibility for getting the flu. Flu shots are generally available in early autumn.

Table 7-19

COMMONLY PRESCRIBED DRUGS IN RESISTIVE PULMONARY DISEASES AND ASTHMA[62]

Bronchodilators Short-acting medications, including albuterol, levalbuterol, pirbuterol, and terbutaline, are taken as rescue medications. Long-acting ones, such as salmeterol and formoterol, are used together with an anti-inflammatory drug every day. Using more than one short-acting canister a month or needing it more than 3 to 4 times a day is a red flag. This may mean that the respiratory inflammation is not well controlled.

- They work quickly and last for varying periods of time
- They open narrowed airways and relieve bronchoconstriction (spasms of the airways)
- They do little to reduce the chronic inflammation that makes bronchial tubes overly sensitive
- They help stop asthma attacks once they have begun and are used as needed
- They have side effects that include nervousness, increased heart rate, restlessness, and insomnia.

Slow onset, long-acting bronchodilators (LABA) These drugs provide long-term relaxation of spasms in the airways.

- They work slowly and last a long time
- They must be used on a regular basis to be effective (those with persistent asthma will need to take this medication once or twice daily)
- They are considered a first line of preventive care because they help to prevent asthma attacks from starting
- They do not immediately stop asthma attacks once begun.

Inhaled corticosteroids Dry powder or aerosol are the commonly prescribed forms and can take 1 week or more to start working fully. These medications are the most effective for long-term control over persistent asthma. Examples include beclomethasone, budesonide, flunisolide, fluticasone, and triamcinolone.

- Inhaled corticosteroids are the most effective medications to prevent swelling and irritation in the lining of inflamed airways
- Inhaled corticosteroids may help reduce the need for inhaled bronchodilators
- Inhaled corticosteroids block the chemicals in the body that cause inflammation
- Inhaled corticosteroids are not the same as anabolic steroids used illegally by some athletes.

Inhaled corticosteroids can cause hoarseness or thrush (a fungal infection in the mouth and throat), which can be prevented in some cases by rinsing and gargling with mouthwash after each dose.

Oral corticosteroids Medications taken by mouth are usually considered short-term medications for asthma flare-ups. Side effects of using oral corticosteroids include slight weight gain, increased appetite, menstrual irregularities, cramps, heartburn, or indigestion. Long-term use could lead to ulcers, weight gain, cataracts, weakened bones, high blood pressure, and elevated blood sugar.

Leukotriene modifiers Antileukotrienes, also known as leukotriene inhibitors or modifiers, are among the newest oral anti-inflammatory medications. The body processes leukotrienes, chemicals that cause inflammation, as part of the reaction to an allergen.

- They may be useful as a primary treatment to control mild persistent asthma or as add-on therapy with moderate or severe persistent asthma
- They block the recognition of allergens, thereby avoiding the usual cascade of symptoms
- They include side effects such as headache and nausea, and the medications may interact negatively with other drugs, such as blood thinners
- They are only available as tablets.

(Continued)

Table 7-19 continued

COMMONLY PRESCRIBED DRUGS IN RESISTIVE PULMONARY DISEASES AND ASTHMA[62]

Mast cell stabilizers These work by preventing the release of substances in the body that cause inflammation. Mast cells play an important role in the body's allergic response. In an allergic response, an allergen stimulates the release of antibodies, which attach themselves to mast cells. Following subsequent allergen exposure, the mast cells release substances such as histamine (a chemical responsible for allergic symptoms) into the tissue.

Theophylline preparations This type of oral medication is a bronchodilator. Theophylline is rarely used in asthma treatment today and is noted for significant side effects, including nervousness, hyperactivity, upset stomach, and headaches.

Anti-histamines Anti-histamines can help if the individual has allergies along with asthma. These drugs work by blocking histamine, which is a chemical released by the body to deal with an allergen. These drugs are in 2 categories: sedating (can make some people feel drowsy) and nonsedating (will not cause people to feel drowsy). Possible side effects may include difficulty urinating, constipation, and dry mouth.

Omalizumab This is a new class of therapy known as anti-IgE and is meant for people with allergic asthma. IgE is an antibody in the body that can cause problems for some people. This medication may help reduce allergic reactions by causing free IgE to go away. As a result, the IgE cannot attach to an allergen such as pollen. This medication is given as a shot every 2 or 4 weeks. Doctors prescribe this medication only to those who have moderate to severe persistent allergic asthma and:

- have trouble controlling their asthma through combination treatments
- have trouble due to inhaled or oral steroid use
- go to the hospital often
- have poor quality of life because of their condition.

Table 7-20

COMMONLY PRESCRIBED DRUGS TO PREVENT AND TREAT CEREBROVASCULAR ACCIDENTS

Anti-thrombotic drugs These reduce the risk of blood clot formation, a major cause of ischemic stroke.

Thrombolytic agents These drugs are used to treat an ongoing, acute ischemic stroke caused by an artery blockage. These medications halt the stroke by dissolving the blood clot that is interfering with blood flow to the brain. One thrombolytic substance, recombinant tissue plasminogen activator, can be effective if administered intravenously within 3 hours of the onset of stroke symptoms. It should be used only after a physician has confirmed that the patient has suffered an ischemic rather than a hemorrhagic stroke. These drugs can increase bleeding and, therefore, must be used only after careful patient screening. Thrombolytics, such as tissue plasminogen activators, are effective only if given within 3 hours from the onset of stroke symptoms. Therefore, it is critical to get to the emergency room as soon as possible. This is usually best accomplished by calling 911 and being transported by ambulance.

Neuroprotectants These drugs protect the brain from secondary injury caused by stroke. The FDA has approved only a few of these drugs; others are undergoing clinical trial.

seem to reduce the incidence of postherpetic neuralgia, but recent studies suggest famciclovir may cut the duration of postherpetic neuralgia in half. Side effects of typical oral doses of these antiviral drugs are minor with headache and nausea reported by 8% to 20% of patients. Severely immunocompromised individuals, such as those with AIDS, may require intravenous administration of anti-viral drugs.

Corticosteroids, such as prednisone, may be used to reduce inflammation but they do interfere with the

Table 7-21

COMMONLY PRESCRIBED ANTI-PARKINSONISM DRUGS

Levodopa Levodopa is the preferred drug for Parkinson's and is usually effective, especially for bradykinesia. The body turns levodopa into dopamine. To protect levodopa from degradation before it gets to the brain, it is combined with carbidopa. The combination is marketed as *Sinemet*. Another medication, *Stalevo*, combines carbidopa and levodopa with entacapone, which extends the time that levodopa is active in the brain.

Levodopa can cause nausea, vomiting, dizziness, and occasional heart rhythm disturbances. After it has been used for a while, the medication can cause restlessness, confusion, and abnormal movements. Sometimes these side effects occur just before the next dose is due; at other times they are unpredictable. Changes by the doctor in the amount or timing of each dose can prevent this.

Anticholinergics Doctors may use these drugs to help relieve tremor. However, these medications can cause dry mouth, constipation, urine retention, and blurred vision. In elderly patients, they can cause confusion and hallucinations, which are particular problems with elderly patients.

Dopamine agonists Other chemicals that act like dopamine can enhance the effect of levodopa when given at the same time, but they also enhance levodopa's side effects, along with having side effects of their own.

Catechol-O-methyl transferase (COMT) inhibitors These drugs are taken with levodopa. COMT inhibitors prolong symptom relief by blocking the enzyme that breaks down levodopa.

Selective monoamine oxidase type B These can help delay the need for *Sinemet* when used in the earliest stages of the disease. They can delay the need for *Sinemet* when prescribed in the earliest stage of Parkinson's disease and have also been approved for use in later stages to boost the effects of *Sinemet*. *Eldepryl* may interact with anti-depressants, narcotic painkillers, and decongestants.

Muscarinic antagonists *Symmetrel* may trigger the release of dopamine from storage sites and block the reuptake of dopamine. The drug may help reduce dyskinesia caused by levodopa and help reduce tremor. The drug is widely used by itself with *Sinemet* added later on. However, *Symmetrel* does not work for long in people with advanced disease.

Propranolol and primidone These drugs are sometimes used to control the tremor of Parkinsonism. Propranolol is also used to treat high blood pressure, and primidone is used for certain kinds of seizures.

---

functioning of the immune system. Corticosteroids, in combination with anti-viral therapy, are also used to treat severe infections, such as those affecting the eyes, and to reduce severe pain.

Once the blisters are healed, some people continue to experience pain for months or even years (postherpetic neuralgia). This pain can be excruciating. Consequently, the doctor may prescribe tranquilizers, sedatives, or anti-depressants to be taken at night. As noted previously, attempts to treat postherpetic neuralgia with the antiviral drug famciclovir have shown some promising results. When all else fails, severe pain may require a permanent nerve block.

A newer medication to treat postherpectic neuralgia is pregabalin, to be marketed in the United States under the trade name *Lyrica*. Pregabalin was approved by FDA in September 2004 for the treatment of diabetic neuropathy as well as postherpetic neuralgia. It has been shown to improve patients'

sleep and overall quality of life as well as relieve pain. Its most common side effects are drowsiness, headache, dry mouth, and dizziness.

Decubitus Ulcers

Every year, millions of older people experience burns; suffer from nonhealing wounds; or have acute wounds that become complicated by infection, dehiscence, or problematic scarring. Effective wound treatment requires carefully considered interventions often requiring multiple clinic or hospital visits. There has been a relatively slow growth of new treatment options for wound management. Pharmacological interventions have been gradually emerging, although currently available wound healing therapies are only partially effective. New therapies are emerging that target various aspects of wound repair and promise new therapeutic interventions.[69]

Wounds in the elderly can include cuts, scrapes, scratches, and punctured skin. They often occur as a result of an accident or injury, but surgical incisions, sutures, and stitches also cause wounds. As dicussed in Chapter 3, the skin of an older individual thins and is more fragile and vulnerable to injury. Often the PTA will be the first clinician to identify areas of the skin at risk for breakdown. It is important to scan the older individual daily for signs of breakdown or infection of an existing wound. The PTA should watch for swelling and redness and report any evidence of skin changes to the PT. Pay particular attention to properly maintaining fingernails and toenails, keeping swelling to a minimum, and the use of careful handling techniques to avoid causing skin tears and bruising. Serious and infected wounds require medical attention.

There are numerous wound care products to enhance healing. These include drugs, ointments, skin cleansers, moisterizers, and medicated dressings.[70] Table 7-22 provides the latest wound care drugs and description of the drug's use and effectiveness. Wound care interventions for the PTA are covered in greater detail in Chapter 10.

Drugs to Treat the Vestibular System

Symptoms of vestibular dysfunction may be treated with a variety of oral medicine or through injections[72]. Anti-histamines, like diphenhydramine, meclizine, and cyclizine, can be prescribed to sedate the vestibular system. A barbiturate medication like pentobarbital may be used to completely sedate the patient and relieve the vertigo. Anti-cholinergic drugs, like atropine or scopolamine, can help minimize nausea and vomiting. *Diazepam* has been found to be particularly effective for relief of vertigo and nausea in Meniere's disease. There have been some reports of successful control of vertigo after antibiotics (gentamicin or streptomycin) or a steroid medication (dexamethasone) are injected directly into the inner ear. Some researchers have found that gentamicin is effective in relieving tinnitus as well as vertigo.

A newer medication that appears to be effective in treating the vertigo associated with Meniere's disease is flunarizine, which is sold under the trade name *Sibelium*. Flunarizine is a calcium channel blocker and anti-convulsant presently used to treat Parkinson's disease, migraine headache, and other circulatory disorders that affect the brain.

Antibiotics are mostly used to treat acute otitis media. The most common type of bacteria determines which antibiotic is used in a given community. Antibiotics are chosen among the following groups:

- Sulfa based;
- Penicillins (including amoxicillin and amoxicillin combinations)
- Cephalosporins
- New "mycins" like azithromycin or clarithromycin.

To control pain and fever associated with vestibular conditions, prescription eardrops can be used until the antibiotics begin to work. Oral pain relievers like acetaminophen or ibuprofen can also be used as needed to reduce inner ear inflammation and pain.

DRUGS AND GASTROINTESTINAL PATHOLOGIES

Gastric Ulcers

The following medication classes are most frequently prescribed by physicians for the diagnosis of peptic ulcer disease.[73] Table 7-23 provides those medications often prescribed or purchased over the counter by the individual to relieve discomfort.

- *Antibiotics.* A 1- to 2-week course of antibiotics to kill the *H. pylori* bacteria.
- *Acid blockers.* Also called H_2 *blockers*, these medications block the action of histamine on the cells that produce acid. Acid blockers are available over the counter as well as by prescription. They relieve ulcer-related pain and promote healing of the ulcer.
- *Antacids.* These neutralize the acid in the stomach and provide rapid relief of ulcer-related pain. They are often used with an acid blocker.
- *Proton pump inhibitors.* These shut down the biological "pump" that produces acid in the cells lining the stomach. They tend to be more effective than the acid blockers but are more expensive. One example, *Prilosec*, is available over the counter.
- *Cytoprotective agents.* These are drugs that coat the stomach lining, protect it against acid secretion, and promote healing.

Atrophic Gastritis

The discovery of *H. pylori's* role in development of gastritis and ulcers has led to improved treatment of chronic gastritis[75]. In particular, relapse rates for duodenal and gastric ulcers have been reduced with successful treatment of *H. pylori* infection. Since the infection can be treated with antibiotics, the bacterium can be completely eliminated up to 90% of the time.

Although *H. pylori* can be successfully treated, the treatment may be uncomfortable for patients and relies heavily on patient compliance. In 1998, studies were underway to identify the best treatment method based on simplicity, patient cooperation, and results. No single antibiotic has been found that would eliminate *H. pylori* on its own, so a combination of antibiotics has been prescribed to treat the infection.

Dual Therapy for Gastritis

Dual therapy involves the use of an antibiotic and a proton pump inhibitor. Proton pump inhibitors help reduce stomach acid by halting the mechanism that pumps acid into the stomach. This also helps promote the healing of ulcers or inflammation. Dual therapy has not been proven to be as effective as triple therapy but may be ordered for some patients who can more comfortably handle the use of less drugs and will therefore more likely follow the 2-week course of therapy.

Triple Therapy for Gastritis

As of early 1998, triple therapy was the preferred treatment for patients with *H. pylori* gastritis. It is estimated that triple therapy successfully eliminates 80% to 95% of *H. pylori* cases. This treatment regimen usually involves a 2-week course of 3 drugs. An antibiotic such as amoxicillin or tetracycline and another antibiotic such as clarithomycin or metronidazole are used in combination with bismuth subsalicylate, a substance found in the over-the-counter medication Pepto-Bismol, which helps protect the lining of the stomach from acid. Physicians are experimenting with various combinations of drugs and time of treatment to balance side effects with effectiveness in the elderly. Side effects of triple therapy are not serious,

Table 7-22

COMMONLY PRESCRIBED DRUGS AND PRODUCTS FOR WOUND CARE[71]

Becaplermin *(Regranex)* Used to treat ulcers of the foot, ankle, or leg in patients with diabetes. Becaplermin is a human platelet-derived growth factor, a substance naturally produced by the body that helps in wound healing. It works in combination with good ulcer care (cleaning, pressure relief, and infection control) by bringing the cells that the body uses to repair wounds to the site of the ulcer.

Growth factors Have been found to stimulate wound healing. The growth factors stimulate the continuous synthesis and degeneration of collagen, promoting the remodeling process for closure of a wound. It has been found that growth factors are naturally secreted at a wound site to facilitate natural healing. Adding growth factors has been found to speed healing.[71]

Wound cleansers/debriders Gently cleanses a wound before dressing application. Wound cleansers are applied directly into the wound for purification. They may contain ingredients that absorb drainage and/or deodorize the wound. Cleansers/debriders are used to remove dead tissue while keeping healthy tissue intact. There are numerous cleansing solutions available.

Moisturizers Add moisture to the skin and assist in keeping the skin from cracking or breaking down, which increases the risk of infection.

Ointments Provide a petrolium-based barrier or water-resistant cream protecting the wound from moisture or exposure to environmental contaminants.

Skin sealants Provide some degree of protection from mechanical and chemical injury by providing a protective film on the skin. These usually contain alcohol and need to be used cautiously as they may dehydrate the skin. Adequate hydration and moisturization of the skin should be used in conjuction with skin sealants.

Enzymatic debriding agents Pharmaceutical agents that assist in obliterating necrotic tissue, secretions, and denatured collagen. Many of these agents are applied using medicated dressings.

Medicated dressings Interact with the wound and enhance healing. These dressings include alginate, anti-microbial, charcoal/odor control, collagen, calcium alginates, hydrocollaid guaze, paste and powder dressings, hydrogel, semipermeable foam dressings, and silicone dressings. Each dressing medicates and helps to prevent infection and debride the dead tissues.

but may cause enough discomfort that patients are not inclined to follow the treatment.[76]

Other Treatments for Gastritis

Scientists have experimented with *quadruple therapy*, which adds an anti-secretory drug (ie, one that suppresses gastric secretion) to the standard triple therapy. One study showed this therapy to be effective with only 1 week's course of treatment in more than 90% of patients. Short course therapy was attempted with triple therapy involving anti-biotics and a proton pump inhibitor and seemed effective in eliminating *H. pylori* in 1 week for more

than 90% of patients. The goal is to develop the most effective therapy combination that can work in 1 week of treatment or less. In order to ensure that *H. pylori* has been eradicated, physicians will test patients following treatment. The breath test is the preferred method to check for remaining signs of *H. pylori*.[77]

Treatment of Erosive Gastritis

Since few patients with erosive gastritis show symptoms, treatment may depend on their severity. When symptoms do occur, patients may be treated with therapy similar to that for *H. pylori*,

Table 7-23

DRUG TREATMENTS PRESCRIBED OR PURCHASED OVER THE COUNTER FOR GASTRIC ULCERS

DRUG	TRADE NAME	METHOD OF ACTION
ANTACIDS		
Sodium bicarbonate	*Alka-Selzer*	Neutralization of gastric acid
Aluminum hydroxide	*Basaljel* *Amphojel*	Relief of hyperacidity
Aluminum hydroxide magnesium	*Maalox* *Mylanta*	Neutralizaton of acidity
Magaldrate	*Riopan*	Rapid and uniform buffering action
H₂ RECEPTOR BLOCKERS		
Cimetidine	*Tagamet*	Inhibits histamine at the H-receptors of gastric cells
Ranitidine	*Zantac*	Inhibits histamine at the H-receptors of gastric cells
Famotidine	*Pepcid*	Inhibits histamine at the H-receptors of gastric cells
ANTI-CHOLINERGICS		
Anisotropine	*Valpin*	Treatment of peptic ulcers; anti-cholinergics decrease the activity of acetycholine synapses; used to diminish parasympathetic activity
Atropine	*Dey-Dose*	Multiple uses; in addition to peptic ulcers, it is also used to treat irritable bowel syndrome, neurogenic bladder, bronchospasm, and postmyocardial infarction
Clidinium	*Quarzan*	Used to treat peptic ulcers and irritable bowel syndrome
Homatropine	*Homapin*	
Hyoscyamine	*Levsin*	
Isopropamide	*Darbid*	
SUCRALFATE	*Carafate*	Formation of ulcer adherent complex, which covers the ulcer site and protects it against further attack by acid, pepsin, and bile salts
METOCLOPRAMIDE	*Reglan*	Stimulates motility in the upper GI tract

especially since some studies have demonstrated a link between *H. pylori* and NSAIDs in causing ulcers. Avoidance of NSAIDs will most likely be prescribed.

Other Forms of Gastritis

Specific treatment will depend on the cause and type of gastritis[78]. These may include prednisone or antibiotics. Critically ill patients at high risk for bleeding may be treated with preventive drugs to reduce the risk of acute stress gastritis. If stress gastritis does occur, the patient is treated with constant infusion of a drug to stop bleeding. Sometimes surgery is recommended but is weighed against the possibility of surgical complications or death. Once torrential bleeding occurs in acute stress gastritis, mortality is as high as 60% and greater.

Pernicious Anemia

Treatment of pernicious anemia requires the administration of lifelong injections of vitamin B_{12}. Vitamin B_{12} given by injection enters the bloodstream directly and does not require intrinsic factor. At first, injections may need to be given several times a week in order to build up adequate stores of the vitamin. After this, the injections can be given on a monthly basis. Other substances required for blood cell production such as iron and vitamin C may also need to be given.

Diarrhea

Table 7-24 provides information on drugs prescribed for diarrhea. Regardless of the cause of diarrhea, gaining control of bowel movements is essential for proper absorption of nutrients and water. Diarrhea results in poor absorption of essential food substances and can lead to extreme dehydration.[79] Diarrhea results from irritable bowel syndrome (IBS), diverticulosis, and colitus, all of which can significantly impact the individual's nutritional status.

Constipation

Laxatives are used to promote the evacuation of the bowel and facilitate bowel movements[80]. *Cathartics* work in a similar fashion, but they are faster acting and are more likely to be employed when there is a bowel obstruction. The use of the terms *laxative* and *cathartic* are often used interchangeably, however, there is a difference in the slow- versus the fast-acting versions of each. *Bulk-forming laxatives* absorb water in the lower intestines. The result of this is to stretch the bowel tract and loosen the bowel to enhance evacuation and decrease discomfort of bowel movements. *Stimulant*

laxatives activate peristalsis by directly irritating the intestinal walls and stimulating contraction. These types of laxatives/cathartics work by increasing fluid retention and softening the hard bowel. *Hyperosmotic laxatives* create an osmotic force by drawing water into the intestines and softening the stool. *Lubricants* and *stool softeners*, like mineral oil, also work to soften the stool and permit the movement of stool through the intestines. These types of laxatives/cathartics also increase the pressure in the bowel to smooth the progress of a bowel movement along the lower intestinal tract. Table 7-25 lists the most frequently prescribed laxatives/catarctics, the method of action, and the potential side effects such as nausea and abdominal discomfort created by contraction of the intestines. Fluid and electrolyte imbalance is also a potential risk. The negative effects are much more common in less mobile, dependent older patients. One of the biggest risks of side effects in the elderly is laxative dependence.

If changes in diet and activity fail to relieve occasional constipation, an over-the-counter laxative may be used for a few days. Preparations that soften stools or add bulk (bran, psyllium) work more slowly but are safer than epsom salts and other harsh laxatives or herbal laxatives containing senna (*Cassia senna*) or buckthorn (*Rhamnus purshianna*), which can harm the nerves and lining of the colon.

A warm-water or mineral oil enema can relieve constipation, and a nondigestible sugar (*lactulose*) or special electrolyte solution is recommended for older adults with stubborn symptoms. If a patient has an impacted bowel, the doctor inserts a gloved finger into the rectum and gently dislodges the hardened feces.

Alternative Treatment

Initially, alternative practitioners[81] will suggest that the patient drink an adequate amount of water each day (6 to 8 glasses), exercise on a regular basis, and eat a diet high in soluble and insoluble fibers. Soluble fibers include pectin, flax, and gums; insoluble fibers include psyllium and brans from grains like wheat and oats. Fresh fruits and vegetables contain both soluble and insoluble fibers. Castor oil, applied topically to the abdomen and covered by a heat source (a heating pad or hot water bottle), can help relieve constipation when used nightly for 20 to 30 minutes.

There are a number of general measures that can be taken to improve bowel function. Controlled trials suggest that fiber supplements like *Metamucil* are effective in constipation-predominant IBS. Medications such as *Imodium AD* control symptoms in diarrhea-predominant IBS. In pain-predominant IBS, 2 classes of medications are effective in reducing pain: the anti-spasmodic agents such as *Donnatal* (belladonna alkaloids with barbiturates), *Bentyl* (dicyclomine), *Librax* (chlordiazepoxide with clidinium), and *Levsin* (hyoscyamine) and the tricyclic antidepressants. Anti-spasmodics prevent or treat painful muscular spasms of hollow tubes within the body, such as the gut. If the gut goes into spasm, severe intermittent pains can develop in the abdomen.

There are many medications used to treat inflammatory bowel disease depending on its severity. Milder cases may be treated with a medication that is a combination of aspirin and a sulfa drug called sulfasalazine. More severe cases require immunosuppressant agents such as corticosteroids, azathioprine, and cyclosporine (also used in transplant recipients to prevent rejection). New classes of medications for refractory disease have been developed within the past several years. One such medication *Remicade* (infliximab) is a monoclonal antibody to tumor necrosis factor (TNF). TNF is an inflammatory mediator in CD. Clinical trials have shown infliximab to be highly effective in the treatment of refractory cases of IBS.

The PTA may play an important role in encouraging self-help strategies in the elderly. Being receptive to and answering an elderly patient's questions about treatments while working together during a therapy session is an important component of therapy. Although not directly a part of the typical physical therapy care plan, optimal bowel function will enhance the older person's well being and ability to participate during therapy.

Urinary Incontinence

Drugs can inhibit contractions of an overactive bladder or relax bladder muscles, leading to more complete bladder emptying during urination[82]. Other drugs tighten muscles at the bladder neck and urethra. Hormone supplements, including estrogen, may help muscles involved in urination to function better. Ask a doctor about the risks and benefits of long-term use of these medications, particularly hormone replacement. Recent studies show hormone replacement can increase incontinence and uterine prolapse, which is the falling down of the uterus into or beyond the vagina[83] (see Table 7-26).

DRUGS AND ENDOCRINE/ METABOLIC DISEASES

The endocrine system includes 8 major glands.[87] These glands make hormones, which act as chemical messengers as they travel through the bloodstream to tissues or organs working steadily and slowly to affect metabolic processes from head to toe. These processes include the following:

- Growth and development
- Metabolism (digestion, elimination, breathing,

Table 7-24

DRUGS USED TO CONTROL AND TREAT DIARRHEA IN THE ELDERLY

DRUG	TRADE NAME	METHOD OF ACTION
Absorbants		
Kaolin Pectin	*Kaopectate* *Kapectolin*	Absorption of excess fluid and causative agent
Bacterial cultures		
Lactobacillus acidophilus *Lactobacillus bulgaris*	(see Table 7-1)	Antibacterial administered to re-establish flora to decrease bacteria
Bismuth salicylate	*Pepto-Bismol*	Stimulates water and electrolyte absorption from the lower GI tract; has an anti-bacterial effect and decreases gastric acid secretion; also has an antacid effect
Opiate derivatives		
Diphenoxylate Loperamide	*Lomotil* *Imodium*	Binds to intestine opiate receptors, decreasing peristalsis and pain; anti-diarrheal drug that directly affects the nerve supply of the GI tract, decreases secretions, and relieves cramping and diarrhea

Table 7-25

LAXATIVES/CATHARCTIC DRUGS TO TREAT CONSTIPATION IN THE ELDERLY

DRUG	TRADE NAME	METHOD OF ACTION	SIDE EFFECTS
Bulk-Forming			
Psyllium methylcellulose	*Metamucil Citrucel*	Absorbs water in the GI tract to form a gelatinous bulk that encourages a normal bowel movement	Powder may cause allergic reaction if inhaled
Perdiem	*Fiberall*	Vegetable mucilages soften stool and provide pain-free evacuation	Laxative dependance, excessive water and body salt loss
Stimulants			
Castor oil	*Fleet-flavored castor oil*	Works directly on small intestine to promote a bowel movement	Laxative dependance, excessive water and body salt loss
Bisacodyl	*Ducolax*	Contact laxative directly on colonic mucosa to produce peristalis through the large intestine	Abdominal cramps
Phenolphthalein	*Modane*	Acts on large intestine to produce semifluid stool	Excess bowel activity, abdominal cramps, weakness, dizziness, heart palpitations
Hyperosmotic			
Lactulose	*Chronolac*	Broken down in the colon to lactic, formic, and acetic acids; causes an increase in stool water content	Intestinal cramps, nausea, vomiting, flatulence
Sodium phosphate	*Fleet's Enema Phospho-soda*	Versatile in action, gentle laxative or purgative	Laxative dependence, sodium loss
Lubricants/stool softeners			
Docusate	*Pericolace Disonate*	Provides general peristaltic stimulation and helps keep stools soft and pain free	Nausea, abdominal cramping, rash, diarrhea
Mineral oil	*Fleet mineral oil enema*	Contact softens and lubricates hard stools	Abdominal pain

blood circulation, and maintaining body temperature)

- Sexual function
- Reproduction
- Mood.

If hormone levels are too high or too low an endocrine disorder develops and affects the homeostasis of the body as a whole. An imbalance of any one hormone will have an effect on the entire body. Endocrine and metabolic diseases also occur if the body does not respond to hormones the way it is supposed to. Stress, infection, and changes in the blood's fluid and electrolytes can also influence hormone levels. The most common endocrine disease in the United States is diabetes. There are many other endocrine and metabolic disorders that occur more frequently as the hormone levels change with age; these are usually treated by controlling how much hormone the body makes. Hormone supplements are sometimes prescribed when there is not enough of a hormone, whereas some drugs counteract the effects of hormones when there is too much. The following is a discussion of the pharmacologic approach to the most common endocrine and metabolic diseases in the elderly (greater detail on each disease is provided in Chapter 4).

Adrenal disorders can cause the adrenal glands to make too much or not enough hormones. With Addison's disease there is too little cortisol, while with Cushing's syndrome there is too much. Some people are born unable to make enough cortisol. Tumors can

Table 7-26

COMMONLY PRESCRIBED DRUGS FOR
URGE AND STRESS INCONTINENCE IN OLDER ADULTS

GENERIC NAME	BRAND NAME	METHOD OF ACTION	SIDE EFFECTS	CONTRAINDICATIONS
URGE INCONTINENCE[84,85]				
Tolterodine	Detrol	Anti-cholinergic, decreases bladder contractility, increases capacity of bladder	Dry mouth, headache, constipation	Urinary retention, pyloric stenosis
Oxybutynin	Ditropan XL Ditropan	Anti-cholinergic, decreases bladder contractility	Dry mouth, constipation, somnolence	Urinary retention, pyloric stenosis, uncontrolled narrow-angle glaucoma
Imipramine	Tofranil	Tricyclic anti-depressant; blocks reuptake of epinephrine and serotonin, increasing bladder capacity and sphincter closure	Dry mouth, constipation, blurred vision, dizziness	Not to be given during the acute phase of myocardial infarction or with MAO inhibitors; urinary retention
Doxazosin	Cardura	Relaxes smooth muscle of urethra and prostatic capsule in men with benign prostatic hypertrophy	Postural hypotension, dizziness, dyspnea, edema	Not to be used in patients with impaired liver function
Terazosin	Hytrin	Relaxes smooth muscle of urethra and prostatic capsule in men with benign prostatic hypertrophy	Postural hypotension, dizziness, nausea	Caution with use of other anti-hypertensives
Tamsulosin	Flomax	Relaxes smooth muscle of urethra and prostatic capsule in men with benign prostatic hypertrophy	Abnormal ejaculation, postural hypotension, dizziness, insomnia, cough	Caution with use of cimetidine
STRESS INCONTINENCE[86]				
Estrogen vaginal cream	Premarin Cream Estrace	Treats atrophic vaginitis	Breast tenderness, uterine bleeding, vaginal candidiasis, headache	Endometrial cancer, impaired renal or liver function
Estradiol	ESTRING	Treats atrophic vaginitis	Headache, leukorrhea, skeletal pain	Caution in patients with impaired liver function
Phenylpropanolamine	Entex LA	Increases urethral smooth muscle contraction	Nervousness, dizziness, insomnia	Uncontrolled hypertension, benign prostatic hypertrophy
Pseudoephedrine	Sudafed	Increases urethral smooth muscle contraction	Central nervous system overstimulation, headache, elevation in blood pressure	Severe or uncontrolled hypertension, benign prostatic hypertrophy, and not for use with MAO inhibitors

also cause disorders in the adrenal glands. Bleeding and infection can cause an adrenal gland problem that can be fatal without quick treatment.

Addison's disease, also called adrenal insufficiency or hypocortisolism, affects the adrenal glands located on the top of the kidneys. The outside layer of these glands makes hormones that help the body respond to stress and regulate blood pressure and water and salt balance. Addison's disease occurs if the adrenal glands do not make enough adrenal hormones.[88] A problem with the immune system usually causes Addison's disease, where the immune system mistakenly attacks its own tissues, damaging the adrenal glands.

Pharmacological treatment of Addison's disease involves the prescription of corticosteroids. Because the body is not producing sufficient steroid hormones, one or more hormones to replace the deficiency may be prescribed. Cortisol is replaced using hydrocortisone *(Cortef),* prednisone, or cortisone. Fludrocortisone *(Florinef)* replaces aldosterone, which controls sodium and potassium levels and keeps the blood pressure normal. In addition, the doctor may recommend treating androgen deficiency with an androgen replacement called dehydroepiandrosterone. Some studies indicate that, for women with Addison's disease, androgen replacement therapy may improve overall sense of well being, libido, and sexual satisfaction. The goal is to take these hormones orally in daily doses that mimic the amount the body normally would make, thereby minimizing side effects. One clinical situation that the PTA should be aware of is an Addisonian crisis, a life-threatening situation that results in low blood pressure, low blood levels of sugar, and high blood levels of potassium. The PTA will note that the individual appears lethargic, complains of dizziness, and becomes energiless and listless. This situation requires immediate medical care. Treatment typically includes intravenous injections of the following:

- Hydrocortisone
- Saline solution
- Sugar (dextrose).

Cushing's syndrome, also called hypercortisolism, is caused by long-term exposure to too much cortisol, a hormone that the adrenal gland makes. Sometimes, taking synthetic hormone medicine to treat an inflammatory disease leads to Cushing's syndrome. Some kinds of tumors secrete a hormone that can cause the body to make too much cortisol. Treatment depends on why there is too much cortisol (eg, if the older adult has been taking synthetic hormones, a lower dose may control symptoms, or if a tumor is the cause, surgery and other therapies may be needed).

Most of the time, Cushing's syndrome is managable and in many cases can be cured.[89]

The most common cause of Cushing's syndrome is the use of oral corticosteroid medication. By contrast, it is rare for the cause to be excess cortisol production by the adrenal gland. Treatments for Cushing's syndrome are designed to return the body's cortisol production to normal. By normalizing or even markedly lowering cortisol levels, noticeable improvements in signs and symptoms occur immediately. Left untreated, however, Cushing's syndrome can eventually lead to death.[90]

The thyroid is a butterfly-shaped gland in the neck just above the collarbone. It is one of the endocrine glands, which make hormones. The thyroid helps set metabolism (ie, how the body gets energy from the foods eaten).

Thyroid disease creates a metabolic situation in which the body uses energy more slowly or quickly than it should. Hypothyroidism is far more common in the elderly. It can result in weight gain, fatigue, and difficulty dealing with cold temperatures. If the thyroid is too active, it makes more thyroid hormones than needed. That condition is hyperthyroidism. Too much thyroid hormone can result in weight loss, speed up the heart rate, and make an individual very sensitive to heat. There are many causes for both conditions. Pharmacological treatment involves trying to reset the body's metabolism to a normal rate.[91]

Anti-thyroid drugs (also called thionamides) are used to treat an overactive thyroid (hyperthyroidism) caused by Graves' disease, an autoimmune condition. These drugs block the synthesis of thyroid hormone by the thyroid gland. They may also help control the disease by indirectly affecting the immune system. Antithyroid drugs may also be used to treat hyperthyroidism associated with toxic multinodular goiter or a toxic adenoma ("hot nodule") and to treat women with hyperthyroidism during pregnancy. Table 7-27 provides information on the function of antithyroid drugs and the types of drugs available. The use of antithyroid drugs has several benefits and few risks.[92]

Most people have 4 pea-sized glands called *parathyroid glands* on the thyroid gland in the neck. Though their names are similar, the thyroid and parathyroid glands are completely different. The parathyroid glands make parathyroid hormone (PTH), which helps the body keep the right balance of calcium and phosphorous.[93]

If the parathyroid glands make too much or too little hormone, it disrupts this balance. If the parathyroids secrete extra PTH, the condition is called hyperparathyroidism (HPT), and the blood calcium rises. In many cases, a benign tumor on a

Table 7-27

DRUGS COMMONLY USED TO TREAT THYROID DISEASE

Iodide Causes a decrease in thyroid function by inhibiting thyroid hormone synthesis; used to treat hyperthyroidism.

Radioactive iodide Destroys thyroid tissue in certain types of hyperthyroidism, like Graves' disease, by reducing thyroid hormone function.

Beta-adrenergic blockers Although associated with the treatment of angina and hypertension, they are used in hyperthyroidism to suppress symptoms such as tachycardia, palpitations, fever, and restlessness; typically used in conjunction with anti-thyroid drugs.

Anti-thyroid drugs Anti-thyroid drugs decrease the production and blood levels of thyroxine (T4) and triiodothyronine (T3).

    Types of antithyroid drugs Two anti-thyroid drugs are currently available in the United States: propylthiouracil (PTU) and methimazole (MMI, Tapazole). Carbimazole (which is converted into MMI in the body) is available in Europe, but not in the United States.

    MMI is usually preferred over PTU because it reverses hyperthyroidism more quickly and has fewer side effects. MMI requires an average of 5.8 weeks to lower T4 levels to normal.

    PTU blocks the conversion of T4 to T3 in nonthyroid tissue, but it does not reverse hyperthyroidism as rapidly as MMI. PTU requires an average of 16.8 weeks to effectively lower T4 levels.

Thyroid hormones Replace deficient thyroid hormones with hypothyroidism.

    Levothyroxine (Synthroid) Alters cellular chemistry making more energy available and increases metabolism in all tissues. Thyroid hormone essential for normal growth and development; this drug replaces the rate of metabolism normally provided by thyroid hormones.

    Liothyronine (Cytomel) Increases cellular metabolism in all tissues, replacing the deficient thyroid hormones.

    Nafarelin (Synarel) Stimulates the pituitary gland to release 2 additional hormones that regulate the production of estrogen by the ovaries; typically used in treating endometriosis.

---

parathyroid gland makes it overactive. Or, the extra hormones can come from enlarged parathyroid glands. Very rarely, the cause is cancer. If there is not enough PTH, the condition is called hypoparathyroidism. In this case the blood will have too little calcium and too much phosphorous. Causes include injury to the glands, endocrine disorders, or genetic conditions. Treatment is aimed at restoring the balance of calcium and phosphorous.[94]

Although surgery is usually recommended for people with HPT (unless they have no symptoms), sometimes other medical problems make surgery too risky and the physician may recommend treatment with medicine alone. Medicines can treat some, but not all, of the symptoms of HPT. A few drugs are used to treat HPT. *Hectorol* is used to lower high parathyroid hormone (PTH) levels, particularly in patients with chronic kidney disease on dialysis. *Calcimimetics* are a new class of drug that turns off secretion of PTH. *Cinacalcet*, a calcimimetic drug that reduces PTH secretion by altering the function of parathyroid calcium-sensing receptors, can be initiated in patients with hypercalcemia due to parathyroid carcinoma,

secondary HPT, and primary HPT. This drug is used alone or with other medications to treat secondary HPT, a condition in which the body produces too much PTH. This occurs in patients with chronic kidney disease and those who are being treated with dialysis. Cinacalcet is also used to treat high levels of calcium in the blood of patients who have parathyroid cancer. Cinacalcet is in a class of medications called calcimimetics. It works by signaling the body to produce less PTH in order to decrease the amount of calcium in the blood.[95]

Intravenous hydration with isotonic sodium chloride solution adequately reduces calcium levels in most patients with hyperparathyroid-induced hypercalcemia. The use of other calcium-lowering agents, such as bisphosphonates, plicamycin, and calcitonin, are used to treat oncologic causes of hypercalcemia and are not used for HPT. For postmenopausal female patients who do not undergo surgery, estrogen may be beneficial to help maintain bone mass.

In addition to closely monitoring this condition, it is important for patients with HPT to drink lots of water, get plenty of exercise, and avoid certain diuretics, such as the thiazides. Immobilization (unable to move) and GI illness with vomiting or diarrhea can cause calcium levels to rise, increasing PTH production.

The major biologic function of vitamin D is to maintain normal blood levels of calcium and phosphorus. Vitamin D aids in the absorption of calcium, helping to form and maintain strong bones. Recently, research also suggests that in hypothyroidism vitamin D may provide protection from osteoporosis, hypertension, cancer, and several autoimmune diseases. Hypoparathyroidism is treated primarily with vitamin D. Dietary supplementation with Ca^{2+} may also be necessary.

Calcitriol is a form of vitamin D that is used to treat and prevent low levels of calcium in the blood. Low blood levels of calcium may cause bone disease. Calcitriol is in a class of medications called vitamins. It works by helping the body to use more of the calcium found in foods or supplements.[96]

The *pituitary gland* is central to well being. It is the master gland of the entire body. It produces (secretes) many hormones that stimulate glands in the body to produce other hormones or to complete certain actions. The pituitary gland makes many different hormones[97]:

- *Prolactin* stimulates milk production from the breasts after childbirth to enable nursing and can affect sex hormone levels from the ovaries in women and the testes in men.

- *Growth hormone (GH)* stimulates growth in childhood and is important for maintaining a healthy body composition and well being in adults. In adults, it is important for maintaining muscle mass as well as bone mass. It also affects fat distribution in the body.

- *Adrenocorticotropin (ACTH)* stimulates production of cortisol by the adrenal glands. Cortisol, a so-called "stress hormone," is vital to survival. It helps maintain blood pressure and blood glucose levels.

- *TSH* stimulates the thyroid gland, which regulates the body's metabolism, energy, growth and development, and nervous system activity. This hormone also is vital to survival.

- *Antidiuretic hormone (ADH)*, also called vasopressin, is stored in the back part of the pituitary gland and regulates water balance. If this hormone is not secreted properly, this can lead to diabetes insipidus (different from diabetes mellitus which affects glucose) because the kidneys are not working well.

- *Luteinizing hormone (LH)* regulates testosterone in men and estrogen in women.

- *Follicle-stimulating hormone (FSH)* promotes sperm production in men and stimulates the ovaries to enable ovulation in women. LH and FSH work together to cause normal function of the ovaries and testes.

Pituitary Tumors

The most frequent cause of pituitary disorders is pituitary tumors[98]. The pituitary gland is made of several cell types. Each cell type releases one of the hormones mentioned previously. Sometimes these cells grow too much or produce small growths or pituitary tumors, which are fairly common in older adults. These are not brain tumors and are not a form of cancer. Cancerous tumors of this sort are extremely rare. Pituitary tumors can interfere with the normal formation and release of hormones, however. In addition, some pituitary tumors make too much of the type of hormone produced by the pituitary cells forming the tumor.

Two types of tumors exist: secretory and nonsecretory. Secretory tumors produce too much of a hormone. Nonsecretory tumors cause problems because of their large size or because they interfere with normal function of the pituitary gland. These conditions must be treated differently. The problems caused by pituitary tumors fall into 3 categories: hypersecretion, hyposecretion, and tumor mass effects.

In *hypersecretion,* too much hormone is secreted into the body. This is usually caused by a secretory tumor. Common secretory tumors make too much prolactin. Other tumors make too much of the pituitary hormones that stimulate growth, the adrenal gland, or the thyroid. Tumors making too much of the hormones stimulating the ovaries or testes are extremely rare.

With *hyposecretion,* too little hormone is secreted into the body. This is usually caused by a nonsecretory tumor, which interferes with the ability of the normal pituitary gland to make hormones. It can also be caused by a secretory tumor that is large. It can also result from therapy of a tumor with surgery and/or radiation treatment.

In *tumor mass effect,* as the tumor grows and presses against the normal pituitary gland or other areas in the brain, complications such as headaches, vision problems, or hyposecretion occur. Tumor mass effects can be seen in any type of pituitary tumor that grows large enough. Injuries, certain medications, and other conditions can also affect the pituitary gland. Loss of normal pituitary function has been reported after major head trauma. The prolonged use of steroid medications such as prednisone can suppress levels of ACTH and result in adrenal insufficiency (ie, a lack of cortisol production) if abruptly discontinued, which must be replaced until ACTH and adrenal function returns. A number of psychiatric medications can lead to an increase in prolactin levels.

Treatment for a pituitary tumor depends on the type of tumor, its size, and how far it has grown into the brain. Age and overall health are also factors. Because pituitary tumors can cause serious problems by putting pressure on the brain, treatment is often necessary. Early detection of pituitary tumors is key to successful treatment. Doctors generally use surgery, radiation therapy, and medications, either alone or in combination, to treat a pituitary tumor and return hormone production to normal levels.

Treatment with medications may help to block excess hormone secretion and sometimes shrink certain types of pituitary tumors.

Prolactin-Producing Tumors (Prolactinomas)

The drugs bromocriptine (*Parlodel*) and cabergoline (*Dostinex*) can treat prolactinomas by decreasing prolactin secretion and often reducing the size of the tumor. These drugs are often so effective in treating these types of tumors that surgery is not necessary.

Growth Hormone-Producing Tumors

Two classes of drugs are available for GH-producing tumors. Drugs known as *somatostatin* analogs (*Sandostatin*, etc) cause a decrease in growth hormone production and may decrease the size of the tumor. Pegvisomant (*Somavert*) blocks the effect of excess growth hormone on the body. These medications are especially useful if surgery has been unsuccessful in normalizing growth hormone production.

If a pituitary tumor has resulted in decreased hormone production or if removal of a pituitary tumor has lowered hormone production, you may need to take replacement hormones to maintain normal hormone levels.

The Pancreas and Diabetes

The *pancreas* is a gland behind the stomach and in front of the spine. It produces juices that help break down food and hormones that help control blood sugar levels. Problems with the pancreas can lead to many health problems.[99] These include pancreatitis, or inflammation of the pancreas, which occurs when digestive enzymes start digesting the pancreas itself; pancreatic cancer; and cystic fibrosis, a genetic disorder in which thick, sticky mucus can also block tubes in the pancreas.

The pancreas also plays a role in diabetes. In type I diabetes, the beta cells of the pancreas no longer make insulin because the body's immune system has attacked them. In type II diabetes, the pancreas loses the ability to secrete enough insulin in response to meals. As a result of either type of diabetes, the blood glucose (sugar) levels are too high. Glucose comes from the foods eaten. *Insulin* is a hormone that helps the glucose get into cells to give them energy. With type I diabetes, the body does not make insulin. With type II diabetes, the more common type, the body does not make or use insulin well. Without enough insulin, the glucose stays in the blood and leads to serious complications (see Chapter 4). Over time, having too much glucose in the blood can damage the eyes, kidneys, and nerves. Diabetes can also cause heart disease, stroke, and even the need to remove a limb due to ulceration, infection, or gangrene.

Exercise, weight control, and sticking to a meal plan that decreases sugar intake can help control diabetes, in addition to frequent monitoring of the blood glucose levels and the use of prescription drugs summarized in Table 7-28. Table 7-29 provides more detail regarding each of the drug groups listed. As the PTA will work with many diabetic patients, a thorough understanding of medications is important. While some people with type II diabetes can control their disease with diet and exercise, most need medication. Treatment can include oral medications, insulin injections, or both. Most oral medications increase insulin production, decrease glucose production, or help the body to respond to its own insulin better.[100]

DEPRESSION

There are several treatment options available for depression. In many cases, a combination of treatments is most successful.[102]

Anti-depressant Drugs

Many anti-depressant medicines are available to treat depression. Most of the available anti-depressants are believed to be equally effective in elderly adults, but the risk of side effects or potential reactions with other medicines must be carefully considered. For example, certain traditional anti-depressants, such as amitriptyline and imipramine, can be sedating and result in a sudden drop in blood pressure when a person stands up, which can lead to falls and fractures. Anti-depressants may take longer to start working in older people than they do in younger people. Since elderly people are more sensitive to medicines, doctors may prescribe lower doses at first. Another factor may be forgetting (or not wanting) to take medication. Many elderly patients take many drugs, which can lead to increased complications and side effects. In general, the length of treatment for depression in the elderly is longer than it is in younger patients.[103] Table 7-30 provides information regarding commonly prescribed drug when treating depression

All medicines have side effects, but some medicines can cause or worsen depression symptoms. Among the commonly used medicines that can create such problems are some pain medicines (codeine, darvon), some drugs for high blood pressure (clonidine, reserpine), hormones (estrogen, progesterone, cortisol, prednisone, anabolic steroids), some heart medications (digitalis, propanalol), anticancer agents (cycloserine, tamoxifen, nolvadex, velban, oncovin), some drugs for Parkinson's disease (levadopa, bromocriptine), some drugs for arthritis (indomethacin), some tranquilizers and anti-anxiety drugs (valium, halcion), and alcohol.[104]

Multisystem Involvement and Polypharmacy and Adverse Effects of Drugs in the Elderly

The major concern for all cases of polypharmacy is the prospect of adverse drug reactions and serious drug-drug interactions. In some instances, it is therapeutically necessary to use multiple agents to treat certain conditions. It is the responsibility of

Table 7-28

COMMONLY PRESCRIBED DRUGS FOR TREATMENT OF DIABETES[101]

DRUG	TRADE NAME	MECHANISM OF ACTION
ORAL HYPOGLYCEMIC DRUGS		
Sulfonylureas	*Diabeta, Diabinese, Diamicron*	Stimulates the pancreas to produce more insulin
	Meglitinides	Rapid acting; stimulates the pancreas to produce more insulin
Biguanides	*Metformin*	Helps the body to use glucose more efficiently
Thiazolidinediones	*Actos, Avandia*	Controls blood glucose by making the muscle cells more sensitive to insulin
Alpha-glucosidase	*Glucoside*	Retards glucose entry into the systemic circulation
Acarbose	*Prandase*	Prolongs the absorption of carbohydrates after a meal
INJECTED THERAPEUTIC INSULIN		
Rapid-acting insulin	*Humulin R, Novolin R, Velsulin Human[H] Iletin I or II, Velsulin*	Administered to complement other drugs (oral hypoglycemics) and to supplement endogenous insulin release
Prompt insulin zinc	*Semilent Insulin, Semilente Iletin I[A]*	Supplement endogenous insulin release
Intermediate-acting	*Humulin N, Novolin H, NPH, Insulin, Isophane Insulin Insulatard NPH[H], NPH, Iletin I, NPH Iletin II[A]*	Complementary to other drugs and supplements endogenous insulin release
Insulin zinc	*Humulin L, Novolin L[H] Lente Insulin, Lente Iletin I or II[A]*	Supplements endogenous insulin release
Long-acting	*Ultralente Insulin*	Supplements endogenous insulin release
Extended insulin zinc	*Ultralente Iletin I[A]*	Supplements endogenous insulin release
Protamine zinc insulin	*Protamine Zinc and Iletin I[A] Protamine Zinc and Iletin II[A]*	Supplements endogenous insulin release

[H] *indicates insulin from human sources (biosynthetic; recombinant DNA);* [A], *insulin from animal sources.*

Table 7-29

TYPES OF DRUGS PRESCRIBED FOR THE TREATMENT OF DIABETES

Sulfonylureas Stimulate the beta cells of the pancreas to release insulin. Sulfonylurea drugs have been around since the 1950s. Chlorpropamide is the only first-generation sulfonylurea still used. All these medications work similarly on blood glucose levels, yet they differ in their side effects depending on how often they are taken and how they interact with other drugs. Low blood glucose (hypoglycemia) is the most common side effect.

Meglitinides Stimulate beta cells to release insulin. Because sulfonylureas and meglitinides stimulate the release of insulin, a patient might develop hypoglycemia, or low blood glucose levels.

Biguanides Lower blood glucose levels by decreasing how much glucose the liver makes. Biguanides help lower blood glucose levels by making muscles more sensitive to insulin, allowing glucose to enter cells. A side effect may be diarrhea.

Thiazolidinediones Help insulin work better in muscle and fat, and also reduce glucose production in the liver. Thiazolidinediones can have a rare but serious effect on the liver. Regular blood tests should be performed to check the liver. Thiazolidinediones can cause fluid accumulation, swelling of the legs (edema), and lead to heart failure.

Alpha-glucosidase inhibitors Help lower blood glucose levels by blocking the digestion of starches (such as bread, pasta, and potatoes) in the intestine. These medications can also slow the breakdown of some sugars consumed in the diet. Alpha-glucosidase inhibitors slow the rise in blood glucose levels after you eat. Side effects may include gas and diarrhea.

Insulin Is taken by many people with type II diabetes to control blood sugar (glucose) levels. Insulin cannot be taken by mouth because it would be destroyed by digestion. Many people get their insulin shots with a syringe and needle. Other methods include insulin pens, insulin jet injectors, and insulin pumps. Some insulin medications are fast-acting, only taking 5 to 15 minutes to start working and finishing in 3 to 4 hours. Intermediate-acting ones take as long as 2 to 4 hours to begin acting and continue to act for 8 to 12 hours. Long-acting insulin may not finish until more than 24 hours later. More than 20 types of insulin products are available.

pharmacists to assess patients with multiple medication regimens and to make recommendations when necessary.

Researchers have shown that more than 75% of adverse drug reactions that result in hospitalization are related to known pharmacologic agents and are partly due to inadequate monitoring, inappropriate prescribing, and lack of patient education and compliance.[105] Research also suggests that the potential for an adverse drug reaction to occur is 6% when an individual takes 2 medications; it increases to 50% when 5 medications are taken concomitantly and it rises to 100% when more than 8 medications are prescribed.[106]

Screening in cases of polypharmacy, particularly in the elderly patient population, is crucial because adverse drug events can often imitate other geriatric syndromes or precipitate confusion, falls, incontinence, urinary retention, and malaise. These side effects in turn may cause a physician to prescribe another agent to treat them.[107]

If elderly patients take several medications at the same time, they are at a high risk for drug-related problems. Elderly patients are particularly susceptible to polypharmacy issues not only because aging affects how their body handles medications, but because they take more medications than younger patients.[108] In the United States, people over 65 make up approximately 13% of the population but use about 30% of all written prescriptions.[109] At any given time, an elderly patient takes, on average, 4 or 5 prescription drugs and 2 over-the-counter medications.[110]

An elderly patient is also more likely to take a medication that has been prescribed inappropriately—one that is unnecessary, ineffective, or potentially dangerous—and to suffer an adverse drug event. In a study of more than 150,000 elderly patients, 29% had received at least 1 of 33 potentially inappropriate drugs.[111] A study of approximately 27,600 Medicare patients documented more than 1,500 ADEs in a single year.[112]

As the elderly population in the United States continues to grow, so will the incidence of ADEs. The PTA can help elderly patients avoid the negative consequences of polypharmacy by understanding how aging affects

Table 7-30

COMMONLY PRESCRIBED DRUGS FOR THE TREATMENT OF DEPRESSION

DRUG	GENERIC (TRADE)	USE OF DRUG	COMMON SIDE EFFECTS
Tricyclics	*Imipramine (Tofranil)* *Amitriptyline (Elavil)* *Nortriptyline (Pamelor)* *Desipramine (Norpramin)*	Work on chemical imbalances in the brain. Reduce symptoms such as extreme sadness, symptoms of hopelessness, and absence of energy.	Dry eyes, drowsiness, weight gain, dry mouth, constipation
Serotonin and norepinephrine reuptake inhibitors (SNRIs)	*Venlafaxine (Effexor, Effexor XR)* *Duloxetine (Cymbalta)*	First-line Rx in the elderly and can help those who have not responded well to other medications.	Fewer side effects than tricyclics and MAO inhibitors (see below); nausea, problems sleeping, sweating, dry mouth, gas, constipation, vomiting
Selective serotonin reuptake inhibitors (SSRIs)	*Fluoxetine (Prozac)* *Paroxetine (Paxil)* *Escitalopram (Lexapro)* *Sertraline (Zoloft)* *Citalopram (Celexa)* *Fluvoxamine (Luvox)*	Increase brain's serotonin levels to improve mood and make serotonin available to the receiving nerve by preventing the return of the chemical serotonin to the sending nerve. Serotonin may help control moods, appetite for sweets, body temperature, and sleep.	Side effects may include sexual problems, which might not go away unless the medication is stopped. Side effects that usually go away may include increased anxiety, restlessness, excessive sleepiness, and heartburn.
Monoamine oxidase inhibitors (MAOIs)	*Phenelzine (Nardil)* *Isocarboxazid (Marplan)* *Tranylcypromine (Parnate)* *Selegiline patch (EnSam)*	MAOIs are the oldest class of anti-depressants. Not often prescribed in the elderly due to side effects.	Unusual signs: high blood pressure, chest pain, large pupils, change in heartbeat, headache, sensitivity to light, heavy sweating, vomiting, and stiff or sore neck. Common: Blurred vision, sexual problems, less urine excretion, dizziness or lightheadedness, feeling tired, mild headache, increased hunger or weight gain, muscle twitching during sleep, nausea, restlessness, sweating, trembling, tiredness, trouble sleeping *(Continued)*

Table 7-30 continued

COMMONLY PRESCRIBED DRUGS FOR THE TREATMENT OF DEPRESSION

DRUG	GENERIC (TRADE)	USE OF DRUG	COMMON SIDE EFFECTS
Other medications prescribed for depression	Bupropion (Wellbutrin XL, Wellbutrin SR and Wellbutrin)	A newer anti-depressant that acts on the neurotransmitters dopamine and norepinephrine; causes fewer side effects than tricyclics and MAO inhibitors	Weight loss, loss of appetite, dry mouth, skin rash, sweating, ringing in the ears, shakiness, stomach pain, agitation, trouble sleeping, anxiety, dizziness, muscle pain, nausea, fast heartbeat, sore throat, and urinating more often
	Mirtazapine (Remeron)	First drug in a new class to target specific serotonin receptors. Along with being able to treat moderate to severe depression, mirtazapine can help with anxiety, motor retardation, and cognitive and sleep problems associated with depression.	Side effects include drowsiness, increased appetite, weight gain, and dizziness; while some side effects decrease, the weight gain can be a continuing problem
	Nefazodone (Serzone)	Inhibits serotonin reuptake and blocks one type of serotonin receptor; fewer side effects and treats moderate to severe depression. Can improve depression-related anxiety and relieve depression-related insomnia.	Blurred vision or other changes in vision, clumsiness and unsteadiness, lightheadedness or fainting, ringing in the ears, skin rash or itching; does not cause weight gain

the body's reaction to medications, which drugs are the most problematic for older patients, and how to spot a drug-related problem and intervene.

Among the first signs that a drug may not be working properly in an older person is a change in mood, energy, attitude, or memory. Too often, these alterations are overlooked, ignored, or chalked off to "old age" or senility. Older people may think their depressed mood is caused by something external such as the death of a friend or simply boredom. Nothing could be farther from the truth. Virtually every heart medication, blood pressure drug, sleeping pill, and tranquilizer has been known to trigger depressive symptoms.[115]

When a psychological symptom appears in an older person, examine his or her medication or drug use first. Consider, too, factors like alcohol intake, poor nutrition, and hormone imbalance. Never dismiss the possibility that a real psychological problem has developed and may itself require medication. Any older person with feelings of hopelessness,

worthlessness, unexplained crying, thoughts of suicide, and similar symptoms could be among the 5% of the elderly who have a treatable, reversible depression. Tables 7-31 through 7-37 provide summaries of the drugs that may cause side effects in the elderly. Tables 7-38 through 7-46 provide information on herbs, dietary supplements, and alternating drug therapies for the treatment of various conditions. As these seemingly safe additions to an elder's drug regime may increase the risk for ADEs, these tables also provide the possible side effects of usage.

Safe Medication Use for the Aged

Safe medication use for the elderly requires vigilance on the part of the older person and those assisting him or her. It is especially important to keep track of maintenance drugs and make sure they are taken regularly. For a chronic condition, such as high blood pressure, these medications are a key to

Table 7-31

COMMON DRUGS THAT CAUSE POSTURAL HYPOTENSION

Tricyclic anti-depressants (depression)

Amitriptyline *(Elavil, Endep)*

Desipramine *(Norpramin, Pertofrane)*

Doxepin *(Adapin, Sinequan)*

Imipramine *(Tofranil)*

Nortriptyline *(Aventyl, Pamelor)*

Protriptyline *(Vivactil)*

Trimipramine *(Surmontil)*

Tranquilizers (insomnia, psychosis)

Thiothixene *(Navane)*

Haloperidol *(Haldol)*

Narcotic analgesics (pain)

All

Calcium channel blockers

Nicardipine *(Cardene)*

Isradipine *(DynaCirc)*

Nitrates (angina)

Nitroglycerin *(Nitro-dur or Nitro-Bid)*

Erythrotyl tetranitrate *(Cardilate)*

Isosorbide dinitrite *(Dilatrate SR)*

Anti-hypertensive drugs (hypertension)

Sympatholitics

Methyldopa *(Aldomet)*

Guanethidine *(Esimil)*

Peripheral α-blockers

Phenoxybenzamine *(Dibenzyline)*

Phentolamine *(Regitine)*

Prazosin *(Minipress)*

β-adrenoreceptor blockers

Atenolol *(Tenormin)*

Pindolol *(Visken)*

Metroprolol *(Lopressor)*

Timolol *(Blocadren)*

Verapamil *(Calan, Isoptin)*

Anti-arrhythmic drugs (cardiovascular disease)

All

Sedative-hypnotics (insomnia, anxiety)

Benzodiazepines

Florazepam *(Dalmane)*

Temazepam *(Restoril)*

Triazolam *(Halcion)*

Anti-Parkinsonians

Levodopa

ACE inhibitors

Captopril *(Capoten)*

Enalapril *(Vasotec)*

Vasodilators

Nifedipine *(Procardia)*

Diuretics (hypertension, congestive heart failure)

All

maintaining good health. Remember, too, that perfectly ordinary medications can lead to unexpected results—especially in the elderly. The PTA needs to be alert for gradual changes that may signal an unwanted side effect and guard against harmful drug interactions by making sure prescribing physicians know about all the medicines the older person is taking, including any over-the-counter drugs.

CONCLUSION

PTs and PTAs have the most frequent contact with an older patient than other caregivers and health care providers. They may be the first to identify confusion, complaints of fatigue, changes in muscle tone, slurred speech, and other side effects of medications. It is important that PTAs understand how an older individual is managing his or her drug regimes. The proper use of medications will directly affect an older person's functional status and physiological responses to increasing level of activity.

This chapter has reviewed drugs commonly prescribed for older adults; changes in absorption, metabolism, and excretion of drugs with age; polypharmacy; self-medications; and side effects of the most frequently prescribed drugs. It is important for the PTA to familiarize him- or herself with current

Table 7-32

COMMONLY PRESCRIBED DRUGS THAT CAUSE DEPRESSION

Anti-hypertensives

Sympathlolytic Drugs

Methyldopa *(Aldomet)*

Clonidine *(Catapres)*

Guanabenz *(Wytensin)*

Receptor Blockers/α-Blockers

Prazosin *(Minipress)*

Receptor Blockers/β-Blockers

Nadolol *(Corgard)*

Propranolol *(Inderal)*

Atenolol *(Tenormin)*

Metaprolol *(Lopressor)*

Pindolol *(Viskin)*

ACE Inhibitors

Guanethidine *(Esimil)*

Reserpine *(Various derivatives)*

Anti-Parkinsonians

Levodopa

Levodopa-carbidopa *(Sinemet)*

Amantadine *(Symmetrel)*

Bromocriptine *(Parlodel)*

Diuretics

Acetazolamide *(Diamox)*

Methazolamide *(Neptazane)*

Hydrochlorothiazide and deserpidine *(Oreticyl)*

H₂ Receptor Antagonist

Cimetidine *(Tagamet)*

Anti-Mycobacterial

Ethambutol *(Myambutol)*

Vasodilators

Hydralazine *(Apresoline)*

Anti-Inflammatories

NSAIDs

Naproxen *(Naprosyn)*

Tolmetin *(Tolectin)*

Indomethacin *(Indocin)*

Meclofenamate *(Meclomen)*

Peroxicam *(Feldene)*

Steroidals

Prednisolone *(Meticortelone)*

Sedative-Hypnotics

Glutethimide *(Elrodorm)*

Barbiturates

Phenobarbital *(Nembutal)*

Benzodiazepines

Flurazepam *(Dalmane)*

Temazepam *(Restoril)*

Triazolam *(Halcion)*

Alcohol

Table 7-33

COMMONLY PRESCRIBED DRUGS THAT CAUSE DEHYDRATION IN THE ELDERLY

Cardiovascular Drugs

Diuretics
Furosemide *(Frusemide, Lasix)*
Ethacrynic acid *(Edecrin, Edecril)*
Chlorothiazide *(Diuril, Chlotride)*
Hydrochlorothiazide *(Esidrix, Esidrex)*
Bumetanide *(Bumex)*

Cardiotonic Glycosides
Digoxin *(Lanoxin)*
Digitoxin *(Crystodigin, Digitox)*

Calcium Channel Blockers
Verapamil *(Isoptin)*
Ciltiazem *(Cardizem)*
Nifedipine *(Procardia)*

Beta Blockers
Atenolol *(Tenormin)*
Metoprolol *(Lopressor)*
Propanolol *(Inderal)*
Nadolol *(Corgard)*
Timolol *(Blocadren)*
Pindolol *(Visken)*
Dipyridamole *(Cardoxine)*

Vasopressors/Sympathomimetics
Dopamine *(Intropin)*
Dobutamine *(Dobutrex)*
Isoproterenol *(Isuprel)*

Coronary Vasodilators
Nitroglycerin *(Glyceryl, Trinitrate)*
Isosorbide dinitrate *(Sorbitrate, Iso-Bid)*
Erythrityl *(Cardilate)*
Verapamil *(Calan, Calan SR)*
Pentaerythritol tetranitrate *(Vasodiatol)*

Peripheral Vasodilators
Hydralazine *(Apresoline)*
Diazoxide *(Hyperstat)*
Nitroprusside *(Nipride)*

Cardiovascular Drugs (continued)

Anti-Arrhythmic Drugs
Quinidine *(Quinaglute)*
Procainamide hydrochloride *(Procan)*
Lidocaine *(Xylocaine)*
Disopyramide phosphate *(Norpace)*
Quinidine gluconate *(Duraquin)*
Quinidine polygalacturonate *(Cardioquin)*

Pain Medications

NSAIDs
Indole acetic acids *(Tolectin, Clinoril, Indocin)*
Fenamic acids *(Meclomen, Ponstel)*
Propionic acids *(Motrin, Nalfon, Naprosyn)*
Phenylacetic acids *(Voltaren)*
Oxicams *(Feldene)*

Gastrointestinal drugs

H_2 Receptor Blockers
Cimetidine *(Tagamet)*
Ranitidine *(Zantac)*
Famotidine *(Pepcid)*

Anti-Diarrheal Absorbants
Kaolin, Pectin *(Kaelin)*

Hyperosmotic Laxatives
Lactulose *(Chronolac)*
Sodium phosphate *(Phosphosoda)*

Psychotropic Agents

Benzodiazepines
Clorazepate *(Tranxene)*
Alprozolam *(Xanax)*
Prazepam *(Centrax)*

Nonbenzodiazepine
Buspironic *(Buspar)*

Tricyclic Anti-Depressants
Doxepine *(Sinequan)*
Amitriptyline *(Elavil)*
Imipramine *(Tofranil)*
Nortriptyline *(Pamelor)*
Trimipramine *(Surmontil)*
Protriptyline *(Vivactil)*

MAO Inhibitors
Isocarboxazid *(Marplan)*
Maprotiline *(Ludiomil)*
Phenelzine *(Nardil)*

Phenothiazine Derivatives
Chlorpromazine *(Thorazine)*
Trifluoperazine *(Stelazine)*
Fluphenazine *(Prolixin)*
Mesordazine *(Serentil)*
Promethazine *(Phenergan)*
Thioridazine *(Mellaril)*

Thioxanthene Derivatives
Tiothixene *(Navane)*

Butyrophenone Derivatives
Haloperidol *(Haldol)*

Table 7-34

COMMONLY PRESCRIBED DRUGS THAT CAUSE CONFUSIONAL STATES IN THE ELDERLY

Cardiac Glycosides

Digitoxin *(Cardigin)*

Digoxin *(Digacin)*

Anti-Inflammatories

Indomethasin *(Indosin)*

Salicylates *(Bufferin, Anacin)*

Phenylbutazone *(Butazolidin)*

Oxyphenbutazone *(Oxalid)*

Diuretics

Methyclothiazide *(Aquatensen)*

Hydrochlorothiazide *(Hydro-Ciuril)*

Furosemide *(Lasix)*

Analgesics

Hydromorphone *(Dilaudid)*

Meperidine *(Demerol)*

Methadone *(Fenadone)*

Pentazocine *(Talwin)*

Anti-Parkinsonians

Benztropine *(Cogentin)*

Levodopa

Trihexylphenidyl *(Artane)*

Amantadine *(Symmetrel)*

Bromocriptine *(Parlodel)*

Hypoglycemic Agents

Tolazamide *(Tolinase)*

Tolbutamide *(Orinase)*

Beta Blockers

Propranolol *(Inderal)*

Metroprolol *(Lopressor)*

Atenolol *(Tenormin)*

Acebutolol *(Sectrol)*

Tricyclic Anti-Depressants

Amitriptyline *(Elavil, Endep)*

Desipramine *(Norpramin, Pertofrane)*

Doxepin *(Adapin, Sinequan)*

Imipramine *(Tofranil)*

Nortriptyline *(Aventyl, Pamelor)*

Protriptyline *(Vivactil)*

Trimipramine *(Surmontil)*

Anti-cholinergics

See Table 7-36

H$_2$ Receptor Antagonists

Cimetidine *(Tagamet)*

Sedative-Hypnotics

Benzodiazepine

Flurazepam *(Dalmane)*

Temazepam *(Restoril)*

Triazolam *(Halcion)*

Barbiturates

Phenobarbital *(Nembutal)*

Secobarbital *(Pramil)*

Table 7-35

COMMONLY PRESCRIBED DRUGS THAT CAUSE DRUG-INDUCED PARKINSONISM

Anti-Psychotics

Phenothiazines

Chlorpromazine *(Thorazine)*

Fluphenazine *(Permatil)*

Mesoridazine *(Serentil)*

Perphenazine *(Trilafon, Triavil)*

Prochlorperazine *(Compazine)*

Thioridazine *(Mellaril)*

Trifluoperazine *(Stelazine)*

Triflupromazine *(Vesprin)*

Butyrophenone

Haloperidol *(Haldol)*

Dehydroindolone

Molondone *(Moban)*

Dibenzoxazepine

Loxapine *(Loxitane)*

Sympatholytics

Centrally Acting

Methyldopa *(Aldomet)*

Presynaptic Adrenergic Inhibitors

Reserpine *(Crystoserpine)*

Table 7-36

DRUGS THAT CAUSE AN ANTI-CHOLINERGIC ACTION

Tricyclic Anti-Depressants

Amitriptyline *(Elavil, Endep)*

Amozapine *(Asendin)*

Doxepin *(Adapin, Sinequan)*

Imipramine *(Tofranil)*

Maprotiline *(Ludiomil)*

Nortryptyline *(Pamelor, Aventyl)*

Protriptyline *(Vivactil)*

Triipramine *(Surmontil)*

Anti-Histamines

Diphenhydramine *(Benadryl)*

Anti-Psychotics

Benztropine *(Cogentin)*

Biperiden *(Akineton)*

Chlorpromazine *(Thorazine)*

Molindone *(Moban)*

Thioidazine *(Mellaril)*

Anti-Parkinsonians

Orphenadrine *(Disipal)*

Trihexyphenidyl *(Artane)*

Table 7-37

COMMONLY PRESCRIBED DRUGS THAT MAY CAUSE DIZZINESS

Anti-hypertensives

Vasodilators

Diltiazem (Cardizem)

Nifedipine (Procardia)

Hydralazine (Apresoline)

Beta Blockers

All

Sympatholytics Acting on the CNS

Clonidine (Catapres)

Guanabenz (Wytensin)

Methyldoap (Aldomet)

Sympatholytics acting on PSN

Guanethidine (Esimil)

Phenoxybenzamine (Dibenzyline)

Alpha Receptor Blockers

Phentolamine (Regitine)

Prazosin (Minipress)

Anti-Hypertensives (continued)

Beta Andrenoreceptor Blockers

Atenolol (Tenormin)

Metaprolol (Lopressor)

Timolol (Blocadren)

ACE Inhibitors

Enlalapril (Vasotec)

Captoril (Capoten)

Lisinopril (Zestril, Prinvil)

Cardiovascular Anti-Lipemic Agents

Gemifibrozil (Lopid)

Colestipol (Cholestid)

Clofibrate (Atromid-S)

Sedative-Hypnotics

Barbituates

All

Benzodiazepines

All

Alcohol

All

Analgesics

NSAIDs

Naproxen (Naprosyn)

Tolmetin (Tolectin)

Indomethiacin (Indocin)

Meclofenamate (Meclomen)

Peroxicam (Feldene)

PSN indicates postganglionic sympathetic neurons

drugs and gain a better understanding of how pharmacological considerations may impact an elderly individual's functional outcomes in rehabilitation.

Pearls

- Many older adults take one or more medications; the greater the number of medications taken, the greater the risk of side effects.

- The PTA must be familiar with the side effects of any prescription and over-the-counter drugs or herbal supplements that an elderly person is taking.

- Polypharmacy is the use of multiple drugs for the same condition.

- Multipharmacy is the use of multiple drugs to treat multipathology and conditions associated with aging.

- Pharmacokinetics is the study of how drugs work in the body and examines the time required for drugs to be absorbed, how they are distributed in the body, how long they remain effective, and how they are eliminated.

- Pharmodynamics is how the body responds to a drug from a physiologic and biochemical perspective.

- Changes in kidney and liver function with age change the way drugs are metabolized. The organs become less effective in clearing drugs and risk toxicity.

- Changes in the digestive system may affect the absorption of drugs.

- If there are changes in short-term memory, the schedule of doses can be affected.

- During therapy sessions, a patient's tolerance to exercise must be closely monitored. Heart medications will typically alter the heart's response and blood pressure.

- The PTA may play an important role in encouraging self-help strategies in the elderly. Being receptive to and answering an elder's questions, while working together during a therapy session, is an important component of therapy.

- Good communication is important between all members of the health care team; information and details related to any observed adverse effects that the PTA identifies is exceedingly important.

References

1. Williams C. Using medications appropriately in older adults. *Am Fam Phys.* 2002;66:1917-1924.
2. Merle L, Laroche ML, Dantoine T, Charmes JP. Predicting and preventing adverse drug reactions in the very old. *Drugs Aging.* 2005;22:375-392.
3. Gingsberg G, Hattis D, Sonawane B. Pharmacokinetic and pharmacodynamic factors that affect sensitivity to neurotoxic sequele in elderly individuals. *Enb Health Persp.* 2005;13:1243-1249.
4. Jorgenson T, Johanssonn S, Kennerfalk A, Waalander MA, Svardsudd K. Prescription drug use, diagnosis and health-care utilization among the elderly. *Ann Pharmacother.* 2001;35:1004-1009.
5. Lidjakupu T, Hartikainen S, Kluukka T, et al. Use of medications and polypharmacy are increasing in the elderly. *J Clin Epidemiol.* 2002;55:809-817.
6. National Center of Health Statistics. *Chartbook on Trends in the Health of Americans 2005.* Hyattsville, MD: National Center for Health Statistics; 2005.
7. Kaufman DW, Kelly JP, Rosenberg L, Anderson TE, Mitchell AA. Recent patterns of medication use in the ambulatory adult population of the United States: the Slone Survey. *JAMA.* 2002;287:337-344.
8. Moxey ED, O'Conner JP, Novielli KD, Teutsch S, Nash DB. Prescription drug use in the elderly: a descriptive study. *Health Care Fin Rev.* 2003;24:127-141.
9. Sloane PD, Zimmerman S, Brown LC, Ives TJ, Walsh JF. Inappropriate medication prescribing in residential care/assisted living facility. *J Am Geriatr Soc.* 2002;50:1001-1011.
10. Hanlon JT, Lindblad CI, Hajjar ER, McCarthy TC. Update on drug-related problems in the elderly. *Am J Geriatr Pharmacother.* 2003;1:38-43.
11. Conry M. Polypharmacy: Pandora's medicine chest? 2000. www.geriatrictimes.com/g001028.html. Accessed May 16, 2007.
12. Zahn C, Sangl J. Potentially inappropriate medication use in the community-dwelling elderly. *JAMA.* 2001;286:2823-2829.
13. Beers MH. Aging as a risk factor for medication-related problems. 1999. www.ascp.com/public/pubs/tcp/1999/dec/aging.shtml. Accessed May 16, 2007.
14. Merle L, Laroche ML, Dantoine T, Charmes JP. Predicting and preventing adverse drug reactions in the very old. *Drugs Aging.* 2005;22:375-392.
15. McLean AJ, LeCouteur D. Aging biology and geriatric clinical pharmacology. *Pharmacol Rev.* 2004;56:163-184.
16. Turnheim K. When drug therapy gets old: pharmacokinetics and pharmacodynamics in the elderly. *Exp Gerontol.* 2003;38:843-853.
17. Caskie GI, Willis SL. Congruence of self-reported medications with pharmacy prescription records in low-income older adults. *Gerontologist.* 2004;44:176-179.
18. Amoako EP, Richardson-Campbell L, Kennedy-Malone L. Self-medication with over-the-counter drugs among elderly adults. *J Gerontol Nurs.* 2003;29:10-15.
19. Cuddy ML. Geriatric pharmacology topics: age related drug dosage adjustment. *J Pract Nurs.* 2004;54:11-16.
20. Routledge PA, O'Mahoney MS, Woodhouse KW. Adverse drug reactions in elderly patients. *Brit J Clin Pharmacol.* 2004;57:121-126.
21. Chang CM, Yeh Liu PY, Yang YHK, Yang YC, Wu CF, Lu FH. Use of the Beers criteria to predict adverse drug reactions among first-visit elderly outpatients. *Pharmacotherapy.* 2005;25:831-838.
22. Simoni-Wastila L, Strickler G. Risk factors associated with problem use of prescription drugs: the elderly. *Am J Pub Health.* 2004;94:266-268.

23. Pringle KE, Ahern FM, Heller DA, Gold CH, Brown TV. Potential for alcohol and prescription drug interactions in older people. *J Am Geriatr Soc.* 2005;53:1930-1936.

24. Gurwitz JH, Field TS, Harrold LR, et al. Incidence and preventability of adverse drug events among older persons in the ambulatory setting. *JAMA.* 2003;289:1107-1116.

25. Fick DM, Cooper JW. Updating the Beers criteria for potentially inappropriate medication use in older adults. *Arch Intern Med.* 2003;163(22):2716-2717.

26. Hilmer SN, McLachlan DJ, Le Couteau DG. Clinical pharmacology in the geriatric patient. *Fundam Clin Pharmacol.* 2007;2:217-230.

27. Fosnight SM, Holder CM, Allen KR, Hazelett S. A strategy to decrease the use of risky drugs in the elderly. *Cleveland Clin J Med.* 2004;71:561-568.

28. Beers MH, ed. *The Merck manual of geriatrics.* 3rd ed, Section 1: basics of geriatric care; chapter 6, clinical pharmacology. 2005. www.merck.com/mrkshared/mmg/sec1/ch6/ch6a.jsp. Accessed May 16, 2007.

29. Turnheim K. Drug therapy in the elderly. *Exp Gerontol.* 2004;39:1731-1738.

30. McLean AJ, Le Couteur DG. Aging biology and geriatric clinical pharmacology. *Pharmacol Rev.* 2004;56:163-167.

31. American Geriatric Society Panel on Chronic Pain in Older Persons. The management of chronic pain in older persons. *J Am Geriatr Soc.* 1998;46:635-651.

32. Greenberger NJ. Update in gastroenterology. *Ann Intern Med.* 1997;127:827-834.

33. Bennett GJ, Dworkin RH, Nicholson B. Anticonvulsant therapy in the treatment of neuropathic pain. Treatment update. Medscape Web site 1999. http://www.medscape.com/medscape/Neurology/TreatmentUpdate/1999/tu04/public/toc-tu04.html. Accessed July 17, 2007.

34. Fam AG. Recent advances in the management of adult myositis. *Expert Opin Investig Drugs.* 2001;10:1265-1277.

35. Rubin CD. Treatment considerations in the management of age-related osteoporosis. *Am J Med Sci.* 1999;318:158-170.

36. Reginster JY, Abadie E, Delmas P, et al. Recommendations for an update of the current (2001) regulatory requirements for registration of drugs to be used in the treatment of osteoporosis in postmenopausal women and in men. *Osteoporosis Int.* 2006;17:1-7.

37. Dougados M. How can one develop disease-modifying drugs in osteoarthritis? *Curr Rheumatol Rep.* 2005;7:22-28.

38. Pressman A, Forsyth B. Ettinger B. Initiation of osteoporosiss treatment after bone mineral density testing. *Osteoporosis Int.* 2001;12:337-342.

39. Kawai S. Current drug therapy for rheumatoid arthritis. *J Orthop Sci.* 2003;8:259-263.

40. Suematsu A, Tajiri Y, Nakashima T, et al. Scientific basis for the efficacy of combined use of antirheumatic drugs against bone destruction in rheumatoid arthritis. *Mod Rheumatol.* 2007;17:17-23.

41. Huising MO. The molecular evolution of the interleukin-1 family of cytokines; IL-18 in teleost fish. *Developmental and Comparative Immunology.* 2004;28:395-413.

42. Baumhakel M, Bohm M. Cardiovascular pharmacotherapy in the aged. *Internist.* 2003;44:943-950.

43. Dornbrook-Lavender KA, Roth MT, Pieper JA. Secondary prevention of coronary heart disease in the elderly. *Ann Pharmacother.* 2003;37:1867-1876.

44. Chandra KK, Malhotra S, Gupta M, Grover A, Sharma N, Pandhi P. Changing trends in the hospital management of unstable angina: a drug utilization analysis. *Int J Clin Pharmacol Ther.* 2004;42:575-580.

45. Vasil'ev AP, Strel'tsova NN. Aerobic and hemodynamic mechanisms of the antianginal effect of drugs in patients with angina pectoris. *Klin Med.* 2004;82:55-59.

46. Malhotra S, Grover A, Verma NK, Bhargava VK. A study of drug utilisation and cost of treatment in patients hospitalised with unstable angina. *Eur J Clin Pharmacol.* 2000;56:755-761.

47. Wichter T, Paul TM, Eckardt L, et al. Arrhythmogenic right ventricular cardiomyopathy: antiarrhythmic drugs, catheter ablation, or ICD? *Herz.* 2005;30:91-101.

48. Fananapazir L, McAreavey D. Therapeutic options in patients with obstructive hypertrophic cardiomyopathy and severe drug-refractory symptoms. *J Am Coll Cardiol.* 1998;31:159-264.

49. Grigorian Shamagian L, Varela Román A, Virgos Lamela A, Rigueiro Veloso P, García Acuña JM, González-Juanatey JR. Long-term trends in drug prescription for hospitalized patients with congestive heart failure: influence of type of dysfunction. *Rev Esp Cardiol.* 2005;58:381-388.

50. De Bruin ML, van Puijenbroek EP, Bracke M, Hoes AW, Leufkens HG. Pharmacogenetics of drug-induced arrhythmias: a feasibility study using spontaneous adverse drug reactions reporting data. *Pharmacoepidemiol Drug Saf.* 2006;15:99-105.

51. Federman AD, Halm EA, Zhu C, Hochman T, Siu AL. Association of income and prescription drug coverage with generic medication use among older adults with hypertension. *Am J Manag Care.* 2006;12:611-618.

52. Grassi G. Sympathetic and baroreflex function in hypertension: implications for current and new drugs. *Curr Pharm Des.* 2004;10:3579-3589.

53. Bradley L, Kirker SG. Secondary prevention of arteriosclerosis in lower limb vascular amputees: a missed opportunity. *Eur J Vasc Endovasc Surg.* 2006;32:491-493.

54. Fagiolino P. The influence of cardiac output distribution on the tissue/plasma drug concentration ratio. *Eur J Drug Metab Pharmacokinet.* 2002;27:79-81.

55. Uemura K, Kamiya A, Hidaka I, et al. Automated drug delivery system to control systemic arterial pressure, cardiac output, and left heart filling pressure in acute decompensated heart failure. *J Appl Physiol.* 2006;100:1278-1286.

56. Neralla S, Meyer KC. Drug treatment of pneumococcal pneumonia in the elderly. *Drugs Aging.* 2004;21:851-864.

57. MacDougall C, Guglielmo BJ, Maselli J, Gonzales R. Antimicrobial drug prescribing for pneumonia in ambulatory care. *Emerg Infect Dis.* 2005;11:380-384.

58. Burrill PD. Drug management of COPD. *BMJ.* 2007;334:864.

59. Breekveldt-Postma NS, Koerselman J, Erkens JA, Lammers JW, Herings RM. Enhanced persistence with tiotropium compared with other respiratory drugs in COPD. *Respir Med.* 2007;101:1398-1405.

60. Nafti S. COPD treatment by drugs. *Rev Mal Respir.* 2006;23:10858-10860.

61. Rogers DF. Mucoactive drugs for asthma and COPD: any place in therapy? *Expert Opin Investig Drugs.* 2002;11:15-35.

62. Holgate ST, Bousquet J, Chung KF, et al. Summary of recommendations for the design of clinical trials and the registration of drugs used in the treatment of asthma. *Respir Med.* 2004;98:479-487.

63. Koennecke HC. Secondary prevention of stroke: a practical guide to drug treatment. *CNS Drugs.* 2004;18:221-241.

64. Weinberger J. Adverse effects and drug interactions of antithrombotic agents used in prevention of ischaemic stroke. *Drugs.* 2005;65:461-471.

65. Karlsson I. Drugs that induce delirium. *Dement Geriatr Cogn Disord.* 1999;10:412-415.

66. Someya T, Endo T, Hara T, Yagi G, Suzuki J. A survey on the drug therapy for delirium. *Psychiatry Clin Neurosci.* 2001;55:397-401.

67. Burns A, O'Brien J, Auriacombe S, et al. Clinical practice with anti-dementia drugs: a consensus statement from British Association for Psychopharmacology. *J Psychopharmacol.* 2006;20:732-755.

68. McGirr G, Compton SA. Drugs for dementia: the first year. An audit of prescribing practice. *Ulster Med J.* 2000;69:123-127.

69. Meier K, Nanney LB. Emerging new drugs for wound repair. *Expert Opin Emerg Drugs.* 2006;11:23-37.

70. Mulder GC, Fairchild PA, Jeter KF. *Clinicians' Pocket Guide to Chronic Wound Repair.* 5th ed. Long Beach, CA: Wound Healing Institute; 2005.

71. Perricone N, Kerstein MD, Kirsner RS, Norman RA, Phillips TJ. How to approach acute and chronic would healing in the elderly. *Wounds.* 1999;11:145-151.

72. Yacovino DA, Hain TC. The pharmacology of vestibular disorders. *Rev Neurol.* 2004;39:381-387.

73. Sakamoto C. The role of mucoprotective drugs in gastric ulcer treatment: with specifical reference to their effects on gastritis mucosa. *Nippon Rinsho.* 2004;62:566-570.

74. Lai KC, Hui WM, Wong BC, Hu WH, Lam SK. Ulcer-healing drugs are required after eradication of *Helicobacter pylori* in patients with gastric ulcer but not duodenal ulcer haemorrhage. *Aliment Pharmacol Ther.* 2000;14:1071-1076.

75. Berspalov VG, Shcherbakov AM, Kalinovski VP, et al. Study of the antioxidant drug "Karinat" in patients with chronic atrophic gastritis. *Vopr Onkol.* 2004;50:81-85.

76. Lahner E, Bordi C, Di Giulio E, et al. Role of *Helicobacter pylori* serology in atrophic body gastritis after eradication treatment. *Aliment Pharmacol Ther.* 2002;16:507-514.

77. Lieber CS. Gastric ethanol metabolism and gastritis: interactions with other drugs, *Helicobacter pylori*, and antibiotic therapy (1957-1997)—a review. *Alcohol Clin Exp Res.* 1997;21:1360-1366.

78. Sakamoto C. The role of mucoprotective drugs in gastric ulcer treatment: with specifical reference to their effects on gastritis mucosa. *Nippon Rinsho.* 2004;62:566-570.

79. Wang K. Application of the drugs for expelling the pathogenic wind in treatment of chronic diarrhea. *J Tradit Chin Med.* 2003;23:263-246.

80. Baun RF, Levy HB. Treating chronic constipation in elderly patients. *Ann Pharmacother.* 2007;41:309-313.

81. Bosshard W, Dreher R, Schnegg JF, Büla CJ. The treatment of chronic constipation in elderly people: an update. *Drugs Aging.* 2004;21:911-930.

82. Hattori T. Drug treatment of urinary incontinence. *Drugs Today.* 1998;34:125-138.

83. Andersson KE. Drug therapy for urinary incontinence. *Baillieres Best Pract Res Clin Obstet Gynaecol.* 2000;14:291-313.

84. Kafri R, Langer R, Dvir Z, Katz-Leurer M. Behavioral vs drug treatment for urge urinary incontinence in older women: a randomized controlled trial. *JAMA.* 1998;280:1995-2000.

85. Burgio KL, Locher JL, Goode PS, et al. Rehabilitation vs drug therapy for urge urinary incontinence: short-term outcome. *Int Urogynecol J Pelvic Floor Dysfunct.* 2007;18:407-411.

86. Hampel C, Gillitzer R, Pahernik S, Melchior SW, Thüroff JW. Drug therapy of female urinary incontinence. *Urologe A.* 2005;44:244-255.

87. Tokita S, Takahashi K, Kotani H. Recent advances in molecular pharmacology of the histamine systems: physiology and pharmacology of histamine H3 receptor: roles in feeding regulation and therapeutic potential for metabolic disorders. *J Pharmacol Sci.* 2006;101:12-18.

88. Longui CA. Primary adrenal insufficiency. *Arq Bras Endocrinol Metabol.* 2004;48:739-745.

89. Sonino N, Fava GA. CNS drugs in Cushing's disease: pathophysiological and therapeutic implications for mood disorders. [published correction appears in *Prog. Neuro-Psycol. Biol. Psychiatry.* 2002;261011-1018]. *Prog Neuropsycholpharm Biol Psychiatry.* 2002;26:763-771.

90. Di Somma C, Colao A, Pivonello R, et al. Effectiveness of chronic treatment with alendronate in the osteoporosis of Cushing's disease. *Clin Endocrinol.* 1998;48:655-662.

91. Zantut-Wittmann DE, Ramos CD, Santos AO, et al. High pre-therapy [99mTc]pertechnetate thyroid uptake, thyroid size and thyrostatic drugs: predictive factors of failure in [131I] iodide therapy in Graves' disease. *Nucl Med Commun.* 2005;26:957-963.

92. Laurberg P. Anti-thyroid drug therapy. *Eur J Endocrinol.* 2006;155:783-786.

93. Wang L, Orhii PB, Banu J, Kalu DN. Effects of separate and combined therapy with growth hormone and parathyroid hormone on lumbar vertebral bone in aged ovariectomized osteopenia. *Bone.* 2001;28:202-207.

94. Cunningham J. Management of secondary hyperparathyroidism. *Clin Calcium.* 2005;15(suppl 1):217-224.

95. Quarles LD. Cinacalcet HCl: a novel treatment for secondary hyperparathyroidism in stage 5 chronic kidney disease. *Kidney Int Suppl.* 2005;1:S24-S28.

96. Koiwa F, Hasegawa T. Indication of parathyroid intervention. *Clin Calcium.* 2007;17:760-766.

97. Seilicovich A, Pisera D, Sciascia SA, et al. Gene therapy for pituitary tumors. *Curr Gene Ther.* 2005;5:559-572.

98. Oshino S, Saitoh Y, Kasayama S, et al. Short-term preoperative octreotide treatment of GH-secreting pituitary adenoma: predictors of tumor shrinkage. *Endocr J.* 2006;53:125-132.

99. Panikar V, Chandalia HB, Joshi SR, Fafadia A, Santvana C. Beneficial effects of triple drug combination of pioglitazone with glibenclamide and metformin in type 2 diabetes mellitus patients on insulin therapy. *J Assoc Physicians India.* 2003;51:1061-1064

100. Hermansen K, Davies M, Derezinski T, Martinez Ravn G, Clauson P, Home P. A 26-week, randomized, parallel, treat-to-target trial comparing insulin detemir with NPH insulin as add-on therapy to oral glucose-lowering drugs in insulin-naive people with type 2 diabetes. *Diabetes Care.* 2006;29:1269-1274.

101. Oiknine R, Mooradian AD. Drug therapy of diabetes in the elderly. *Biomed Pharmacother.* 2003;57:231-239.

102. Scholz H, Schautzer F. Integration of drug therapy and psychotherapy concepts in treatment of depression. *Wien Med Wochenschr.* 1998;148:364-369.

103. Nagayama H. Drug therapy for patients with depression. *Seishin Shinkeizaku Zasshi.* 2001;103:596-601.

104. Hallager K. Preventive drug therapy of depression. *Uzeskr Laeger.* 2003;165:2968-2969.

105. Roberts J, Snyder D. Geriatric pharmacology. *Aging.* 1997;9,443-445.

106. Wehling M. Geriatric pharmacology. *Internist.* 2003;44:935.

107. Lim WK, Woodward MC. Improving medication outcomes in older people. *Aust J Hosp Pharm.* 1999;29:103.

108. Ugalino JA. Understanding the pharmacology of aging. *Hospital Physician Medical Practice for Staff & Residents*, Geriatric Medicine Board Review Manual. 1st ed. 2001;1.

109. Williams CM. Using medications appropriately in older adults. *Am Fam Physician.* 2002;66:1917.

110. Beers MH. Aging as a risk factor for medication-related problems. www.ascp.com/public/pubs/tcp/1999/dec/aging.shtml. Accessed August 2, 2007.

111. Simon S, Chan KA. Potentially inappropriate medication use by elderly persons in U.S. health maintenance organizations, 2000-2001. *J Am Geriatr Soc.* 2005;53:227.

112. Gurwitz JH, Field TS. Incidence and preventability of adverse drug events among older persons in the ambulatory care setting. *JAMA.* 2003;289:1107.

113. Corcoran ME. Polypharmacy in the older patient with cancer. 1997. www.moffitt.usf.edu/pubs/ccj/v4n5/article5.html. Accessed May 16, 2007.

114. Lin P. Drug interactions, a method to the madness. *Perspectives in Cardiology.* 2004;20:20-29.

115. Fulton MM, Allen J. Polypharmacy in the elderly: a literature review. *J Am Acad Nurse Pract.* 2005;17:123-126.

Table 7-38

HERBS, DIETARY SUPPLEMENTS, AND DRUGS USED TO TREAT SLEEP DISORDERS AND INSOMNIA

ACTIVE HERB, SOURCE, FORM, AND DOSAGE	THERAPEUTIC EFFECT AND MECHANISM OF ACTION	SIDE EFFECTS, DRUG INTERACTIONS, CAUTIONS
Herbs for Sleep		
Valerian root[64,65] Volatile essential oils (monoterpenes and sesquiterpenes) from dried root and rhizome *Source:* 400- to 900-mg capsules, 2 to 3 g powdered leaf, or 3 to 5 mL of tincture *Dosage:* 2 to 3 times daily and before bed	Restlessness, sleeping disorders based on nervous conditions, muscle relaxant; reduced sleep latency; improved perception of sleep quality; delayed onset of action: 2 to 4 weeks therapy to achieve results; weakly binds GABA and benxodiazepine receptors in vitro	Mild headache, excitability, and uneasiness Overdose may cause severe headache, nausea, morning grogginess, blurry vision Do not take with sedatives, anxiolytics, or alcohol Use caution when driving or operating machinery
Dietary Supplements for Sleep		
Melatonin[66,67] Synthetic preparations include sublingual tablets, ordinary tablets, and capsules *Dosage:* 0.2 to 5 mg taken at bedtime Results are variable; Melatonin does not work for everyone Large first-pass effect through liver Half-life is 30 to 60 minutes	Induces sleep but does not maintain sleep; may alter patient's circadian rhythms and/or have a direct sleep-inducing effect; also associated with a decrease in body temperature	Should not be used when person is malnourished or frail, in people taking steroids, or those with severe allergies or autoimmune diseases
5-Hydroxytryptophan (5-HTP)[68,69] Commercially produced by extraction from seeds of *Griffonia simplicifolia* *Dosage:* 50 mg 3 times a day with meals, or 100 to 300 mg before bedtime Well absorbed, 70% ends up in bloodstream Crosses blood-brain barrier without transport molecule	Increased sleep compared to placebo (600 mg dose); at high doses (2500 mg) sleep decreased; precursor to serotonin, a neurotransmitter associated with sleep	Possible GI upset, nausea, diarrhea, and cramping Do not use with antidepressants Rare possibility of an eosinophilia myalgia syndrome (EMS)
Drugs Prescribed for Sleep[6]		
Benzodiazepines	Effective in short-term management of insomnia; reduces sleep-onset latency; decreases the number and duration of awakenings; increases total sleep time	Used cautiously and with appropriate behavioral treatment programs
Flurazepam *(Dalmane)*	Effective in inducing and maintaining sleep for up to 1 month of consecutive usage Decreases daytime alertness, increases daytime sedation	Rapidly absorbed: half-life 48 to 120 hours Accumulation with nightly use; washout slow after termination of use *(Continued)*

Table 7-38 continued

HERBS, DIETARY SUPPLEMENTS, AND DRUGS USED TO TREAT SLEEP DISORDERS AND INSOMNIA

ACTIVE HERB, SOURCE, FORM, AND DOSAGE	THERAPEUTIC EFFECT AND MECHANISM OF ACTION	SIDE EFFECTS, DRUG INTERACTIONS, CAUTIONS
Temazepam *(Restoril)*	Good for sleep maintenance problems; best used for late-life insomnia	Minimal tolerance for up to 3 months of use Intermediate absorption, half-life is 8 to 20 hours; moderate accumulation with multiple dosing
Triazolam *(Halcion)*	Reduces sleep-onset latency and increases total sleep time Allows maximal daytime alertness May be associated with early morning awakening and daytime anxiety	Fast absorption, short half-life (2 to 6 hours); minimal accumulation during multiple dosing
Zolpidem tartrate *(Ambien)*	Decreases sleep-onset latency, but does not decrease number or duration of awakenings Slow wave sleep well preserved	Rapid onset and short duration Therapeutic gains maintained 5 weeks No next-day residual effects of rebound insomnia

Table 7-39

HERBS USED TO TREAT HEADACHES[82,83]

ACTIVE HERB, SOURCE, FORM, AND DOSAGE	THERAPEUTIC EFFECT AND MECHANISM OF ACTION	SIDE EFFECTS, DRUG INTERACTIONS, CAUTIONS
Feverfew Sesquiterpene lactones (parthenolide), and flavonoid glycosides *Dosage:* 125 mg of dried leaf preparation, containing at least 0.2% parthenolide	Inhibits prostaglandin systhesis in vitro; inhibits serotonin release from platelets; may produce an anti-migraine effect in a manner similar to Sansert	Rebound symptoms may occur after discontinuation; side effects when chewed include mouth ulceration, inflammation of the oral mucosa and tongue, often with lip swelling and loss of taste Long-term safety has not been established
Peppermint oil Oil obtained by steam distillation from freshly harvested flowering sprigs (yields 0.1% to 10% of volatile oil composed primarily of menthol)	Applied externally for myalgia and neuralgia Exhibits spasmolytic activity on smooth muscle	When used topically, no known side effects or interactions with other drugs

Table 7-40

HERBS AND DRUGS USED TO TREAT DEPRESSION AND ANXIETY DISORDERS

ACTIVE HERB, SOURCE, FORM, AND DOSAGE	THERAPEUTIC EFFECT AND MECHANISM OF ACTION	SIDE EFFECTS, DRUG INTERACTIONS, CAUTIONS
Herbs for Depression and Anxiety		
St John's wort[70,71,72] Anthraquinone derivatives hypercin and pseudohypercin; also contains flavonoids, glycosides, phenols, carotenoids, organic acids, choline, pectine, tannins, and long chain alcohols Flowers provide active constituents Klamath weed or goatweed harvested and dried Daily dose: 200 to 1000 mg alcohol abstract, taken 2 to 3 times per day	Mild to moderate depression Under investigation as a treatment for AIDS and other viruses Exact mechanism of action unknown Thought to exert anti-depressant effects by inhibiting serotonin reuptake by postsynaptic receptors Some reports suggest MAO antagonism as another probable mechanism	Side effects are rare but include gastrointestinal reaction (0.6%), allergic reactions (0.5%), fatigue (0.4%), restlessness (0.3%) No known drug interactions, but not recommended to be used with other anti-depressants, effects of reserpine antagonized; rash caused by photosensitivity rare
Kava-kava[70,73] Kava pryrones (kawain) found in rhizome (root); other complex chemical components include 7 kava lactones Kava extract standardized to 55% to 70% kava lactones (kava alpha-pyrones) *Dose:* for anxiety, 45 to 75 mg 3 times a day; for sedation, 135 to 210 mg 1 hour before bedtime	Sedative and sleep enhancement (CNS depressant effect) Reduced nonpsychotic type anxiety Masticated kava causes numbness of the mouth Mechanism of action unknown	May adversely affect motor reflexes and judgment for driving; side effects include dry, flaking, discolored (yellow) skin; scaly rash; red eyes; puffy face; some muscle weakness Contraindicated if using alcohol, barbiturates, or psychoactive agents
Prescription Medications for Depression[6]		
Selective Serotonin Reuptake Inhibitors (SSRI) Fluoxetine *(Prozac)*; Sertraline *(Zoloft)*; Paroxetine *(Paxil)*		May cause nausea, GI distress, anxiety, nervousness, change in appetite or weight, fatigue, drowsiness, and sexual dysfunction
Tricyclic Anti-depressants (TCAs) Tofranil *(Imipramine)*; Anafranil *(Clomipramine)*; Elavil *(Amitriptyline)*		Dry mouth, constipation, blurry vision, increased sensitivity to sunlight, increased sweating, weight gain
Bupropion *(Wellbutrin)*		Increased restlessness, agitation, anxiety, insomnia
Venlafaxine *(Effexor)*		Nausea, headache, sweating, anxiety, insomnia
Prescription Medications for Anxiety[6]		
Benxodiazepines Diazepam *(Valium)*; Alprazolam *(Xanax)*; Chlordiazepoxide *(Librium)*		Habit forming, withdrawal symptoms, drowsiness, dizziness, inability to concentrate, increased salivation, constipation, weight gain, blurred vision, decreased sex drive, impotence
Buspirone *(BuSpar)*		Mild headache, drowsiness, nausea, dry mouth

Table 7-41

HERBS AND DIETARY SUPPLEMENTS:
MEMORY, ALZHEIMER'S DISEASE, AND COGNITIVE FUNCTION

ACTIVE HERB, SOURCE, FORM, AND DOSAGE	THERAPEUTIC EFFECT AND MECHANISM OF ACTION	SIDE EFFECTS, DRUG INTERACTIONS, CAUTIONS
Herbs and Cognitive Function		
Ginkgo biloba[50,51,52,74]		
Standardized extract from leaves contains 24% flavone glycosides and 6% terpene lactones *Dosage for dementia:* 120 to 240 mg per day, taken in 2 to 3 separate doses for a minimum of 8 weeks	Treatments for cerebrovascular insufficiency (causing anxiety, memory, concentration and mood impairment, hearing disorders), dementia, circulatory disorders (see Table 7-30) Anti-oxidant inhibits platelet activating factor (PAF)	Possible side effects may include headache, dizziness, GI and dermatologic reactions, heart palpitations; ginkgo seeds are toxic; contact with fruit pulp causes allergic dermatitis; may potentiate the effects of anti-coagulants

HORMONES,[75,76] VITAMINS,[76-81] NUTRACEUTICALS,[76-81] AND DRUGS[6,76] FOR COGNITIVE FUNCTION

SUBSTANCE	REPORTED BENEFITS	MECHANISM OF ACTION
Estrogen (ERT)	Associated with reduced risk of Alzheimer's disease; enhanced response to tacrine in women with AD	May have direct effects on neurotransmitter development and activity, enhancing the growth of cholinergic neurons; may act as an antioxidant; reduces generation of β-amyloid peptides
Vitamin E (alpha-tocopherol) *Dosage:* 2,000 IUs daily for 2 years	Slowed functional deterioration seen in moderately severe Alzheimer's patients	Antioxidant; inhibits lipid peroxidation and reduces cell death associated with β-protein
Selenium	Deficiency signs include confusion	Co-factor for anti-oxidant enzymes
Phosphatidylserine (PS)	Exerted mild benefit in age-related cognitive decline and in patients with early symptoms of Alzheimer's disease Preparation used was extracted from bovine brain cortex[48]	A major phospholipid in the brain; involved with neurotransmitter release and supports signal transduction
Docosahexanoic acid (DHA)	Epidemiological correlation between low levels of serum DHA and dementia, depression, and memory loss	DHA can make up 20% to 30% of the phospholipids in the graymatter of the brain
Lecithin	Studies failed to find significant memory improvement with choline or lecithin supplementation in Alzheimer's patients[46,47]	Contains choline, the precursor to acetylcholine; also used to make phosphatidyl choline
Vitamin B$_{12}$ and folic acid	Deficiency symptoms include depression and dementia	Methyl donors add metylmoities to monoamine neurotransmitters (dopamine and serotonin)
Acetyl-L-carnitine[76,81] (component of choline)	Improved cognitive function and memory in patients with age-related dementia and slowed rate of deterioration in patients with Alzheimer's disease	Crosses the blood-brain barrier and produces cholinergic effects; also increases cerebral blood flow
NSAIDs[76]	Slowed functional deterioration and cognitive impairment of Alzheimer's patients Reduced risk of developing Alzheimer's disease	Reduces inflammation in the brain due to the deposition of amyloid protein

Table 7-42

HERBS USED TO TREAT CARDIOVASCULAR DISORDERS[61,64,83]

ACTIVE HERB, SOURCE, FORM, AND DOSAGE	THERAPEUTIC EFFECT AND MECHANISM OF ACTION	SIDE EFFECTS, DRUG INTERACTIONS, CAUTIONS
Garlic *(Allium sativum)* Garlic bulbs, consisting of fresh or carefully dried bulbs, as well as its preparations in effective dosage Garlic contains alliin, which is converted to allicin and other sulfur-containing compounds *Dosage:* 2 to 4 g fresh garlic (1 to 2 cloves) or its equivalent in commercial product with daily intake of 10 mg alliin or total allicin potential of 4 mg, taken for at least 1 to 3 months	Supportive to dietary measures that lower elevated levels of total and LDL cholesterol and for prevention of atherosclerosis May help reduce systolic and diastolic blood pressure in patients with mild hypertension,[1] but effect is not adequate for specific antihypertensive therapy in patients with high blood pressure Inhibits platelet aggregation by interfering with thromboxane synthesis; prolongs bleeding and clotting time; enhances fibrinolytic activity	Side effects rare, but include GI symptoms, changes to flora of intestines, allergic reactions, and hypotensive circulatory reactions May potentiate the effect of antihypertensive and anti-coagulant medications The odor of garlic may pervade the breath and skin
Ginkgo biloba Standardized extract from leaves contains 24% flavone glycosides and 6% terpene lactones *Dosage:* 40 mg 3 times daily should be taken consistently for 12 weeks to be effective	Supportive treatment for peripheral arterial disease; protects against cardiac ischemia reperfusion injury, adjusts fibrinolytic activity, in combination with aspirin treats thrombosis; inhibits binding of platelet-activating factor to membrane receptors	Possible side effects include headache, dizziness, heart palpitations, GI, and dermatologic reactions
Guggul *(Commiphora mukul)* Standardized extract known as Guggulipid contains 25 mg of guggulsterones per gram *Dosage:* 500 mg for 12 weeks	Appears to lower total and LDL cholesterol and increase HDL Stimulates thyroid-stimulating activity	No significant adverse effects reported in clinical studies, any symptoms are GI in nature
Hawthorn leaf with flower Leaf with flower, consisting of dried flowering twig tips Main constituents are flavonoids, prodyanidins, catechins, and other compounds *Dosage:* 160 to 900 mg aqueous alcoholic extract with a designated content of flavonoids (4 to 30 mg) or oligomeric procyanidins (30 to 160 mg) per day, for at least 6 weeks	Heart failure and coronary insufficiency, as described in functional Stage II of New York Heart Association[2]; not appropriate for more advanced stages; exercise improves cardiac performance Peripheral vasodilator and positive inotropic agent (associated with lengthening of the refractory period) to stabilize heart rhythm	Side effects are mild, may include nausea, headache, swelling of the lower extremities

(Continued)

Table 7-42 continued

HERBS USED TO TREAT CARDIOVASCULAR DISORDERS[61,64,83]

ACTIVE HERB, SOURCE, FORM, AND DOSAGE	THERAPEUTIC EFFECT AND MECHANISM OF ACTION	SIDE EFFECTS, DRUG INTERACTIONS, CAUTIONS
Digitalis *(Digitalis purpurea)* Leaves and seeds of wild varieties contain at least 30 different cardiac glycosides including digoxin and digitoxin	Used in treatment of CHF; improves cardiac conduction, thereby improving the strength of cardiac contractility	Narrow therapeutic margin and high potential for severe side effects
Horse chestnut seed Dry extract manufactured from seeds, adjusted to a content of 16% to 20% triterpene glycosides (calculated as anhydrous aescin) *Dosage:* 100 mg aescin corresponding to 250 to 300 mg twice daily in delayed release form	Chronic venous insufficiency (eg, pain and a sensation of heaviness in the legs, swelling of the legs) Anti-exudative and vascular tightening effect by reducing vascular permeability	Noninvasive treatment measures (eg, leg compresses, support hose, cold H_2O therapy) should be used Side effects may include pruritis, nausea, and gastric complaints

[1]*All of the blood pressure trials used the same dried powder preparation (Kwai), which has a standardized allicin content, in the dose range 600 to 900 mg daily. This is the equivalent of 1.8 to 2.7 g/day fresh garlic. The median duration of therapy was 12 weeks.*

[2]*Stages I and II of the New York Heart Association refer to stages of heart disease in the NYHA's 1994 Revisions to Classification of Functional Capacity and Objective Assessment of Patients with Disease of the Heart: Patients With Cardiac Disease but without resulting limitations of physical activity. They are comfortable at rest. Ordinary physical activity results in fatigue, palpitation, dyspnea, or anginal pain.*

Table 7-43

HERBS USED TO TREAT IMMUNE AND RESPIRATORY SYSTEM DISORDERS[61,64,83]

ACTIVE HERB, SOURCE, FORM, AND DOSAGE	THERAPEUTIC EFFECT AND MECHANISM OF ACTION	SIDE EFFECTS, DRUG INTERACTIONS, CAUTIONS
Echinachea *(E purpurea, E pallida)* Common name: cone flower 0.1R caffeic acid glycoside (echinacoside) and many other complex substances; no single compound appears to be responsible for plant's activity *Dosage:* 15 drops/day, equivalent to 900 mg Do not use for more than 8 weeks (Parenteral: no longer than 3 weeks)	Supportive treatment of recurrent infections of upper respiratory tract and lower urinary tract; appears to shorten duration/frequency of the common cold Immune stimulant; stimulates phagocytic activity, release of interleukin I, tumor necrosis factors, and interferon; increases number of WBC and spleen cells; may elevate body temperature	No known side effects Contraindicated in patients with progressive systemic diseases, such as tuberculosis, leukosis, multiple sclerosis, collagen disorders, and other autoimmune diseases, or HIV Metabolic condition in diabetes can decline upon parenteral application
Ephedra *(Ephedra sinica)* *Common name:* Ma Huang, Mormon tea, sea grape, yellow horse Main alkaloid is ephedrine Standard preparations have supplanted the use of the crude drug in most countries *Dosage:* herb preparation corresponding to 0.5 mg total alkaloid per kg body weight *Maximum daily dosage:* 300 mg total alkaloid, calculated as ephedrine Should only be used short-term (1 week)	Clears up respiratory congestion, relaxes airways (bronchodilator) Stimulates the sympathomimetic and CNS	Side effects: insomnia, motor restlessness, irritability, headaches, nausea, vomiting, disturbances of urination, tachycardia In higher dosages: drastic increase in blood pressure, cardiac arrhythmia, can develop dependency Contraindicated in patients with anxiety and restlessness, high blood pressure, glaucoma, enlarged prostate Do not use with cardiac glycosides, MAOIs, guanethidine
Ginseng *(Panax ginseng)* *Common name:* Korean ginseng Whole root used, contains triterpenoid saponin glycosides Wide range of commercial products available Proper dose and duration remain poorly defined *Dosage:* 2 to 3 g is standard in capsules	Reported effective as an adaptogen: to increase physical, chemical, and biological stress, and to build up vitality	Not usually associated with serious adverse effects Common side effects: nervousness and excitation; both side effects usually resolve after first few days of use; may also have hypoglycemic effect
Eleutherococcus *(Acanthopanax seticosus)* *Common names:* Siberian ginseng, devil's shrub, eleuthera, eleuthero, touch-me-not Contains electherosides, glucose, sucrose, and a variety of dyestuffs Leaves contain saponins normally found in ginseng roots *Dosage:* 2 to 3 g/day limited to 3 months	Immunomodulator; increases absolute number of T cells Used as a tonic to counteract fatigue and weakness, as a restorative for declining stamina and impaired concentration, and as an aid to convalescence	Rare reported side effects have included slight languor or drowsiness immediately after taking Contraindicated in hypertension

Table 7-44

HERBAL TREATMENTS FOR WOUNDS, SKIN, AND ORAL HEALTH[61,64,83]

ACTIVE CONSTITUENTS: SOURCE, FORM, DOSAGE	THERAPEUTIC ACTION	SIDE EFFECTS, DRUG INTERACTIONS, CAUTIONS
Echinacea *(Echinacea angustifolia, E purpurea, E pallida)* *Common names:* cone flower, black susans, comb flower, Kansas snakeroot, Indian head Semisolid preparation containing at least 15% pressed juice, do not use more than 8 weeks	Used externally for poor healing wounds and chronic ulcerations	No reported side effects or interactions
Gotu Kola *(Centella asiatica)* *Common names:* hydrocotyle, Indian pennywort, talepetrako Contains active principle madecassol, asiatic acid, and glycoside asiaticoside	Promotes wound healing, used in patients with surgical wounds, fistulas, and gynecological lesions; helpful in treating psoriasis	Contact dermatitis reported in some patients
Tea tree oil *(Melaleuca alternifolia)* *Common names:* desert essence, tea tree oil soap Essential oil obtained by steam distillation of leaves, main constituent is terpin-4-ol (~30%)	Anti-microbial effects without irritating sensitive tissues; effective against tinea pedia (athlete's foot) and acne Can be added to baths or to vaporizers to help treat respiratory disorders	Use has resulted in allergic contact eczema and dermatitis Harmful if ingested
Aloe *(Aloe vera, A ferox)* *Common names:* Cape, Zanzibar, Socotrine, Curacao, Barbados aloe, aloe vera Aloe gel is a clear, thin, gelatinous material obtained by crushing the mucilaginous cells found in the inner tissue leaf; contains the polysaccharide glucomannan	Minor burns and skin irritations Moisterizing effect, which helps prevent air from drying the wound; also accelerates wound healing	Not associated with adverse reactions when used topically
Oil of Evening primrose *(Oenothera biennis)* *Common name:* Efamol Rich in gamma-linolenic acid Available in capsule form; maximum dose 4 g/day	Treats itching associated with atopic dermatitis and eczema	Mild GI upset, headache, and nausea possible
Goldenseal *(Hydrastis canadensis)* *Common names:* eye balm, ground raspberry, Indian dye, jaundice root, orange root, tumeric root Contains hyrastine and berberine	Topically, as eye wash Astringent and weak antiseptic properties that are effective in treating oral problems	Small amounts of the plant can be ingested (as in tea) with no side effects; large doses can be toxic; should not be taken during pregnancy

(Continued)

Table 7-44 continued

HERBAL TREATMENTS FOR WOUNDS, SKIN, AND ORAL HEALTH[61,64,83]

ACTIVE CONSTITUENTS: SOURCE, FORM, DOSAGE	THERAPEUTIC ACTION	SIDE EFFECTS, DRUG INTERACTIONS, CAUTIONS
Myrrh *(Commiphora molmol, C abyssinica)* *Common names:* African myrrh, myrrh, gum myrrh, bola, gal, bol, heerabol Oleo-gum-resin that contains from 15% to 17% of volatile oil (40% commiphoric acid and 60% of gum yields a variety of sugars upon hydrolysis	Mild astringent properties; may exert anti-microbial activity; also helpful in treating canker sores Added to mouthwashes, used in fragrances, and as a food flavoring	Generally considered to be nonirritating, though several cases of dermatitis have been reported
Sage *(Salvia officinalis)* *Common names:* garden sage, true sage, meadow sage, scarlet sage Contains 1% to 28% of a volatile oil	Topical use as an antiseptic and astringent Exerts anti-microbial activity against *Staphylococcus aureus*	Reports of cheilitis and stomatitis in some cases following ingestion of sage tea; large amounts may cause dry mouth or local irritation
Bloodroot *(Sanguinaria cana densis)* *Common names:* red root, red puccon, tetterwort, Indian red plant, Indian plant, sanguinaria Many isoquinoline derivatives, including sanguinarine and berberine Contains a negatively charged ion that binds to dental plaque	In toothpastes and oral rinses to help reduce and limit the deposition of dental plaque; effective against common oral bacteria	Should not be ingested, as it can induce CNS depression and may also produce nausea and vomiting

Table 7-45

HERBAL TREATMENTS FOR GASTROINTESTINAL SYSTEM AND LIVER HEALTH[61,64,83]

ACTIVE CONSTITUENTS: SOURCE, FORM, DOSAGE	THERAPEUTIC ACTION	SIDE EFFECTS, DRUG INTERACTIONS, CAUTIONS
Gentian (*Gentiana lutea*) *Common names:* Stemless genitian, bitter root, pale gentian, gall weed Dried rhizome and roots, quickly dried Approved for food use; usually consumed as tea prepared by gently boiling root in water	Used as bitter tonic to stimulate appetite and improve digestion May stimulate taste buds and increase flow of saliva and stomach secretions	May cause headache and gastric irritation, resulting in vomiting and nausea
Ginger (*Zingiber officinale*) Rhizome of plant contains volatile oil that is responsible for characteristic aroma and oleoresin *Dosage:* 2 to 4 g/day	Possesses carminative, diuretic, stimulant, anti-emetic properties Symptomatic relief in pregnant women suffering from hyper-emesis gravidarum (250 mg, 4 four times day)	No reports of toxicity Large overdoses carry potential for causing CNS depression and cardiac arrhythmias
Chamomile (*Matricaria chamomilla*) *Common names:* German, Hungarian, or genuine chamomile Flower head contains essential oil; teas contain small amount of oil, but used over long periods of time may have cumulative effect	Gastrointestinal anti-spasmodic	May cause contact dermatitis, anaphylaxis, and other hypersensitivity reactions in persons allergic to ragweed, asters, and chrysanthemums May delay drug absorption from gut
Peppermint oil (*Mentha x piperita*) Complex chemistry; volatile oil composed primarily of menthol As a tea: 1 cup of boiling water over 1 tablespoon of leaves (3 to 4 cups daily with meals)	Anti-spasmodic (carminitive) effects on smooth muscle Used in treatment of irritable bowel and abdominal pain	Persons with hiatal hernia may experience worsening of symptoms due to its relaxing effect on lower esophageal sphincter Do not use during pregnancy or in presence of gallstones
Turmeric root (*Curcuma aromatica, C domestica, C longa*) *Common names:* Tumeric, curcuma, Indian saffron Rhizome, contains volatile oil consisting of 60% Sesquiterpene ketones known as turmerones *Dosage:* 1.5 to 3 g/day	Digestive aid Stimulated production of bile Possesses anti-hepatotoxic effects	No side effects reported Contradicted in obstruction of bile passages

(Continued)

Table 7-45 continued

HERBAL TREATMENTS FOR GASTROINTESTINAL SYSTEM AND LIVER HEALTH[61,64,83]

ACTIVE CONSTITUENTS: SOURCE, FORM, DOSAGE	THERAPEUTIC ACTION	SIDE EFFECTS, DRUG INTERACTIONS, CAUTIONS
Psyllium seen *(Plantage psyllium)* *Common names:* psyllium, Indian Plantago seed, psyllium seed, flea seed, black psyllium Dried ripe seed, containing mucilages *Dosage:* 75 g of seed or 1 teaspoon husks, mixed into 8 oz glass of water or juice (consumed quickly)	Chronic constipation; irritable bowel; acts as a bulk laxative; mixed with water, produces a mucilaginous mass; regulates intestinal peristalsis May lower cholesterol levels	Varying degrees of psyllium allergy including anaphylaxis, sneezing, chest congestion, and watery eyes Take with adequate fluid to avoid blockages May inhibit absorption of lithium and carbamazepine
Cascara *(Rhamnus purshiana)* *Common names:* Buckthorn, cascara sagrada, chittem bark, sacred bark Dried bark contains not less than 7% total hydroxyanthracene derivatives calculated as cascaroside A on a dried basis Available as ingredient in OTC laxatives; if using capsules of powdered bark, dose is 1 g	Stimulant laxative, used for constipation Inhibits stationary and stimulating propulsive contractions in colon, resulting in accelerated intestinal passage, and reduction in liquid absorption	Reduce dosage if cramp-like discomfort occurs Contraindicated in acute intestinal inflammation (eg, Crohn's disease, colitis, abdominal pain of unknown origin), children under 12, and if pregnant or nursing
Senna *(Cassia acutigolia, Cassia senna)* *Common names:* senna leaf, black draught granules, *Senokot* Leaves contain anthraquinones and sennosides Should not be used over extended period of time (1 to 2 weeks) without medical advice *Dosage:* 20 to 30 mg hydroanthracene derivatives daily, calculated as sennoside B; individually correct dosage is the smallest amount necessary to maintain a soft stool	Potent laxative effect Decreases intestinal transit time	Contraindications: same as Cascara above Aggravates loss of potassium if on diuretics Cautions: chronic use may result in "laxative dependency syndrome" characterized by poor gastric motility in the absence of repeated laxative administration; abuse may result in diarrhea, altered electrolytes (which may enhance effectiveness of cardiac glycosides), cachexia, and reduced serum globulin levels May decrease absorption of oral medications *(Continued)*

Table 7-45 continued

HERBAL TREATMENTS FOR GASTROINTESTINAL SYSTEM AND LIVER HEALTH[61,64,83]

ACTIVE CONSTITUENTS: SOURCE, FORM, DOSAGE	THERAPEUTIC ACTION	SIDE EFFECTS, DRUG INTERACTIONS, CAUTIONS
Aloe *(Aloe vera, A ferox)* *Common names:* Cape, Zanzibar, Socotrin, Curacao, Barbadoes aloe, aloe vera Anthraquinone glycosides aloin A and B *Dosage:* 20 to 30 mg hydroanthracene derivatives daily, calculated as anhydrous aloin	Potent laxative used for acute constipation	Contraindications and cautions: see previous
Bilberry fruit *(Vaccinium myrtillus)* *Common names:* bilberries, bog bilberries, blueberries (variety of), whortleberries Contains tannins, anthocyans, flavonoids, plant acids, inverted sugars and pectins; must be dried to obtain tannins, which come about by condensation of tannin precursors during drying process	Supportive treatment of acute nonspecific diarrhea	Effects of ingesting large doses unknown; no known side effects or interactions with other drugs
Licorice root *(Glycyrrhiza glabra)* *Common names:* licorice, Spanish or Russian licorice Dried rhizome and roots contain at least 4% triterpene glycoside; on hydrolysis, glycyrrhizin loses its sweet taste and is converted to glycyrrhetic acid	Treatment of peptic ulcers (but not as effective as cimetidine) Anti-inflammatory properties	Side effects include headache, lethargy, sodium and water retention (eg, contraindicated in high blood pressure); excessive excretion of potassium Potentiates toxicity to cardiac glycosides such as those in digitalis due to potassium loss in urine; should not be used with spironolactone or amiloride; or with corticoid treatment
Milk thistle *(Silybum marianum)* *Common names:* Holy thistle, lady's thistle, Marian thistle, Mary thistle, St Mary thistle, silybum From fruits (seeds), 70% contains silymarin, a mixture of 4 isomers, including main constituent silybin (silibinin) Dosages: 12 to 15 g; formulations equivalent to 200 to 400 mg silymarin, calculated as silybinin Poorly soluble in water, so aqueous preparations (eg, teas) ineffective; best administered parenterally or as a capsule containing concentrated extract due to poor absorption from GI tract	Dyspeptic complaints For supportive treatment in chronic inflammatory liver disease and hepatic cirrhosis; also used in *Amanita phalloides* poisoning Alters structure of outer cell membrane of hepatocytes to prevent penetration of liver toxin into interior of cell and/or stimulates regenerative ability of the liver and formation of new hepatocytes Acts as an antioxidant	No known contraindications or side effects

Table 7-46

HERBS USED TO TREAT IMMUNE AND RESPIRATORY SYSTEM DISORDERS: COUGH REMEDIES[61,64,83]

HERB (BOTANICAL NAME)	PREPARATION
Anti-tussives (Cough Suppressants)	
Marshmallow root (*Althaeae officinalis*) and Mallow leaf (*Malvae folium*)	• Consumed in tea, 1 to 2 teaspoons (5 to 10 g) in 150 mL water (daily dose: 6 g) *Note:* absorption of oral drugs taken simultaneously may be delayed
Iceland moss (*Lichen islandicus*)	• 1% to 2% infusion (1 to 2 teaspoons/150 mL), drink 1 cup 3 times daily; do not use in large quantities over extended period of time (can be toxic)
Mullein flowers (*Verbascum thapsus*)	• 3 to 4 teaspoons or 1.5 to 2 g used to prepare tea, drink several times a day
Plantain (*Plantago lanceolata*)	• Tea prepared from 2 to 3 g of herb and 150 mL water; used also for inflammatory conditions of the oral cavity
Slippery elm (*Ulmus rubra*)	• Lozenges most effective form
Expectorants	
Horehound (*Marrubium vulgare*)	• Tea prepared from 2 teaspoons cut herb steeped in 1 cup boiling water or hard candy used as a cough lozenge
Thyme (*Thymus vulgaris*)	• Tea prepared from 1 teaspoon herb per cup water, drink up to 3 times daily; may be sweetened with honey, which also acts as a demulcent
Eucalyptus leaves (*Eucalyptus globulus*)	• Tea prepared from ½ teaspoon leaves in about 150 mL hot water, drink freshly prepared 3 times daily The volatile oil is commonly incorporated into a variety of nasal inhalers and sprays, balms, and ointments for external application and mouthwashes
Licorice (*Glycyrrhiza glabra*)	• 1 to 2 g fried root taken 3 times daily
Senega snake-root (*Polygala senega*)	• Decoction prepared from 0.5 g and 1 cup water daily, dose should not exceed 3 g due to tendency to cause upset stomach, nausea, and diarrhea

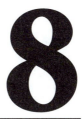

Settings of Care in Geriatrics: The Role of the Physical Therapist Assistant

The practice of physical therapy is conducted by a PT and the assisting PTA in the provision of care in all geriatric care settings. The PTA can assist the PT in data collection and physical therapy interventions as designed by the supervising PT. The PTA can only follow the selected interventions prescribed by the PT. Any change in treatment plan or goals must be done as part of patient management by the PT. With practice, a good educational background, and clinical experience, PTAs develop the ability to recognize the need to alter or change treatment procedures and make recommendations to intervention changes that might benefit the individual in progressing in rehabilitation. With increasing demand to provide excellence in physical therapy services in geriatric settings and to contain the costs of care while maintaining quality, there is increasing responsibility of the PTA to communicate with the PT and actively participate in the care delivered to older adults in every health care setting. It is important to examine the role the PTA plays in each of the geriatric settings that a PTA might choose for employment.

This chapter addresses the role that the PTA plays in various settings of care. It discusses the level of supervision required for both the PTA and the student PTA in each respective care setting. PTs' and PTAs' perspectives on the management and delivery of physical therapy services are provided in preparation for the restructuring of health care services with future health care reform and changes in public policy that will impact care in each of the practice settings for the elderly.

THE ROLE OF THE PHYSICAL THERAPIST ASSISTANT

The PTA is a skilled, technical health care worker who implements treatment programs under the direction and delegation of the PT.[1,2] Some duties of the PTA include reading patients' charts; transferring patients; applying physical agents such as heat, cold, and electrical stimulation to specific muscles; instructing patients in functional skills; and observing and reporting changes in a patient's condition to the PT. PTAs work in settings where PTs are employed. PTAs work in hospitals, outpatient clinics, private practices, rehabilitation centers, nursing homes, school systems, and other qualified agencies.

The PTA assists in data collection, implementation, and modification of interventions prescribed by the PT under a plan of care, participation in discharge planning and follow-up care, documentation of the care provided, and education of those involved in the care of each patient (eg, PT and PTA students, aides, family members and caregivers, volunteers). Depending on the specific settings and circumstances of care, the PTA may participate in patient care with other health care professionals.

Bottomley J. *Geriatric Rehabilitation: A Textbook for the Physical Therapist Assistant* (pp 233-242).
© 2010 SLACK Incorporated

SUPERVISION

The PTA provides physical therapy services under the supervision and direction of the PT. The PT is responsible for determining when to utilize a PTA for selected interventions. The decision to incorporate the PTA in patient care often depends on the stability and complexity of the patient's medical status as well as the PTA's expertise, skill level, and ability to predict consequences of interventions.

Depending on state law, which dictates the practice of physical therapy, the PT may or may not be required to be present or on site for supervising a PTA. State law dictates the specific nature of supervision required by the PT in overseeing the work of the PTA. The vast majority of states require *general supervision*. The descriptive terminology of this legislative regulation states that the PT must maintain a level of general supervision by being immediately available via phone, beeper, or nearby office or clinic setting. Additionally, supervision occurs through regularly scheduled meetings between the PT and PTA to review patient care plans. Factors that might also influence the level of supervision might include the severity and stability of the patient's medical status; availability, accessibility, and proximity of the PT; and the type of environment in which service is provided. Specifics on supervision in various home settings of care are explained in greater detail under each geriatric environment described next.

Student PTAs require *continuous onsite supervision* by the PT or PTA mentor guiding the student through incorporation of knowledge and skills acquired in the academic setting into clinical practice. Regardless of the practice setting or clinical expertise in physical therapy, this level of supervision is required during clinical training, cooperative education, and service learning experiences. This prohibits students from making a visit at a patient's home unless a PT or PTA is there. PTAs may practice problem solving and treatment techniques only when the PT (includes the faculty member overseeing clinical experiences from the academic setting) or PTA is onsite. If the licensed physical therapy practitioners are not in the clinical setting for any reason, the student can observe but cannot provide care. Supervision of the student PTA cannot be assumed by a nurse, physician, aide, or any other health care practitioner.

GUIDE FOR CONDUCT AND STANDARDS OF CARE AND STATE LICENSURE

The American Physical Therapy Association (APTA) Code of Ethics is a part of the Guide for Conduct and

Standards of Care established by the APTA. The APTA provides a code of ethics specific to the PTA. This document is available on the APTA Web site www.apta.org. Professional organizations establish their own codes of conduct to protect the rights of patients. In addition, this document establishes the standards for autonomy and supervision, defines standards for peer review and reimbursement for services, and outlines professional expectations and responsibilities for licensed PTs and PTAs.

State physical therapy practice acts may differ from state to state. Each state has jurisdiction over the definition and legal requirements for the practice of physical therapy in each state. To obtain a copy of a specific state's physical therapy practice acts, refer to the *Quick Reference Dictionary for Physical Therapy*, which also provides a listing of state physical therapy chapters, which are excellent resources for standards of care in physical therapy that may be state specific.[3]

PRACTICING IN GERIATRIC REHABILITATION SETTINGS

There is no question that the population worldwide is aging. The result is the need for care in all health care settings increasingly includes the elderly. The role of the PTA is becoming more prominent in all facilities that provide care to the elderly. Employment of PTAs is expected to grow much faster in geriatric settings than all other health care occupations through 2014.[4] The Bureau of Labor Statistics predicts the demand for PTAs will continue to rise in accordance with the increasing number of elderly and individuals with disabilities or limited function in all settings of care. PTs are expected to increasingly use PTAs to reduce the cost of therapy services. The growing number of elderly is predicted to be vulnerable to chronic and debilitating conditions and require a variety of therapeutic services. With the backdrop of a current shortage of licensed PTs throughout the United States and the increasing need for rehabilitation services for older patients, the role of PTAs becomes even more critical.

Academic preparation for working with older adults includes course work in lifespan growth and development. Due to the medical complexity in most elder individuals, it is important that special attention to education specific to treating geriatric clients be included in the curriculum.[5] It is important to understand the stages of cognitive, emotional, and physical development across the life cycle. By recognizing the stages of individual development, the PTA will be better prepared to deal with different stages and personalities and understand various spiritual and moral dimensions that accompany the aging process. Additionally, sensitivity to various cultural influences on life span development assists the PTA in changes or modifications in his or her own behavior required to effectively interact with the individual and in a group setting.

Older people are seen for physical therapy in a variety of settings or rehabilitation-based programs. Acute care and subacute hospitals, rehabilitation facilities, outpatient rehabilitation, long-term care skilled nursing facilities, assisted living environments and other group housing, home- and community-based care, as well as hospice settings, industrial rehabilitation settings, fitness centers, and health promotion programs are some examples that may involve the provision of physical therapy services. The following section of this chapter will discuss various models of care existent in the US health care system that may employ PTAs for rehabilitation services.

PTs play an increasingly important role in the care of older adults in all settings of care. Proper patient selection; a thorough medical, social, and functional history; and a physical examination emphasizing the functional and physical status of the older adult are cornerstones of the evaluation process. Treatment is individualized and goal driven regardless of setting. The PT's unique intervention may ultimately allow an elder person to remain in his or her home by preventing falls and other accidents.[6] For instance, safety proofing the home environment, gait training that challenges balance, and the use of assistive devices for safe mobility may ensure that an older adult can live out the rest of his or her life at home.

MODELS OF CARE IN THE US HEALTH CARE SYSTEM

Rehabilitation rarely is conducted in only one care setting. Especially now, with the emphasis on reducing the length of stay in high-cost inpatient settings, rehabilitation spans a continuum of care in order to be cost effective, yet complete. The rehabilitation care settings have become more complicated than they were 15 years ago. Care for adults with significant functional limitations usually begins in the acute care hospital. In acute care, the where and when of admission and discharge are identified. Persons needing post acute rehabilitation have several options, including the following:

- Traditional inpatient rehabilitation unit of a hospital

- Free-standing rehabilitation hospital
- Subacute rehabilitation, which usually is located in a skilled nursing facility
- Rehabilitation in the home
- Rehabilitation in an outpatient clinic.

Patients may be transferred to any of these settings in any order. From the acute care setting, several alternative settings exist providing a range of intensities of treatment, resources available, and costs to be incurred. Triage should result in selecting the right patient for the right treatment setting at the right time. The ultimate goal at completion of rehabilitation is the patient's return to living in the community, which could mean living at home independently, living with family, receiving home health care, or living in an assisted living residence.

In order to render cost-effective care, a method for anticipating probable resource needs and outcomes would be helpful to determine, at the time of admission to acute care, what might be expected of each patient after acute care discharge. The continuum of care has become increasingly complex, ranging from high-cost and high-intensity care in acute care hospitals to lower-cost and lower-intensity care in outpatient settings. Adding to the complexities are insurance payment systems that vary across clinical settings. The demographics of an aging population means an increasing prevalence of chronic health conditions requiring a rational system for linking assessments of patients from the acute care hospital to the rehabilitation program and into outpatient and home-based programs. Assessment of patients across the continuum of care should be understandable, meaningful, cost effective, and manageable.

There are many settings in which health care and rehabilitation services may be provided and in which PTAs might be employed along the continuum of care. It is important to know what services are available to older individuals, especially related to rehabilitation, and how services may differ from setting to setting in terms of geriatric physical therapy.[7]

An older person might present with multiple clinical problems for which multiple services are required. For instance, the therapist may find, in addition to the clinical problems being addressed in rehabilitation, that there is also a need for psychological or social services. In some of these settings, the PTA may be the first to recognize such a situation. It is crucial that he or she knows when to communicate with the referring PT to initiate referral to other health care or social service professionals. Another example, in home care, recognizing problems such as poor nutrition may necessitate the referral to nutrition programs within the community (see Chapter 6).

Home Care Settings

Rehabilitation for older people has acquired an increasingly important profile for both policymakers and service providers within health and social care agencies. This growing demand for rehabilitation services has generated an increased interest in the use of alternative home care environments (eg, services provided in the patient's own home or comprehensive care home environments like assisted living or congregate housing for older persons where rehabilitation is a part of the amenities provided).[8]

At a time when there is pressure on policymakers and service providers to explore the use of such care settings for the provision of rehabilitation for older people, there still exists a limited number of PTs and PTAs available to provide these services. Reimbursement for services in home care is often capped, making goal attainment difficult. The decision of the PT to incorporate the PTA in patient care in the home depends on the skill level and ability of the individual PTA, his or her proficiency and clinical experience, the supervising PT's assessment of the PTA's ability to predict consequences of interventions and respond appropriately, and the elder individual's medical complexity and overall health and physical status.[9]

Nonetheless, adequately trained and capable PTAs often *do* provide care for elderly individuals, as directed by a PT and they do so without incident. It is important to discuss the provision of home care in various home care settings and provide the PTA with types of residences that constitute home care.

A perpetual shortage of PTs providing home care has increased the employment of the PTA in this setting in order to meet the increasing need for physical therapy services. Utilizing the PTA in the delivery of care potentially allows the PT to oversee and manage the care of more people.[10] Essential in every PT/PTA partnership is communication for providing the best physical therapy service in home care settings.

In the home setting, PT services need to be provided in a safe and effective manner under the general supervision of a skilled PT. The Centers for Medicare and Medicaid Services (CMS) describe general supervision in the following way:

- CMS requires that the initial direction and periodic reassessment be completed by a PT
- Supervision of a PTA in the home setting does not need direct (eg, physically present or on the premises) supervision by the PT
- The PTA may perform interventions specifically prescribed by the PT

- Changes in treatment protocol can only occur as prescribed by the PT following interactions and communication between PTA and PT or onsite reinspection by the PT
- The PTA is responsible for the documentation of each treatment session
- The PT must complete the discharge summary prior to discharging a patient from home care services.

The Elder's Own Home

Ask any older adult where he or she would like to be through the last phases of his or her life, and most will choose his or her own home.[11] There are some problems inherent in being at home, and living arrangements are often not conducive to safely living there. The elder may live alone, live in a home where safety and environmental obstacles are a concern, live with a spouse with his or her own health issues, or live in remote settings where family and services are not readily accessible. Staying at home may not be a reasonable option in the long run.

There are significant limitations on available home care services and agencies, and Medicare (as well as other third-party payers) limits reimbursement for services. Currently, CMS restricts the number of treatments or caps payment for health care services in the home setting. Many required services become out-of-pocket expenses for elderly individuals. This makes needed home interventions inaccessible and financially untouchable. As CMS requirements are fluid, it is advisable to keep current practice laws up-to-date by checking www.cms.gov on a regular basis. Updates and changes are usually posted at www.apta.org as well.

The role of the PTA in the home setting is quite unique. It is recommended that the PTA and referring PT, as well as the agency providing home health services, review the CMS guidelines and pay attention to any variations in state administration of Medicare laws. With strict adherence to the practice acts and the requisite evaluations and periodic reassessments by a PT, as well as general supervision and direction by a PT, a PTA working autonomously in the home setting must have the skills and experience to practice without the direct support of other health care professionals. The elder's or family member's home is an example of a setting in which know-how and experience in many different settings prior to assuming a position in home care may serve the PTA well. In other words, home care could indeed be risky for the inexperienced new PTA graduate without qualified mentors close at hand.

Several other settings and living environments in geriatric practice are defined as home care environments. The PTA may practice in any of these home settings including congregate housing and retirement or group homes; senior communities, senior hotels; foster care; or assisted living communities.

Congregate Housing, Retirement Homes, or Group Homes and Communities

There are increasing opportunities for older individuals to move into homes where other seniors reside. Congregate or group homes provide the option for older adults to assist each other. These environments are often based on the cooperative housing trend where individuals live together to share expenses and chores. Abilities of one elder may complement the abilities of others living in the group setting; therefore, the model is one of seniors assisting seniors. The principles of rehabilitation in the home setting previously described would also be applicable in this sort of living arrangement.

Senior Hotels and Housing Facilities

Another model for home care is the senior hotel or senior housing facilities. Often old hotels are converted into senior housing or apartment complexes are built specifically to accommodate the elderly population in a given community. In the hotel settings, daily maid service and restaurants (including room service) are often provided. In the senior housing apartments, a common area is frequently turned into a cafeteria or dining room, and meals are provided for the residents of the housing complex as part of their monthly rental fees. Both the hotel and the apartment models are typically subsidized for low-income elders, making them attractive alternatives to more expensive independent living environments. Visiting health care services, including rehabilitation services, are generally provided. Sometimes, rather than treating the elder in his or her hotel room or apartment, an exercise or therapy room is provided by the management of the building to accommodate rehabilitation needs of the residents. The PTA may also be involved in providing group exercise or educational programs in addition to seeing patients on an individual basis. The laws regarding supervision requirements in the senior hotels or housing facilities are typically the same as in the home setting although they may vary by state. When a group program is provided solely by the PTA, requirements regarding supervisory responsibilities may require more frequent reassessment and onsite visits by the PT, or the presence of another individual, such as an aide or nurse, in the event of an emergency. It is important that the PTA review his or her state's practice acts as supervisory regulations for group programs may be different from state to state. Often there are other individuals at a senior housing facility or senior hotel that are adequate to meet these state regulations. Nonetheless, for the most part, supervisory requirements will be identical to the home care setting as previously described.

Elder Foster Care

The same concept of *foster care* in the care of children applies to foster care settings with the elderly. Elders are *adopted* into family environments. As with fostering children, each foster home must meet state regulatory standards in order to be considered for fostering an older individual. State stipends for caring for an older individual are often an incentive to become a foster caregiver and, as in children, need to be monitored for potential abuse.

Assisted Living, Life Care, and Continuing Care Communities

Housing settings that generally have all levels of living, from independent apartments or housing units to assisted living for those who need minimal to moderate assistance with ADL, are found in assisted living, life care, and continuing care communities. In many comprehensive care communities, skilled nursing home facilities are also available. Comprehensive services, such as house cleaning, laundry, restaurants or dining amenities, transportation services, grocery and/or drug and specialty stores, fitness, and other recreational settings are often provided onsite. Additionally, social and medical care is typically available onsite 24 hours a day, 7 days a week. Physical and occupational therapy services are often a part of the services offered for individuals residing in these communities. In fact, the fitness and rehabilitation amenities are frequently hubs of facility activity throughout the day. Onsite physical therapy services are frequently integral to the benefits available in these community-based settings, though some assisted living environments will be served by visiting nurses or consulting rehabilitation services from contracting agencies.

Depending on the size of the facility and average number of residents who receive therapy services, rehabilitation services are often provided by a stationary team of physical, occupational, and speech therapists. With this therapeutic situation, the PT and PTA are located within the same building and supervision requirements are not usually an issue. However, it is not uncommon for PTAs to travel between 2 or more residences on any given day, providing physical therapy services to a few older individuals at each site. In the latter circumstance, supervisory requirements are consistent with those in a skilled nursing facility where care is provided in more than one building. Again, effective communication, both verbal and written, is vital to a successful and coordinated PT/PTA partnership and optimal patient care.

Hospital-at-Home: An Emerging Model of Care

Providing acute hospital-level care in an elderly patient's home is a developing trend and appears to be a feasible, safe, and efficacious option for some patients. It reduces costs and decreases hospital-acquired diseases and complications.[12] The need for hospital-at-home care arises because, for older people, the acute hospital is not always the ideal care environment. They are exposed to germs to which they would otherwise not be exposed, and it is easy for them to develop acute confusion. The consequences can be devastating and result in the need for nursing home placement, hospice care, or death. Patients treated at home may receive oxygen therapy, intravenous antibiotics, or nebulizers/misters and bronchodilators. Patients in the hospital-at-home are less likely to develop delirium or receive sedative medication, dramatically improving functional abilities. In a study completed at John Hopkins, older adults treated at home experienced fewer critical complications and fewer deaths. Length of stay was significantly shorter in the hospital-at-home group and costs significantly reduced. During the 8 weeks after admission, there were no differences in the number of emergency department visits, inpatient hospital readmissions, admissions to skilled nursing facilities, or home health visits.[5]

Acute Care Settings

In the inpatient setting, elderly individuals are acutely ill or often admitted as the result of a fall or other accident. Acute care stays may involve surgery or stays in intensive care units, greatly impacting function quickly. Acute care stays are frequently short stays as the result of diagnostic related groups (DRGs), which limit the time Medicare will cover services in the acute care setting based on diagnosis. Due to DRG constraints, physical therapy primarily focuses on evaluation and projecting discharge needs and discharge planning. Intervention will only be possible for a very brief period of time (eg, 2 to 3 days) before the patient is transferred to another less costly setting.

Role changes for PTs in patient care delivery in the acute care facility include shifting toward increased utilization of PTAs to maximize time and efficiency of time-limited intervention. Once evaluation has been completed, the PTA is frequently responsible for prescribed care of elderly patients, focusing immediately on discharge goals established by and for the elderly individual. This shift provides more effective utilization of support staff and family members in assisting with patient care and accomplishing favorable discharge outcomes.[13]

Patients' functional activity and mobility are essential to recovery and minimization of the risks associated with immobility in hospitalized elders. In practice, however, there is a tendency to not fully consider the rehabilitation perspective of an older adult until the time of discharge. An interdisciplinary approach upon admission. including nursing and physical and occupational therapy, would assist in preventing functional decline during an acute illness. Early intervention and an increased awareness of the need to increase patient activity would reduce the incidence of immobility-associated complications.[14]

Physical therapy services provided by the PTA in a hospital setting are those services that can be safely and competently performed under the general supervision of a PT. Medicare does not specify regulations for supervision in inpatient hospitals or delineate the required direction of the PT with relation to the PTA's role. Most acute care facilities defer to state practice acts, so it is important that the physical therapy department establish the level of supervision necessary and provide this in the policy and procedure manual for the department.

Subacute Care Settings

Subacute rehabilitation units are either a part of the acute care hospital or a part of a skilled nursing facility.[15] It is intended to be a relatively short (2 to 4 weeks), intensive rehabilitation admission as a transition to home care. Care is limited for needed services with limits on days of admission as well as a cap on reimbursement for rehabilitation and other needed services.[16]

Certified rehabilitation agencies that provide subacute care must follow Medicare guidelines in addition to the state law governing the aspects of patient management that may include the PTA. For example, the PT must perform the initial examination and evaluationl; establish the plan of care and goals; and conduct periodic reassessment of functional status, progress of care, and goals. Depending on state practice acts and the policy of the facility, the PTA can practice with general supervision in most subacute services. The PTA may also supervise services provided by other support practitioners (eg, teaching a certified nursing attendant how to manage safe transfers or move the patient in bed).

Many postacute care providers are concerned about the effects of the prospective payment system in subacute facilities. One of the best ways to enhance and develop physical therapy services within the financial constraints is to increase the appropriate utilization of the PTA.[17] Although believed by some to be underutilized, the PTA may play a pivotal role in the delivery of cost-effective rehabilitation services in subacute settings.[18] It is common for a PTA to work with the patient once the PT determines the plan of care and establishes goals until a re-evaluation is needed or the goals/plan of care need revision. This requires clear lines of communication between the PT and PTA and meticulous documentation.

Subacute settings are effective for improving older patient outcomes and reducing undesirable health care use after an acute illness by more intensively addressing rehabilitation issues as quickly after the acute event as possible. The likelihood of admission to nursing home settings is reduced by the utilization of subacute rehabilitation.[18]

Skilled Nursing Facilities

Skilled nursing facilities (SNFs) are specific units within nursing homes or specially designated wings of acute or subacute facilities that have certified Medicare beds and provide rehabilitation services and long-term care. For many elderly, these settings are their last home and entered only as a last resort. The older adults admitted to SNFs are usually older, frailer, and more medically complex. Provision of physical therapy interventions for this population is a challenge due to the medical complexity, presence of comorbidities, and substantially higher levels of disability in the SNF patient, requiring a highly competent PTA.

Higher therapy intensity has been associated with better outcomes as they relate to length of stay and functional improvement for patients who have stroke, orthopedic conditions, cardiovascular and pulmonary conditions and are receiving rehabilitation in the SNF setting.[19] PTAs will frequently be involved in orthopedic, cardiac rehabilitation, respiratory, and neuromuscular interventions—all in the same patient. Geriatrics will challenge all of a PTA's learned physical therapy skills.

Dependent on state laws, skilled physical therapy services provided by the PTA are made available with general supervision (in most states) of the PT. As in the acute and subacute environment, the initial evaluation and subsequent reassessments, as well as the development of a plan of care and establishment of goals, must be completed by the PT. Any changes in the direction of care must be initiated by the PT, though the PTA will play a crucial role in communicating patient status changes requiring treatment and/or goal modification. For most states, the level of supervision required by Medicare in a SNF is that of general supervision. The supervising PT need not always be physically present or on the premises when the PTA is providing services but should be available via telecommunications as needed.

Outpatient Settings

Outpatient physical therapy services might be provided in an outpatient hospital-based setting, a comprehensive outpatient rehabilitation facility (CORF), a PT-owned private practice, or as an adjunct to services in a physician's office. The outpatient center of care is an area of evaluation for the utilization of PTAs. However, a recent examination of PTA utilization in outpatient clinics indicates that the use of these care extenders tends to decrease the efficiency and lengthen the time of care when frequent communication between the PT and PTA did not occur.[20] When more frequent and ongoing communication with the PT by the PTA occurred, the care extender helped to facilitate more rapid and quicker goal obtainment and more favorable functional outcomes. This clearly demonstrates that more aggressive rehabilitation approaches, more frequent re-evaluations by the PT, and discharge planning upon initiation of treatment, in addition to ongoing communication between the PT and PTA from the outset, must be implemented to improve and expedite favorable outcomes. This will assist in providing effective, efficient therapy and possibly decreasing the likelihood of Medicare-imposing caps on reimbursement for outpatient services.

Many of these settings are not geriatric-specific and result in a lack of comprehensive interdisciplinary care often need by elderly patients. Reimbursement restrictions may limit the number of visits, and education toward self-care is key in the provision of physical therapy services.

In each setting, physical therapy must be furnished by qualified physical therapy professionals.[21] In CORF settings, depending on state law, PTs need not be on the premises when PTAs provide patient care as long as they have direct phone or beeper communication capabilities for consultation and assistance during the hours of operation of the outpatient setting. In the event that an unqualified staff member, such as an aide, is providing interventions, the PT or PTA must be on the premises during the time that the therapy treatment is being done. This is true for any unlicensed support staff. No form of intervention can be initiated unless a licensed PT or PTA is physically on site. Additionally, only nonskilled services, such as readying the treatment space or preparing a hot pack, can be rendered by an unlicensed support staff member. Any direct patient care can only be provided by licensed PTs or PTAs.

In the outpatient hospital-based setting, the same supervision recommendations that apply to the inpatient setting are applicable. Therefore, attention needs to be given to the directives provided in state practice acts. Private practice settings require that physical therapy services can only be provided with direct supervision by the PT. Direct supervision means that the supervising PT must be present at the clinic when service is provided by the PTA. Provision of physical therapy in a physician's office also requires direct supervision under Medicare. A physician cannot legally bill for services provided by a PTA, and billable services are only those billed using the Medicare provider number of the supervising PT. The PT must be onsite in the office suite when an older recipient of care is receiving therapy services by a PTA or when supportive personnel are assisting.[22]

Hospice and Palliative Care

PTAs are often involved in palliative care of the elders at the end of their lives. Care may be in a formal hospice care setting or may occur in the home setting. Terminal care involves comfort measures, such as positioning, gentle range of motion, ambulation for functional distances, assistance with ADL, and management of pain.

Hospice care is the support and care for people in the last phase of an incurable disease so that they may live as fully and comfortably as possible. *Palliative care* is given to improve the quality of life of patients who have a serious or life-threatening disease. The goal of palliative care is to prevent or treat, as early as possible, the side effects caused by interventions and treatment of a disease. The primary function in palliative care, however, is to provide psychological, social, and spiritual support for the problems the patient and their families encounter in relation to the disease, the treatment, and end-of-life issues. As such, hospice care is an organized program for delivering palliative care.

The catalog of services PTs can offer patients at the end of life is extensive, including everything from pain management and relief, positioning to prevent pressure sores and enhance respiratory health, therapeutic exercise, edema management, equipment training, home modifications, and family education.[23] The PT's and PTA's role in hospice care is basically rehabilitation in reverse; they do not intervene to reach functional goals or improve physical status rather, as a patient's abilities diminish through the course of the disease, they assist in maintaining the most function possible and provide relief of pain. In essence, touch and comfort is provided, allowing a patient to retain some dignity and control at the end of his or her life.[24]

Supervision of the PTA or student PTA in hospice settings is dependent on the location of home. If it is in a care facility or at home, the SNF or the Home Care Medicare regulations apply, respectively.

Community-Based Senior Centers

Senior centers are set up by local communities and provide a place for older residents of a town or city to gather for social interaction, meals, scheduled events and trips, and the provision of services as required. The social worker is usually an employee of these centers and may make referral to PTs when functional deficits, risk for falls, or other rehabilitation issues arise. Senior centers are excellent environments for holding community health screening programs, educational programs including health promotion and wellness programs, and establishing group fitness programs. Screening of physical status often results in referral for outpatient physical therapy services.

Supervision requirements for the PTA working in a senior center are consistent with those that are required in the home settings of care for the elderly. Specifically, depending on the state practice act, the PTA may participate at a senior center without the PT on premises in a general supervision state to provide intervention and education and participate in data collection after the PT has completed the examination and evaluation and established a plan of care and goals.

Health Clubs and Fitness Centers

Fitness and health clubs are utilizing physical therapy services in many instances. Especially with the exercising elderly, the availability of physical therapy services is a wonderful adjunct to membership in these clubs. Fitness centers provide another wonderful environment for screening and educational programs. Supervisory levels are those applied in private practice outpatient settings. Once again, the level of supervision is dependent upon state practice acts. Typically, these services are provided on a cash basis so that state law and standards of practice dictate the practice expectations for the PT/PTA partnership consistent with outpatient practice settings.

Industrial Rehabilitation Settings

An increasing number of elders return to work after retirement, therefore, more and more companies that employ older workers are establishing industrial rehabilitation programs. Additionally, many companies provide fitness centers at the worksite. Physical therapy positions, including those for PTAs, are opening in industries across the United States to address the special physical and functional needs of their older workers.

Industrial rehabilitation may involve work hardening or conditioning, as well as ergonomic screening and worksite modification required to prevent undue postural stresses and injury. These involve educating the worker, which is a role the PTA fulfills beautifully.

INTERDISCIPLINARY COLLABORATION: WORKING AS A TEAM

In all geriatric settings of care, the PTA becomes a part of an interdisciplinary team whose primary goal is to maximize patient outcomes, namely, to be able to participate in self-care and move about as comfortably as possible. The many facets of care and needed services of an elderly, medically complex individual could hardly be met by a single professional. Collaboration with other PTs and therapy support staff, occupational therapists, nurses, speech pathologists, social workers, case managers, clerical staff, and numerous other health care and social disciplines is required to address every aspect of care. In addition to the professional members of the team, the patient, family, and others involved in an elder's life are integral members of the patient's team.

Establishing mutual goals, so that each team member is on the same path with a patient-centered focus, is crucial to achieving positive outcomes. Building strong relationships, cooperation, and communication with each team member is also an important adjunct to physical therapy interventions. The PTA is often involved in teaching other health care providers, family members, and the older care recipient skills that are learned and practiced during physical therapy sessions. Follow-through by other caregivers of proper transfer and bed mobility techniques; ambulation incorporating proper gait training needed to achieve independence; reinforcement of balance, strengthening, flexibility, and endurance exercises; and allowing maximum independence in all ADL are important adjuncts to reaching physical therapy objectives. Conversely, the PTA may also serve to support therapeutic contributions of other health care providers. For instance, working collaboratively with a *wound care team* to facilitate wound healing or participating as a member of an interdisciplinary team for screening and establishing risks for falls supports team efforts toward achieving maximal function and medical status, and ultimately, discharge.

Socioeconomic status, cultural and ethnic background, language barriers, educational levels, as well as physical and functional components, are incorporated into holistic patient care when interdisciplinary alliances are instituted. It is important that each team member is sensitive to every component of the elder's life, so that realistic targets of achievement and expected outcomes can be reached. The health care and social service systems are incredibly complex and often difficult to navigate. Focus on discipline-specific care serves only one aspect of an individual's needs. Interdisciplinary collaboration creates a system that assists in meeting the complex needs of an older patient. Effective team approaches involve the following[25]:

- A patient-centered focus
- Case management
- Coordinated intervention and treatment
- Referrals to other health care professionals, social services, and agencies to meet the patient's needs
- Frequent, clear, and effective communication with all team members
- Procedures that enhance sharing of information and resources available to each patient
- Establishing available services for the patient
- Providing access to health care, social, and community services
- Establishing mechanisms for linking patient with other service providers
- Continual outcome-oriented evaluations.[25]

Communication, both verbal and written, is fundamental to the building of an effective interdisciplinary team. Clear and concise written communication should include all team members. Each discipline should provide its perspective and treatment concerns to the rest of the team. Listen open-mindedly to each colleague's input. If the message is not understandable or seems inconsistent with team goals, ask questions for clarification.

PTAs should always put themselves in the other disciplines' shoes. Each health care provider has perspectives unique to his or her educational, personal, and clinical experiences. Each discipline views a given circumstance or situation from its own set of lenses. Effective teamwork hinges on perspective and actions toward others. Developing skills to work as a team member requires that the PTA eliminate potential pre-existing stereotypes, biases, or ideas about other professional groups, patients, gender, ethnic group, or age. Acknowledging biases is a first step in doing away with them so that they do not impede the ability to listen openly to other professional viewpoints. The complexity of the current social service and health care system and the diversity of the patient population requires coordinated, interdisciplinary collaboration to ensure the access to and provision of comprehensive services to our older patients.

CONCLUSION

The impact of restructuring health care services in rehabilitation on a day-to-day basis needs to be examined. The changing scope of practice affects the locations where physical therapy takes place. Limited resources often impact who is providing services. Therapists' perspectives need to shift toward the utilization of PTAs in the provision of geriatric services. It is also important to encourage the resetting of our lenses both academically and clinically to prepare for the future increasing role of the PTA in geriatric settings. Refocusing on maintaining the highest potential functional levels, in addition to playing a role in the prevention of disability, alters the way a PT has practiced for decades. There is an absence of the *rehabilitation* perspective in geriatrics at many levels of care, including acute care and outpatient facilities, and sadly, even in geriatric-specific facilities of care, like SNFs or assistive living environments. Physical therapy practitioners need to improve the breadth of geriatric-focused education and care; they need to ensure that physical therapy services in geriatric settings be provided only by licensed PTs and PTAs. We need to shift toward an interdisciplinary management paradigm that ensures effective and efficient use of limited health care resources in rehabilitation as the nation ages.

The PT of 2020, with an increased responsibility and an expanded role in the health care community, will need a highly qualified individual to assist in providing physical therapy services. The preferred provider relationship that now exists between the PT and PTA must not only continue, but expand. As evidence-based practice becomes the standard and the knowledge base in health care continues to grow, the educational requirements will need to keep pace. A highly qualified assistant will allow an efficient and effective utilization of PT services in geriatric settings.

REFERENCES

1. Robinson AJ, DePalma MT, McCall M. Physical therapist assistants' perceptions of the documented roles of the physical therapist assistant. *Phys Ther.* 1995;75:1054-1064.
2. Robinson AJ, McCall M, DePalma MT, et al. Physical therapists' perceptions of the roles of the physical therapist assistant. *Phys Ther.* 1994;74:571-582.
3. Bottomley JM, ed. *Quick Reference Dictionary for Physical Therapy.* 2nd ed. Thorofare, NJ: SLACK Incorporated; 2003.
4. Bureau of Labor Statistics. http://www.bls.gov. Accessed March 15, 2008.
5. Rivard A, Hollis V, Darrah J, Madill H, Warren S. Therapists' perspective on the management and delivery of occupational therapy and physical therapy services. *Health Manage Forum.* 2005;18:9-13.
6. Richards S, Cristian A. The role of the physical therapist in the care of the older adult. *Clin Geriatr Med.* 2006;22:269-279.
7. Cress C. *Handbook of Geriatric Management.* Gaithersburg, MD: Aspen; 2001.
8. Ward D. Drahota A, Gal D, Severs M, Dean TP. Care home versus hospital and own home environments for rehabilitation of older people. *Cochrane Database Syst Rev.* 2008;4:CD003164. http://www.medscape.com/medline/abstract/1884364. Accessed April 4, 2010.
9. Hollis V, May L. Managerial and professional collaboration in the provision of home care rehabilitation. *Health Manage Forum.* 2005;18:13-15.
10. Roach JP, Cook LM. Physical therapist assistant in a California home health agency. *Phys Ther.* 1981;61:1281-1283.
11. Lynch JS. The cycle of relocation: one family's experience with elder care. *Topics Adv Practice Nursing.* 2006;6:1-8.
12. Leff B. Hospital-at-home care for elderly deemed safe and effective. *Ann Intern Med.* 2005;143:798-808,840-841.
13. Lopopolo RB. The effect of hospital restructuring on the role of physical therapists in acute care. *Phys Ther.* 1997;77:918-932.
14. Markey DW, Brown RJ. An interdisciplinary approach to addressing patient activity and mobility in the medical-surgical patient. *J Nurs Care Qual.* 2002;16:1-12.
15. Gulick G, Jett K. Applying evidence-based findings to practice: caring for older adults in subacute care. *Geriatr Nurs.* 2006;27:280-281.
16. Bode RK, Heinemann AW, Semik P, Mallinson T. Relative importance of rehabilitation therapy characteristics on functional outcomes for persons with stroke. *Stroke.* 2004;35:2537-2542.
17. Stahl DA. Subacute care: creating alternatives. Reengineering: the key to survival and growth under PPS. *Nurs Manage.* 1998;29:14-17.
18. Kauh B, Polak T, Hazelett S, Hua K, Allen K. A pilot study: post-acute geriatric rehabilitation versus usual care in skilled nursing facilities. *J Am Med Dir Assoc.* 2005;6:321-326.
19. Jette DU, Warren RL, Wirtalla C. The relation between therapy intensity and outcomes of rehabilitation in skilled nursing facilities. *Arch Phys Med Rehabil.* 2005;86:373-379.
20. Resnik L, Feng Z, Hart DL. State regulation and the delivery of physical therapy services. *Health Serv Res.* 2006;41:1296-1316.
21. Druss BG, Marcus SC, Olfson M, Tanielian T, Pincus HA. Trends in care by nonphysician clinicians in the United States. *N Engl J Med.* 2003;348:130-137.
22. Culver L. Understanding APTA positions on the use of personnel. *PT: Magazine of Physical Therapy.* 2000;8:28-33.
23. Woods EN. Quality of life: physical therapy in hospice. *PT-Magazine of Physical Therapy.* 1998;6:38-45.
24. Mueller K. *Seasons of Loss: A Guided Experiential Process for Understanding the Transitions of Illness and End of Life.* Thorofare NJ: SLACK Incorporated; 2006. http://www.slackbooks.com/view.asp?slackCode=47670. Accessed April 4, 2010.
25. Curtis KA, Newman PD. *The PTA Handbook: Keys to Success in School and Career for the Physical Therapist Assistant.* Thorofare, NJ: SLACK Incorporated; 2005.

9

Treatment Rationale and Design in Geriatrics

As the professional title implies, much of physical therapy management, examination, evaluation, assessment, and intervention focuses on the physical nature of a condition; the mainstay of treatment approaches consists of appraising an older person's abilities and difficulties in performing functional tasks, such as transfers on and off a chair or bed, and general mobility. Physical therapy evaluation and subsequent treatment design is established by identifying underlying impairments. For example, decreased strength, limited flexibility and balance problems, or psychological barriers such as a fear of falling, depression, as well as potential social issues such as limited community resources or lack of family support, may be identified as impairments that will be addressed in the treatment program. A comprehensive review of an older person's entire life circumstance is a necessary element in designing and providing quality physical therapy interventions and obtaining favorable treatment outcomes

This chapter addresses the rationale for designing interventions based on inclusive, interdisciplinary evaluations; outcome measures; and interdisciplinary care planning in geriatric settings (specific treatment approaches will be discussed in greater detail in Chapter 10). In this chapter, the rationale for treatment design, care plan, and intervention goals based on the outcome measures obtained through assessment tools, with consideration of the medical complexity of an elderly patient, will be explored.

Fundamental Principles of Treatment Prescription in the Elderly

A PTA working with older people will use every skill acquired during his or her academic experiences. A PTA who works in a geriatric setting becomes a "Jack-of-all-trades." It is widely recognized that working with older people is a highly respected clinical area that requires advanced skills and knowledge in all aspects of physical, functional, psychological, and social models of rehabilitation to ensure a holistic, comprehensive, patient-centered approach.[1] Competency is needed in every area of physical therapy, including orthopedics, neurology, cardiopulmonary, integumentary care, as well as the age-related changes that affect function. As previous chapters (Chapters 1 through 8) in this text have explored, the PTA will often be providing therapeutic care for a frail, medically complex older adult with age-related changes associated with inactivity, poor nutrition and hydration, multisystem involvement due to chronic conditions, multipharmacy, psychosocial influences, and environmental barriers.[2] Yet, the goal will always be to maximize functional capabilities and strive for the highest level of independence.

The fundamental principles on which geriatric physical therapy is based (philosophy discussed in Chapter 1) are as follows:

Bottomley J. *Geriatric Rehabilitation: A Textbook for the Physical Therapist Assistant* (pp 243-266).

- Disability is generally due to a pathological process or injury and not *prima facie* (old age)

- The effects of aging reduce the efficiency of body systems, although optimum function is obtainable through careful treatment design and comprehensive care plans by an interdisciplinary team

- Physical therapy plays a key role in enabling an older person's ability to regain favorable function and guiding him or her toward enhanced mobility and independence

- When neither improvement nor maintenance of functional mobility is a reasonable goal, physical therapy can contribute to helping older people remain comfortable and pain free

- Prevention of disability in late life can be accomplished through health promotion.

Core standards for treatment rationale and design in geriatric care need to be understood by the PTA.[3] The tenets of geriatric care include consideration of the older patient's autonomy, thorough examination and assessment, realistic goal setting, comprehensive interventions, team-based treatment approaches working in concert with other disciplines and caregivers, providing education for the patient and any person involved in care, and ensuring quality of services through ongoing review and case management.

Any human, regardless of age, desires to regain or maintain personal *autonomy*. It is crucial in geriatric rehabilitation that we aim for increasing the older adult's personal responsibility for recovery and recognize when a patient is not satisfied with the quality of his or her life and chooses not to participate in physical therapy initiatives. Accurate *examination, assessment,* and *documentation* of each individual's physical status, taking into account psychosocial and environmental needs, are inherent in treatment planning and development. Older patients tend to progress slower with rehabilitation efforts than younger individuals, making periodic and continued *reassessment* and *review* an absolute must in establishing treatment strategies. *Goal setting* is based on the older individual's aspirations; incorporates caregivers' objectives; establishes sensible timeframes; and includes frequent review, discussion, and modification. *Treatment prescription* is in response to the strengths and needs of older people and any caregivers. Physical therapy *interventions* consist of a blend of providing advice, teaching, and physical therapy treatment. All involve evaluating and providing skilled services in order to enable patients to recover or maintain the highest level of function and independence. The PT is responsible for managing the care of the person, including the examination, evaluation, goal setting, treatment prescription (ie, plan

of care), and reassessments in order to demonstrate functional changes and make necessary adjustments in the goals and treatment prescription. The PTA is the ideal partner to carry out the plan of care toward goal accomplishment. Specifically, the PTA will provide physical therapy treatment and education to the patient, caregivers, and family, as well as collect ongoing data and measurements in order to ascertain progress toward goals and the need for the PT to reassess.

INTERDISCIPLINARY PERSPECTIVES

Working closely with other team members and sharing skills and discipline-specific knowledge with all of those concerned with the patient's management and support is essential for intervention to be effective, efficient, and patient centered. The team approach should be applied in all geriatric rehabilitation settings, although the model of care may vary from *multidisciplinary* to *interdisciplinary* based on availability of team members and practice setting. The current management model considered ideal is the provision of seamless service for elderly patients. To this end, services need to be provided across the boundaries of *primary* care (clinics and health care community settings), *secondary* care (acute care hospitals), and *tertiary* care (rehabilitation, subacute, home, and community settings; see Chapter 8). The necessary services being provided by a mixture of health care professionals and social service workers, counseling and legal services, private and community agencies, as well as the elderly individual and his or her caregivers, are often required to provide the most holistic type of care to facilitate the highest level of independence and autonomy.[4] In order to provide the most comprehensive services required to meet all of the elder's needs, a host of various health care workers may be required. A PT is frequently a vital member of these health care interdisciplinary teams.

The interface of many disciplines is crucial to reducing the burdens on the caregivers. In addition, it is important to appreciate the vital responsibility of supervising or assisting caregivers to help their loved one with ADL, as well as instrumental activities that will enhance his or her quality of life. The key role of caregivers as members, if not leaders, of the interdisciplinary team should be acknowledged. It follows that caregivers should be consulted about and, if appropriate, involved in all aspects of physical therapy intervention. The PTA is often the provider of this interface. Realistic, supportive physical therapy education strategies give older people and their caregivers the opportunity to help themselves achieve optimal levels of health despite medical, physical, and functional disabilities.[5]

RATIONALE FOR TREATMENT CHOICE, PROGRESSION, AND OUTCOME MEASURES

The PT will perform an initial evaluation to establish a baseline of range of motion, strength, and functional restrictions. He or she will also evaluate soft tissue tightness, pain levels, and motion dysfunctions. From these initial findings, the PT will design a treatment plan that will give an elder the best possible rehabilitation outcome possible and instruct the PTA in the prescribed care plan and expectations. Ongoing review of intervention with older individuals by interdisciplinary team members is necessary to determine whether treatment is effective and efficient. Modifications in treatment approach will follow accordingly. Universally, the evaluation of outcomes of physical therapy interventions has become a priority in the progression of treatment and as a means of monitoring clinical quality and competency of PT practice in any given setting.

An *outcome measure* is a measure of change. Outcome measures are important in gaining an overview of the effect of the therapist's therapeutic input. For example, the PTA is interested in how much the patient's function has changed and whether he or she is progressing toward the goals established for discharge. Third-party payers are concerned about outcome measures, the cost of delivery of care, and if therapy is helpful and not wasteful. Of course, the patient will also be interested in the progress he or she is making toward the discharge home and obtaining independence in function in everyday life. Therefore, what is measured depends on each respective discipline or perspective used to define the outcome of interest—or who wants the information and for what purpose.[6]

Care should be taken to avoid the bad habit of using *generic* measuring tools as an assessment form for all elderly individuals. It is best to use diagnostic-specific outcome measures and tools specific to functional, emotional, and psychosocial assessment.[7,8] Although this chapter is not intended to provide every possible geriatric assessment tool used in rehabilitation, the tools discussed should give the PTA a sense of what the significance of the score indicates from a therapeutic standpoint.

ASSESSMENT TOOLS COMMONLY USED IN GERIATRICS

The assessment tools used with older individuals may vary according to discipline, purpose of the evaluation, and desired outcomes. Assessment of older people varies from that of younger people in that it must take into account the differences in the individual as a result of aging (see Chapter 3). Appropriate care must be taken with some assessment techniques and more time allowed for collecting evaluation information. It is also important that tools specific to a diagnosis be utilized to give the most accurate assessment/evaluation of disease-specific status. For instance, a Bobath, Brunnstrom, or Carr and Shepherd evaluation would provide much more cerebrovascular accident-specific information than a generic assessment tool. The Parkinson's Disability Rating Scale would establish the phase of Parkinson's disease and from that direct the treatment approaches selected. Table 9-1 provides a listing of various physical therapy tests and measures used most often in geriatric rehabilitation. There are many methods used to quantifiably document patient physical and functional status and abilities, cognitive and mental status, depression, pain, and the like. Some tools are global measures that look at functional status or specific outcome measures. These are typically interdisciplinary tools. Certain tools are age specific and others are disease specific. Many tools look at one element of function, such as balance, gait, or cardiovascular status. Other tools might measure emotional status of the patient or caregiver, quality of life, or environmental safety. It is important that the PTA is aware of the assessment and evaluative tools, measures, and devices used for substantiating information, as well as the significance of the scores in establishing treatment protocol. Although this text does not include the actual evaluation forms and specific measurement tools, each tool is described and scoring indicated where appropriate. The reference list at the end of this chapter provides research and resources for obtaining additional information on tools listed in Table 9-1 (see specifically references 9 through 82 as cited in the table).

In additional to physical and functional status, drug history is of importance. Older patients can often be put on medication and left on them without review until the drugs reach toxic levels, or the patients misuse the drug or self-prescribe the dosage schedule to save money. The elderly individual may not report a medical condition that would otherwise alert the therapist as to the type of drugs he or she might be taking; as a result, it is always important to ask. The PTA may

Table 9-1

ASSESSMENTS, TESTS, AND MEASURES IN GERIATRIC REHABILITATION

FEAR OF FALLING SCALES

Activities-Specific Balance Confidence Scale (ABC)[9]

- Self-administered or administered via personal or telephone interview
- The patient is asked to indicate his or her level of confidence in doing the activity without losing balance or becoming unsteady
- Percentage points on the scale form 0% to 100%—an 11-point scale
- Total the ratings (possible range = 0 to 1600) and divide by 16 to get each subject's ABC score

Modified Falls Efficacy Scale[10]

- Completed by clinician or patient
- Very quick—5 minutes (great for screening)
- Scoring on a 10-point visual analog
  - o 0 = Not confident/not sure at all
  - o 5 = Fairly confident/fairly sure
  - o 10 = Completely confident/completely sure
  - o Higher scores reflect less fear of falling (more confidence)
  - o Lower scores reflect more fear of falling (less confidence)

BALANCE ASSESSMENT

Berg Balance Scale[11]

- A scale that measures balance and mobility during 14 functional activities
- Useful in a frailer population
- 5-point scale
- Scoring: A 5-point ordinal scale, ranging from 0 to 4, where 0 indicates the lowest level of function and 4 indicates the highest level of function
- Graded according to ability to do independently without assistance (4), requires supervision to minimal assistance (3), requires moderate assistance (2), requires maximal assistance (1), unable to do (0) on the 5-point scale. Total possible score = 56
- *Interpretation*: 41 to 56 = low fall risk, 21 to 40 = medium fall risk, 0 to 20 = high fall risk

Functional Reach Test[12]

- With a ruler taped to a wall or free-standing tripod, the elder stands/sits at the end of the ruler and reaches as far as he or she can before having to take a step or otherwise catch him- or herself
- The distance obtained on the ruler that is reached is recorded and called functional reach
- Limits of stability during reach in standing and sitting
- Cone of stability shrinks with age
- Forward, sideways, diagonal, and backward stability measured

The Get-Up and Go Test (TUG)[13,14]

- Measures balance, gait, and overall mobility
- The elder is asked to stand up from a chair, stand still, then walk toward a wall and before reaching the wall, turn without touching it and return to the chair

(Continued)

Table 9-1 continued

ASSESSMENTS, TESTS, AND MEASURES IN GERIATRIC REHABILITATION

- Observations are made of steadiness, difficulty in getting into or out of the chair, gait, ability to turn, and strategies for accommodating for balance loss
- Patients are timed (in seconds) when performing the TUG—3 conditions
  1. *TUG alone*: From sitting in a chair, stand up, walk 3 meters, turn around, walk back, and sit down
  2. *TUG cognitive*: Complete the task while counting backward from a number between 20 and 100
  3. *TUG manual*: Complete the task while carrying a full cup of water
- The time taken to complete the task is strongly correlated to level of functional mobility (ie, the more time taken, the more dependent in activities of daily living)
- Older adults who take longer than 14 seconds to complete the TUG have a high risk for falls

Sharpened Rhomberg[15]

- Tests static balance with progressively difficult-to-maintain stances
  o First, with the feet together and eyes opened then closed
  o Next, with feet in semi-tandem and eyes opened then closed
  o Finally, with feet in a full tandem position and eyes opened then closed
- Both sides are tested so it is a 6-part test
- Significant postural sway, a loss of balance, or the inability to stand with the eyes closed is indicative of a cerebellar injury when the feet are together, as well as somatosensory deficits with semi-tandem and tandem stance patterns
- Graded as to amount of sway while standing in a target and corrective maneuvers employed

Sternal Nudge[16]

- The older adult is pushed gently in all directions while standing and balance strategies are observed
- Tests the *cone of stability*

Tinetti Assessment Tool[17,18]

- This tool combines assessment of balance and gait
- A 3-point ordinal scale ranging from 0 to 2
  o 0 = The highest level of impairment and 2 = the level of the individual's independence
- Provides a cumulative score for balance that is rated against a possible 16 total points
  o 16 points indicative of no balance problems
  o Deficits in tested areas are reported as a fraction (eg, 10/16)
- Gait score has a high score of 12 and is reported as a fraction (eg, 8/12)
- A total score for balance and gait uses a fraction of N/28
  o Total balance score = 16
  o Total gait score = 12
  o Total test score = 28
- Interpretation: 25 to 28 = low fall risk, 19 to 24 = medium fall risk, <19 = high fall risk

(Continued)

Table 9-1 continued

ASSESSMENTS, TESTS, AND MEASURES IN GERIATRIC REHABILITATION

GAIT ASSESSMENT

Ambulation Profiles[20]

- Clinical tests of locomotion skill or quantitative methods of assessing ambulatory function that include standing balance, ability to negotiate turns, ability to rise from a chair, and in some profiles, cardiorespiratory or muscular endurance, along with standard gait parameters

Functional Ambulation Profile[21,22]

- A tool that is particularly useful for clients who have suffered from a stroke
- It measures bilateral and unilateral stance time (eyes open and eyes closed), weight transfer from one foot to the other, and ambulation efficiency
- Score is based on time in seconds that is takes the individual to accomplish a task or time he or she maintains balance without loss or protective strategies
  - o Bilateral stance time up to 2 minutes eyes open
  - o Unilateral stance time eyes open
  - o Repeat tests with eyes closed
  - o Record what is needed for *functional ambulation*
  - o Measure off distance—amount of time it takes to ambulate and count number of steps
- Document use of assistive devices
- Cumulative score

Gait Abnormality Rating Scale (GARS)[23,24]

- Developed to detect those at risk for falls and to quantify aspects of gait patterns
  - o Staggering, guardedness, weaving, waddling, staggering
- Easy to use and score
- Numerical value for each item listed
- Scores added to get individual's GARS score
- Score of 18 or more indicates the individual is more likely to fall

MUSCLE STRENGTH MEASURES[25]

Dynamic Muscle Tests[26]

- Isokinetic testing uses a mechanical device that provides electronic outcome information
- Device prevents a moving body segment from exceeding a preset angular speed
- Device is aligned with anatomic axis of the joint being tested and lever arm is attached to the tested limb
- Isokinetic tests measure *torque, work,* and *power*
- Examples: Cybex, Lido, Kinetron

Handheld Dynamometer[27]

- Handheld device uses spring scales or strain gauges to measure applied force in kilograms or pound
- Measures hand grip strength or pinch strength
- Examples of hand dynamometers: Jamar, Nicholas
- Examples of pinch meters: TEC

Manual Muscle Test (MMT)[28]

- Standard positions that attempt to isolate muscle function

(Continued)

Table 9-1 continued

ASSESSMENTS, TESTS, AND MEASURES IN GERIATRIC REHABILITATION

- Resistance to motion is applied throughout the range or at a specific point in the range (break test)
- Muscle is graded numerically or descriptively
- Numerical—descriptive scoring
  - 5/5 = Normal
  - 4/5 = Good
  - 3/5 = Fair
  - 2/5 = Poor
  - 1/5 = Trace

Modified Sphygmomanometer

- Instrumented muscle test used to quantify the resistance used during a manually resisted isometric contraction (ie, a blood pressure cuff)

JOINT RANGE OF MOTION[29]

Attraction or Distraction Methods

- Measuring procedure using a tape measure to record a decrease or increase in distance between 2 points marked on the skin over the spine as it extends or flexes

Goniometer

- A device with an axis aligned with the axis of the joint being measured
- Two long arms aligned with standard landmarks along the moving segments of the extremity

Gravity Protractor

- A fluid-filled disk or a disk-shaped weighted needle indicator
- Measures the plane and range of motion based on the fluid or needle movement

Spinal Inclinometer

- A circular fluid-filled disk with a weighted needle indicator
- Maintained in the vertical
- Placed over the spine and used to measure the degrees of range of motion of spinal movement

CARDIOVASCULAR AND PULMONARY FUNCTION—VITAL SIGN TESTING[30]

Blood Pressure

- Resting and exercise measurements of blood pressure measure the cardiovascular response to changes in position or increasing levels of activity
- 120/80 considered normal blood pressure

Dyspnea Scale

- A scale that has the individual subjectively rate the sensation of difficulty breathing during exercise

Heart Rate

- The easiest way to monitor cardiovascular responses to activity; there is a linear relationship between heart rate, the intensity of aerobic exercise, and oxygen consumption
- Normal considered between 68 and 76 beats per minute

Perceived Exertion[31]

- A rating scale used by the exercising individual that reflects his or her perception of exercise intensity from very, very light to very, very hard

(Continued)

Table 9-1 continued

ASSESSMENTS, TESTS, AND MEASURES IN GERIATRIC REHABILITATION

Pulse Oximeters
• Noninvasive measure of oxyhemoglobin saturation, which is the oxygen saturation of hemoglobin in arterial blood • Resting normal value is generally 95% or more
Pulses

• Palpation of pulses to determine their intensity
  o 0 = No pulse
  o 1+ = Diminished pulse
  o 2+ = Normal
  o 3+ = Bounding and usually visible without palpation

Respiratory Rate

• Counting the number of breaths per minute
  o Resting rate usually 12 to 16 in older adults
  o Can increase in frequency to 36 to 46 breaths per minute during maximal exercise

ENDURANCE TESTING[32]
Balke Test
• A treadmill test in which there is a constant speed with the grade starting at 0% • Increased grade occurs by 3.5% every 2 minutes • Used for individuals with impaired pulmonary or cardiovascular function • All vital signs are monitored for physiologic response to increased work levels
Bicycle Test
• A test using a bicycle ergometer set at a specific workload • Workload is gradually increased based on client response • Vital signs are monitored for response to increasing levels of work
Chair Step Test
• A progressive test with 4 increasing levels of difficulty • Conducted in sitting by placing feet, in a stepping fashion, on increasingly higher levels • Reciprocal arm movements may be added with the stepping in the seated posture • Vital sign are monitored
Functional Activity Test
• The measurement of vital signs during ADL
Graded Exercise Test
• Physical performance of measured, incremental workloads with measurement of physiologic response • Used to assess physiologic response to exercise stress for determination of cardiac and respiratory status
Submaximal Exercise Test
• A test that ends at a predetermined endpoint below the maximal heart rate • Example: A heart rate of 150 beats per minute or the appearance of shortness of breath, cyanosis, claudication, or perceived exertion or exhaustion

(Continued)

Table 9-1 continued

ASSESSMENTS, TESTS, AND MEASURES IN GERIATRIC REHABILITATION

Timed Walk Test
• An indirect means to measure cardiovascular endurance in the clinical setting by noting the distance walked in a fixed period of time such as 1, 3, 6, or 12 minutes • The older individual walks as far and as fast as possible
TESTS OF CIRCULATION
Buerger-Allen Test[33]

• Measures the time it takes for blood to fill the lower extremity vessels when legs go from a horizontal to dependent position, and the time it takes for blood to drain from the legs when they are elevated
• A measure used in rating peripheral vascular involvement
  o Normal circulation draining and filling times range from 10 to 20 seconds
  o Compromised circulation is considered over 20 seconds to 1 minute
  o PVD is over 1 minute draining and filling times

PULMONARY TESTS[34]
Pulmonary Function Tests
• Measures of air flow and air flow resistance, lung volumes, and gas exchange mechanically with instrumentation such as a flow meter
Tidal Volume and Minute Ventilation
• Tidal volume is the volume of air breathed in one inhalation and exhalation • Minute ventilation is the product of the tidal volume times the respiratory rate
PAIN ASSESSMENT[35,36]
McGill Pain Questionnaire

• The most widely used and thoroughly researched assessment tool for pain
• The individual is asked to identify the area of pain on a front/back drawing of the body
• The next part categorizes 102 words that describe different aspects of pain into 20 subclasses
  o The subclasses consist of words that describe:
    • *Sensory* qualities of pain (eg, time, space, pressure, heat, etc)
    • *Affective* qualities of pain (eg, tension, fear, autonomic nervous system properties, etc)
• The next part assesses how the pain changes over time
• The last part rates the *evaluative* qualities of pain (eg, intensity of the pain experience)

Numerical Rating Scale
• A scale that has the individual rate his or her perceived level of pain intensity on a numerical scale from 0 to 10   o An 11-point scale where 0 is no pain and 10 is extreme pain
Oswestry Low Back Pain Disability Questionnaire

• A self-rating scale that illustrates the degree of functional impairment the individual is experiencing
• Consists of 10 questions regarding pain intensity during specific activities
  o Personal care
  o Lifting
  o Walking

(Continued)

Table 9-1 continued

ASSESSMENTS, TESTS, AND MEASURES IN GERIATRIC REHABILITATION

o Sitting
o Standing
o Sleeping
o Sexual activity
o Social life (eg, visiting with others, going to church)
o Leisure activities (eg, golfing, bowling, hiking, canoeing)
o Traveling (eg, driving, riding bus or train, boat or cruise ship, air travel)

Pain Discomfort Scale

- A scale that rates discomfort for 10 statements based on level of agreement from 0 ("This is very untrue for me.") to 4 ("This is very true for me.")

Pain Location, Body Diagrams, and Mapping

- A front/back drawing of the body in which the individual is asked to color or shade areas that correspond to areas of his or her pain

Verbal Pain Rating Scale

- A list of adjectives that describe different levels of pain intensity ranging from no pain to extreme pain
- Similar to numerical rating or visual analogue scales of pain

Visual Analogue Pain Scale

- Another measure used to assess pain intensity; typically consists of a 10 to 15 cm line, with each end anchored by one extreme of perceived pain intensity form "no pain" to "pain as bad as it could be"

NEUROMUSCULAR SYSTEM

Electromyography

- Recording of electrical activity of muscles through the use of needle or surface electrodes[37]

NEUROPHYSIOLOGIC ASSESSMENT[38]

Modified Ashworth Scale for Spasticity[39]

- An objective means to assess the severity of spasticity
- Involves manually moving a limb through the range to stretch specific muscle groups
- The resistance encountered during the passive muscle stretch is graded on a 5-point ordinal scale from 0 to 4, with 0 representing normal tone and 4 depicting severe spasticity

Parkinson's Disability Rating Scale[40]

- Comprehensive physical and functional assessment

Parkinson's Disease Rating Scale[41]

- Combines assessment of signs and symptoms with ADL

Parkinson's: Stage of Disability[42]

- Stage I: Minimal or no functional impairment and unilateral involvement only
- Stage II: Bilateral involvement without any type of balance impairment
- Stage III: Mild to moderate disability; lose righting reflexes; unsteadiness with turns
- Stage IV: Moderate to severe disability; can walk and stand unassisted but not stable
- Stage V: Severe disability; confined to bed or wheelchair

(Continued)

Table 9-1 continued

ASSESSMENTS, TESTS, AND MEASURES IN GERIATRIC REHABILITATION

Pendulum Test for Spasticity/Hypertonicity[43]
• A test for spasticity
• Lower limb is extended to full extension at the knee in a sitting position
Examiner then releases the extremity and allows it to fall free
The leg swings like a pendulum before the motion is damped by the viscoelastic properties of the limb
• *Hypertonicity* is assessed by taking the angular difference between maximum knee flexion and the angle of flexion at which the knee first reversed direction toward extension in the swing

Tendon Reflexes[44]
• Slight stretching of a muscle activates the neuromuscular spindle, which sends an electrical message to the spinal cord via the large muscle spindle afferent exciting the motor neurons and resulting in the contraction of the stretched muscle

MOTOR CONTROL[45]

Ashburn's Physical Assessment for Stroke Patients[46,47]
• Provides an ordinal scale
• Divided into 3 major sections
o Lower limb
o Upper limb
o Balance and movement activities

Bobath Assessment of Hemiplegia[48]
• Postural reactions in response to being moved
• Tests for voluntary movement on request
• Tests for balance and other automatic protective reactions
• Graded subjectively on level of assistance needed, unusual resistance or uncontrolled movement patterns

Brunnstrom Assessment of Stroke[49]
• Motor behaviors in terms of synergies
o Extensor synergy
o Flexor synergy
• Grades according to tone from flaccid to normal

Carr and Shepherd's Motor Assessment Scale[50]
• This scale measures motor function following stroke in 7 tasks
o Supine to side lying onto intact side
o Supine to sitting over side of bed
o Balanced sitting
o Walking
o Upper arm function
o Hand movements
o Advanced hand activities

(Continued)

Table 9-1 continued

ASSESSMENTS, TESTS, AND MEASURES IN GERIATRIC REHABILITATION

- The assumptions are that recovery is characterized by stereotyped movements in synergies and recovery proceeds in a proximal to distal sequence
- Each item is scored on a 7-point scale from 0 to 6
  - 0 = unable; 6 = independent

Fugl-Meyer Assessment[51,52]

- An assessment scale using Brunnstrom's sequence of recovery as a framework in developing an ordinal scale for assessing motor performance in individuals after a stroke
- This tool has 6 components
  - Joint motion
  - Pain
  - Sensation
  - Balance
  - Upper extremity motor function
  - Lower extremity motor function
- Each item is rated on an ordinal 3-point scale for a maximum of 100 points
  - 0 = cannot perform; 1 = partially performs; 2 = performs fully
  - The lower the score, the greater the motor involvement
- Significance of scoring:
  - 50 or less = severe motor impairment
  - 50 to 84 = marked motor impairment
  - 85 to 95 = moderate motor impairment
  - 96 to 99 = slight motor impairment
  - 100 = normal

Montreal Evaluation[53]

- Based on the Bobath approach to hemiplegia and scores objectively
- This tool measures 6 parameters of function
- Each parameter scored on a 4-point scale ranging from 0 for most severe impairment to 3 for normal performance
- The functional parameters measured are mental clarity, muscle tone, reflex activity, voluntary movement, automatic reactions, and pain

Unified Parkinson's Disease Rating Scale[39]

- Assesses mentation, behavior, and mood; ADL; and motor function

SENSORY TESTING[54,55]

Confrontational Visual Testing[56]

- Evaluation for visual field deficits such as homonymous hemianopsia or depth perception
- Individual focuses on a targeted area and a stimulus target is moved in an arc from the periphery
- Individual indicates when the target stimulus comes into view
- For depth perception, the individual identifies which of 2 objects is closer

(Continued)

Table 9-1 continued

ASSESSMENTS, TESTS, AND MEASURES IN GERIATRIC REHABILITATION

Pain[57]
• Assessed by randomly applying the blunt or sharp ends of a pin to the individual's skin for appropriate identification

Proprioception

• Clinical testing for position-sense is done by identifying the position that an extremity is placed in
  o Verbally
  o Physically repeating the position that an extremity has been placed in and then taken out of
  o Reproducing the position of one side on the other side of the body

Semmes-Weinstein Monofilament Test[58]

• Nylon filaments on rods graded by the thickness of the filament determine an objective level of touch-pressure sensation
  o Ability to feel the 4.17 filament indicates normal sensation
  o Ability to feel the 5.07 filament indicates the presence of protective sensation
  o Inability to feel the 6.0 filament indicates a loss of sensation
• Fine gradations of the filaments range between 4.17 and 6.0, so an absolute level of sensation can be determined

Temperature
• Assessed by test tubes of hot and cold water applied randomly to the individual's skin

Vibration Test

• Traditionally, a procedure in which a tuning fork, randomly applied to bony prominences, is graded based on the report of the subject's sensitivity to the vibration of the tuning fork
  o Examiner starts the fork vibration, applies it to the subject, and asks the subject to indicate when the vibration stops
    • If vibration continues to be felt by the examiner's fingertips but the individual reports its sensation, the vibratory sense is recorded as *diminished*
    • If vibration by the subject is not felt, it is graded *absent*
    • If both the examiner and subject report cessation of vibration at the same time (assuming the examiner's vibratory sensation is intact), it is graded as *normal*

LEVELS OF CONSCIOUSNESS[59]

Glasgow Coma Scale (GCS)
• Used to assess level of consciousness following traumatic brain injury • Three aspects of coma are observed independently: eye opening, best motor response, and verbal response • A score of 8 or less indicates coma

Levels of Cognitive Function Scale (LCFS)
• Eight stages of cognitive function and recovery following a traumatic brain injury

MENTAL STATUS/COGNITIVE DISABILITY MEASURES

Allen Cognitive Level[60]
• Test that screens and assesses individual cognitive levels through performance of set tasks • A quick screening assessment of a person's ability to function based on simple to complex activities and rating of 1 to 6, where 1 is the lowest level and 6 the highest

(Continued)

Table 9-1 continued

ASSESSMENTS, TESTS, AND MEASURES IN GERIATRIC REHABILITATION

Dementia Rating Scale
• Measures the differences between demented and normal individuals in the areas of neurological status, behavioral, and cognitive functions
• Includes 36 tasks with 5 subscales for attention, initiation and perseveration, construction, conceptualization, and memory

Mental Status Questionnaire[61]
• Composed of 10 questions and is easy to administer
• Used frequently in research due to its convenience, ease, validity, and reliability
• Lacks sensitivity and may show false positives
o Does not pick up impairment until score is in low range
o Omits domains of reasoning, visual-spatial relationships, and many aspects of language

Mini-Mental State Exam (MMSE)[62]
• A mental status assessment that assesses orientation, the ability to follow verbal and written directions, attention, recall, language, reading, writing, and copying
• Assesses deficits in memory, language, or both
• High correlation with Alzheimer's disease
• Easy to administer and only takes 5 to 10 minutes to complete
• Max score = 30
• Score below 24 indicates impairment
• Correlates to depression—evaluation for depression should occur if the elder gets a score of 19 or below

DEPRESSION

Beck Depression Inventory[63]
• Twenty sets of statements reflecting mood, optimism, motivation, etc
• Scoring from 0 to 3
o Rates from no depression (0) to progressive levels of depression (1 to 3)
• A cutoff score of 13 (summing the entire set of 21) is indicative of depression
• Very popular in geriatric settings

Geriatric Depression Scale[64]
• A 30-item yes-or-no questionnaire
• One point for each response that matches the yes or no answer after the question is tallied
• A score of 8 on this form may indicate depression
• Highly sensitive and picks up ~90% of older adults with clinical depression

Popoff Index of Depression[65]
• A good test for community-dwelling elders as it picks up covert responses
• There is a covert, overt, and healthy response to each of 15 statements
o If an individual selects all overt answers, he or she is considered severely depressed
o If the covert response is chosen most often, the individual is also considered depressed
• Somatize or hide his or her depression with complaints of physical problems
o Healthy responses indicate the absence of depression

(Continued)

Table 9-1 continued

ASSESSMENTS, TESTS, AND MEASURES IN GERIATRIC REHABILITATION

- A very sensitive and reliable tool for assessing depression in older adults
- A score greater than 10 is indicative of depression

Zung Self-Rating Scale[66]

- Composed of 10 negative and 10 positive statements
- Respondent gives an answer that correlates with a 1 to 4 rating
  - o 1 = A little of the time
  - o 2 = Some of the time
  - o 3 = A good part of the time
  - o 4 = Most of the time
- 80 is the highest score and most indicative of severe depression

SELF-PERCEPTION EXAMINATIONS[31]

Additive Activities Profile Test (ADAPT)

- Self-administered test that relates ADL to perceived physical fitness

Borg Perceived Exertion

- A cardiac patient's assessment of his or her own level of exertion on stress tests

SF-36[67]

- Thirty-six questions directed at the assessment of functional capacity versus actual observation of performance
- The questions are in the area of ADL as well as items that reflect depression and quality of life

FUNCTIONAL ASSESSMENT

Barthel Index[68]

- One of the oldest self-care and mobility measures
- Initially developed to measure changes in functional status for an adult undergoing inpatient rehabilitation
- Self-care index includes 9 tasks (includes dressing, eating, grooming, bathing, bowel and bladder functioning) that have a total possible score of 53
- Mobility index is composed of 6 activities (eg, getting in and out of chair, walking 50 yards, propelling wheelchair) with a possible score of 47
- Two groups totaled make up the total Barthel Index with best score at 100 and worst score at 0
- Includes 15 activities rated using a 3-point ordinal scale that are weighted
  - o "Can do by myself," "Can do with help of someone else," or "Can't do at all"
  - o Each activity has a different level of required skills and is scored based on difficulty
- Moderately sensitive screening assessment used mainly in geriatrics

Functional Independence Measure (FIM)[69]

- An assessment used to describe the degree of disability experienced by an older adult
- Evaluates change in functional status over time
- The FIM uses a 7-point scale to evaluate 18 items in areas of self-care, sphincter control, mobility, locomotion, communication, and social cognition
  - o 7 or 6 = Complete to relative independence
  - o Scores 5 and below indicates that assistance is required

(Continued)

Table 9-1 continued

ASSESSMENTS, TESTS, AND MEASURES IN GERIATRIC REHABILITATION

Functional Status Index (FSI)[70]

- A self-report tool in which older adults are asked to rate their performance as well as the degree of pain and difficulty in accomplishing tasks
- Includes 18 items in the area of gross mobility, hand activities, personal care, home chores, and social activities
- Scoring is based on the need for assistance
  - 1 = No help/extremely easy/no pain
  - 2 = Uses equipment/somewhat easy/mild pain
  - 3 = Needs human assistance/neither easy or difficult/moderate pain
  - 4 = Needs human assistance and equipment/somewhat difficult/severe pain
  - 5 = Unable to do/extremely difficult
- Benefit of the FSI is it includes the degree of perceived difficulty, pain, and use of equipment

Katz Index of Activities of Daily Living[71]

- The Katz Index is a short ADL index designed to classify individuals in rehabilitation who have self-care problems
- Helps to predict need for later assistance requirements
- Includes 6 items (bathing, dressing, toileting, transfers, continence, and feeding)
- Each item is scored on a nominal scale of independence or dependence

Minimum Data Set (MDS)[72,73]

- Comprehensive screening tool reflecting quality of life concerns in a skilled nursing facility
- Includes ADL, self-performance, disease diagnosis, and activity pursuits
- Assesses all psychometric variables–depression, cognition, problem solving, and learning
- Requirement for nursing homes using third-party payers (eg, Medicare)
- Resident Assessment Instrument provides baseline of patient status on admission to nursing facility
- Nationwide tool used to periodically measure the functional performance of each nursing home resident
- Identifies problem areas that can be positively influenced with intervention

Outcome Assessment and Information Set (OASIS)[74]

- Comprehensive screening tool reflecting quality of life concerns in the home setting
- Includes ADL, self-performance, disease diagnosis, and activity pursuits
- Assesses all variables of socioeconomic factors and living arrangement, cognition, nutritional status, ability to manage medications, and judgment for safety in home
- Requirement for nursing homes using third-party payers (eg, Medicare)
- Nationwide tool used to periodically measure the functional performance of each home care patient
- Identifies problem areas that can be positively influenced with intervention

ELDERS AND CAREGIVERS ASSESSMENT

Assessment of Living Skills and Resources (ALSAR)[75]

- A multidimensional assessment of the elderly that includes information on balance of functional ability (eg, ability to stay in a community setting versus being institutionalized) and available resources

(Continued)

Table 9-1 continued

ASSESSMENTS, TESTS, AND MEASURES IN GERIATRIC REHABILITATION

Kohlman Evaluation of Living Skills (KELS)[76]
• Standardized test combining interview and task performance in the home
• Used to evaluate an individual's ability to function safely and independently in a community setting
ELDER WORK ASSESSMENT[77,78]
Functional Capacity Evaluations (FCEs)
• Return-to-work functional capacity evaluations that evaluate lower back problems, upper extremity and hand injuries, cervical injuries, and lower extremity injuries
• The physical demand levels are rated as sedentary, light, medium, and heavy work
• Computerized testing is generally used looking at isometric, isoinertional, and isokinetic abilities
Hand Tool Dexterity Test
• A measure of efficiency using regular mechanical tools
• This test measures manipulative skill independence in performing manual tasks
Key Method
• A whole-body assessment that is a standardized, computerized, objective evaluation used for return-to-work decisions
• Twenty-seven functional tests measure weight lifting, pushing and pulling, carrying, work day tolerance, sitting, standing, upper extremity function, walking tolerance, and posture within 4 levels of increasing work intensity
Purdue Pegboard
• Measures dexterity for 2 types of activity, one involving gross movements of the hands, fingers, and arms and the other, primarily fingertip dexterity
Testing, Orientation, and Work Evaluation in Rehabilitation (TOWER)
• First work sampling system, developed in 1936 for individuals with physical disabilities
• It is now used for all types of people, including those with emotional disabilities
• Very helpful in determining older adults' ability to return to work
Work Evaluations Systems Technologies II (WEST II)
• Equipment that simulates work tasks and is used in pre-placement or pre-employment screening, work evaluation, work hardening, and performance on functional capacity evaluation
ENVIRONMENTAL EVALUATION[79-81]
Functional Home Assessment Profile
• A tool developed to allow performance-based environmental risk assessment
• Performance during routine activities is graded and scored for 0 = no risk, 1 = low risk, 2 = moderate to high risk
• The frequency of the activity on a weekly basis is also recorded
Home Assessment Checklist for Fall Hazards[82]
• A tool used to evaluate the safety of an individual's home
Institutional Environmental Evaluation
• A tool used to evaluate the safety of a hospital, nursing home, or other public facility
Multiphasic Environmental Assessment Procedure (MEAP)
• Collection of checklists and questionnaires designed to evaluate the quality of living in a given sheltered care facility
• The assessment focuses on the structural components of the facility, the social atmosphere, programs offered, and the attributes of the resident and staff

be the first to observe and document adverse affects of medications. (Refer to Chapter 7 for a review of the signs and symptoms of adverse effects of commonly used drugs.)

Psychosocial information should also be obtained. Typically, social workers or nurses will gather this information from the elder or his or her family members; however, the PTA may be the sole caregiver in many geriatric settings. The social history becomes vital in the case of an older person. If the person is to be discharged home alone, he or she may need additional services. For instance, he or she may be able to safely ambulate functional distances within the home, however, unable to stand safely to cook a meal or walk long enough to go food shopping.

EVIDENCE-BASED PRACTICE IN PHYSICAL THERAPY TREATMENT

It is important that the PTA work closely with the supervising PT and frequently engage in critical re-evaluation and ongoing assessment regarding the progression of or changes needed in an older patient's plan of care. The concept of *evidence-based practice*[83] is rooted in the need for all health care professionals, regardless of discipline, to assess research and evidence related to the effectiveness or ineffectiveness of treatment interventions being used therapeutically. Decisions made related to patient care need to be made objectively and based on interventions that are supported by investigation. In other words, research needs to be the guide for the prescription of treatment protocol and subsequent evolution of the care plan.

Clinical decision making and problem solving in physical therapy involves the recognition and discovery of the patient's functional and physical problems and the identification of possible solutions.[84] As PTAs are typically delegated to provide physical therapy interventions in geriatric settings, it is important that the PTA continually update his or her own knowledge of studies related to the efficacy and efficiency of commonly prescribed rehabilitation approaches. The PTA is responsible for recognizing and recommending modification of treatment approaches within the PT's established plan of care.

The PTA participates in many clinical problem-solving activities related to the patient's status during treatment and as a part of the interdisciplinary team. The PTA is responsible for the notification of the PT that there is a need to alter or redirect the course of treatment. Frequent reassessment of intervention goals and outcomes achieved is necessary in providing the highest quality of care. All decisions

should be supported by evidence-based studies and validation of acceptable physical therapy practices. Figure 9-1 provides the process through which a PTA may make clinical decisions; problem solve during treatment; and interact with the PT, patient, and other support staff in any geriatric care setting.

ESTABLISHING SHORT-TERM AND LONG-TERM GOALS IN THE ELDERLY

The PTA should be aware of the difference between therapy goals and patient-centered goals. The latter often are achieved through the coordinated efforts and interventions of the interdisciplinary team. For example, a patient's goal may be to walk independently at home with a walker. The physical therapy goal might be to increase lower extremity and trunk strength and posture for safe transfers to standing and to improve balance and endurance. The PT, in concert with every other team member, may work collectively to ensure that the patient walks an optimal amount to increase strength and confidence. The occupational therapist may provide equipment to enable safe transfers and establish goals to ensure that the older individual is able to feed him- or herself in order to provide energy through adequate nutrition for functional activities. The physician might prescribe analgesics to inhibit pain and allow participation in functional activities. The nurses may ensure that the person is able to comply with the medication regime and is well hydrated. The dietitian will seek to guarantee that the older individual is well nourished and understands the importance of a balanced diet and good nutritional status for maintenance of health. The social worker may provide services that aim to ensure that the older adult has the financial and social support services necessary to maintain independence in the home setting following discharge. Each team member contributes an important element to comprehensive care.[85]

Goals should be directed toward the management and improvement of a condition rather than simply caring for the immediate, acute situation without any long-term goals. The therapist needs to identify rehabilitation potential. This is accomplished by establishing which of the patient's presenting features are related to deconditioning, pathology-specific effects on functional skill, or aging. Next, it is important to determine what is reversible, what is a permanent disability, and what is manageable, or something to which the patient can accommodate. Last, goals are directed toward what may be needed to

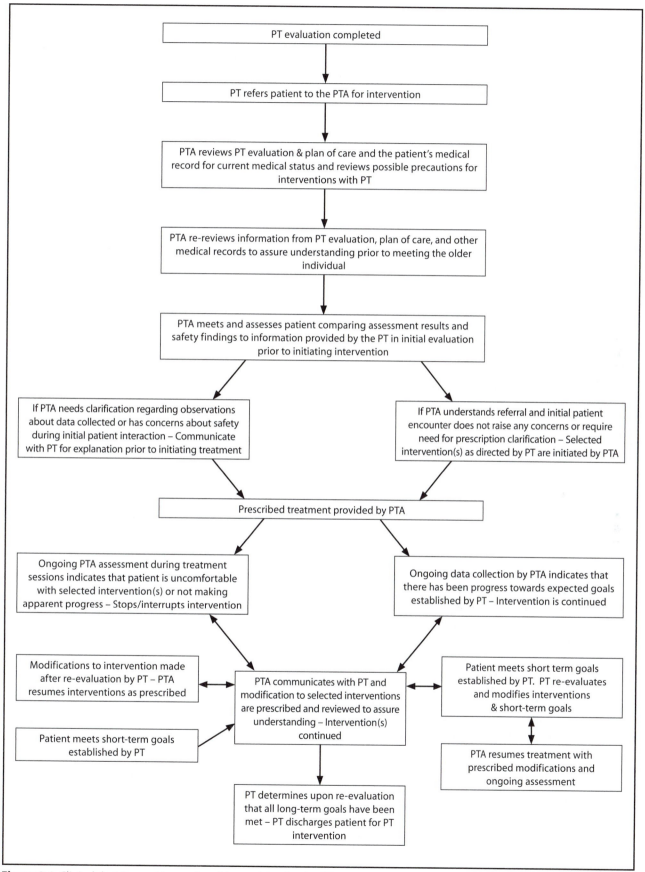

Figure 9-1. Clinical decision making and problem solving for the PTA in geriatric care.

complement and supplement resources at home to obtain optimal safety and maximal functional capacity.[86] To this end, the PTA must have knowledge of what are considered acceptable goals for the older adult. It is also crucial that the *norms* for a specific age group be understood. For example, what is "normal" or expected for an 85 year old related to gait patterns, gait speed, and posture?

The physical therapy personnel should not make decisions without consultation and collaboration with the full team. Decision making needs to include the older person and, when appropriate, the elder's intended caregivers. The older adult's cognitive status and mental condition should be taken into account when decisions are being made related to his or her circumstances.[87] Often, they do not fully understand the ramifications of their physical inabilities. Education and ongoing demonstration and practice of functional skills and motor activities need to be accompanied with frequent teaching to ensure safety and appropriate patient judgment and decision making in different circumstances (see Chapter 11 for further discussion of tools for educating the older adult in role-playing circumstances).

Discharge planning is another important consideration, and goals for discharge need to be established early in the course of physical therapy intervention. A basic idea of what the patient is expecting at the end of the intervention will help the PTA to focus and modify input and instruction constructively. For example, whether the older individual wishes to return to his or her own home, be re-housed, or go into long-term care may influence subsequent goals established for discharge. Each discharge decision and goal establishment will require communication with each of the different team members.[88] Decisions should be based on necessary assessments and evaluations to identify specific skill level and the patient's ability to safely carry out the task in discharge-based environments. For instance, stair climbing assessment may need to determine if the patient is able to climb stairs higher than 7 inches if he or she needs to be able to board a city or town bus where the first stair is frequently over 1 foot high, and each subsequent stair 8 to 9 inches high, and it is his or her only available mode of transport to and from medical appointments or other social events.

Another challenge is to learn specialized communication and motivational skills to engage these older individuals. Many elderly patients are difficult to motivate. They feel the ramifications of aging superimposed on their recent acute illness and often are unable to see the benefits of investing their perceived limited energies on exercises or attempts to increase their functional capabilities. Their perceived future, chronological age, and their mental health will often dictate their willingness to participate in therapy.

When working toward goals with an older adult, the PTA needs to consider the following:

- Does the patient/caregiver understand the meaning of the illness and diagnosis?
- How important is the illness/current diagnosis and its treatment compared to other social, psychological, or physical circumstances?
- What is the elder's style of coping with illness/disability (eg, avoidance, emotional focus, problem solving)?
- What is his or her mood (depression, anxiety)?
- What is his or her cognitive status for participation with rehabilitation efforts?
- Are there hidden energy cost implications in terms of the difficulty of performing exercises?
- How much time will rehabilitation efforts take each day?
- Will treatment cause pain or discomfort?
- Does the patient perceive risks in cooperating with therapy interventions?
- Is progress visible?
- Are there financial implications?

The older person may feel that these considerations outweigh any benefits of exercise. This is very important in the establishment of goals in the care of the elderly patient.

MEDICALLY COMPLEX ELDERS, INTERVENTIONS, AND LEARNING TO PRIORITIZE

It is rare that elderly individuals will present with only one diagnosis. Key areas of difficulty emerge in the care of the older individual. As discussed in previous chapters, the care of the older patient presents a complex puzzle requiring skilled therapeutic problem solving and frequently a great deal of creativity. The elderly patient is characteristically medically complicated and problematic because of pre-existing chronic conditions. For example, the older individual may have been admitted due to an acute illness, such as a severe GI or cardiovascular event, however, he or she may have difficulty functioning due to a previous stroke, have poor endurance as a consequence to an old heart attack, or have significant pain in an osteoarthritic knee from an old injury.

Personal and interpersonal challenges may confound an acute illness. An older person may live alone, making the goal of "discharge home" a tenuous, and possibly unrealistic, aspiration. In addition, the elder may live with a disabled spouse unable to care for him or her in the event that he or she is discharged home. An elderly patient may not have a spouse or family who is willing to accept him or her back into the home setting. Financial burdens, inadequate resources, and insurance limitations may further confound rehabilitation efforts. The greatest challenge occurs when an elderly patient has difficulty in more than one area—physical, psychosocial, cognitive, functional, and environmental. The lack of integration between health care settings is often a problem for providing continuity in care.[89]

CONCLUSION

More comprehensive, interdisciplinary, and accurate evaluation and assessment of older patients could lead to more favorable outcomes for older patients being treated in any geriatric setting. Screening tools, such as the physical and functional assessment tools reviewed in Table 9-1, could potentially identify patients who would benefit from a more comprehensive provision of services. Viewing the patient as a whole through coordinated interdisciplinary care can ultimately influence the quality of life for any older individual.

Because of the day-to-day involvement in care by the PTA, he or she will often be the first professional to identify and recommend a change in intervention course for an older individual. As this chapter has discussed, much of physical therapy assessment and intervention focuses on the physical nature of a condition and the foundation of the treatment approaches are about considering an older person's abilities and difficulties in performing functional tasks, such as transfers on and off a chair or the bed, and general mobility. Physical therapy evaluation and subsequent treatment design are established by identifying underlying impairments, such as weakness, poor endurance, limited mobility and balance difficulties, and environmental or psychological barriers such as a fear of falling or depression, limited community resources, or deficient support for staying at home.

Comprehensive review of an older person's entire life circumstance is a necessary element in designing and providing quality physical therapy interventions and obtaining favorable treatment outcomes. An all-inclusive geriatric assessment is an integral component of care. Interdisciplinary participation provides examination of all factors affecting the course of a

disease or impairment and incorporates the medical complexity experienced by older patients. As reviewed in this chapter, the principal areas of focus of the comprehensive assessment and subsequent rationale for treatment design include the older patient's functional, physical, mental, emotional, pharmacotherapeutic, and socioeconomic status.

In this chapter it was stated that contextual conditions, such as the practice environments and the PTA's training and personal values related to aging, shape the experience of providing care and how difficult the obstacles to be surmounted may seem. Much of the difficulty elders experience could be eliminated by changes in the health care delivery system and in medical education that includes instruction in comprehensive, interdisciplinary intervention and treatment approaches.

We will all be geriatric individuals one day. As we age, we face many physical and emotional challenges that can affect the level of function and well being. As the population ages as a whole, and people live longer, we, as physical therapy professionals, must play a vital and visible role in aiding an older person toward maintaining the highest possible functional independence and address the needs of each older person. PTAs play an integral role in assisting the PT with ongoing assessment, facilitation of the progression and change of the care plan, and communication with other health care professionals. The PTA will often direct and facilitate efforts toward favorable outcomes of treatment and the integration of care for each older individual with whom he or she works. Rehabilitation of geriatric patients is imperative for the patients' well being and has the potential of greatly improving their quality of life.

REFERENCES

1. American Geriatrics Society. *Geriatrics Syllabus for Specialists.* New York, NY: American Geriatrics Society; 2002.
2. Demers L, Desrosiers J, Ska B. Assembling a toolkit to measure geriatric rehabilitation outcomes. *Am J Phys Med Rehabil.* 2005;84:460-472.
3. American Physical Therapy Association. *Normative Model of Physical Therapist Assistant Education. Version '99.* Alexandria, VA: American Physical Therapy Association; 1999.
4. Auger C, Demers L, Desrosiers J, Giroux F, Ska B, Wolfson C. Applicability of a toolkit for geriatric rehabilitation outcomes. *Disabil Rehabil.* 2007;29:97-109.
5. DeLisa JA. *Rehabilitation Medicine: Principles and Practice.* 3rd ed. Philadelphia, PA: Lippincott Williams & Wilkins; 1998.
6. de Rooij SE, Abu-Hanna A, Levi M, de Jonge E. Factors that predict outcome of intensive care treatment in very elderly patients: a review. *Crit Care.* 2005;9:R307-R314.
7. Mukamel DB, Temkin-Greener H, Delavan R, et al. Team performance and risk-adjusted heath outcomes in the Program of All-Inclusive Care for the Elderly (PACE). *Gerontologist.* 2006;46:227-237.

8. Mukamel DB, Peterson DR, Bajorska A, et al. Variations in risk-adjusted outcomes in a managed acute/long-term care programs for frail elderly individuals. *Int J Qual Health Care.* 2004;16:293-301.

9. Powell, LE, Myers AM. The Activities-Specific Balance Confidence (ABC) Scale. *J Gerontol Med Sci.* 1995;50:M28-M34.

10. Chamberlin ME, Fulwider BD, Sanders SL, Medeiros JM. Does fear of falling influence spatial and temporal gait parameters in elderly persons beyond changes associated with normal aging? *J Gerontol A Biol Sci Med Sci.* 2005;60:1163-1167.

11. Berg KO, Maki BE, Williams JI, Holliday PJ, Wood-Dauphinee SL. Clinical and laboratory measures of postural balance in an elderly population. *Arch Phys Med Rehab.* 1992;73:1073-1080.

12. Duncan PW, Studenski SA, Chandlers J, Prescott B. Functional reach: predictive validity in a sample of elderly male veterans. *J Gerontol.* 1992;47:M93-M98.

13. Wall JC, Bell C, Campbell S, Davis J. The Timed Get-Up-and-Go Test revisited: measurement of the component tasks. *J Rehabil Res Dev.* 2000;37:109-113.

14. Hershkovitz A, Brill S. Get up and go—home. *Aging Clin Exp Res.* 2006;18:301-306.

15. Gill-Brody KM, Popat RA, Parker SW, Krebs DE. Rehabilitation of balance in two patients with cerebellar dysfunction. *Phys Ther.* 1997;77:534-552.

16. Horak FB, Henry SM, Shumway-Cook A. Postural perturbations: new insights for treatment of balance disorders. *Phys Ther.* 1997;77:517-533.

17. Bright L. Strategies to improve the patient safety outcome indicator: preventing or reducing falls. *Home Healthc Nurse.* 2005;23:29-36.

18. Cipriany-Dacko LM, Innerst D, Johannsen J, Rude V. Interrater reliability of the Tinetti balance scores in novice and experienced physical therapy clinicians. *Arch Phys Med Rehabil.* 1997;78:1160-1167.

19. Wolfson L, Whipple R, Amerman P. Gait assessment in the elderly: a gait abnormality rating scale and its relation to falls. *J Gerontology.* 1990;45:M14.

20. Criak RL, Oatis CA. *Gait Analysis: Theory and Application.* St. Louis, MO: Mosby-Year Book; 1995.

21. Wolf SL, Catlin PA, Gage K, Gurucharri K, Robertson R, Stephen K. Establishing the reliability and validity of measurements of walking time using the Emory Functional Ambulation Profile. *Phys Ther.* 1999;79:1122-1133.

22. Liaw LJ, Hsieh CL, Lo SK, Lee S, Huang MH, Lin JH. Psychometric properties of the modified Emory Functional Ambulation Profile in stroke patients. *Clin Rehabil.* 2006;20:429-437.

23. VanSwearingen JM, Paschal KA, Bonino P, Chen TW. Assessing recurrent fall risk of community-dwelling, frail older veterans using specific tests of mobility and the physical performance test of function. *J Gerontol A Biol Sci Med Sci.* 1998;53:M457-M464.

24. VanSwearingen JM, Paschal KA, Bonino P, Yang JF. The modified Gait Abnormality Rating Scale for recognizing the risk of recurrent falls in community-dwelling elderly adults. *Phys Ther.* 1996;76:994-1002.

25. Bohannon RW Alternatives for measuring knee extension strength of the elderly at home. *Clin Rehabil.* 1998;12:434-440.

26. Wieser M, Haber P. The effects of systematic resistance training in the elderly. *Int J Sports Med.* 2007;18:59-65.

27. Wang CY, Olson SL, Protas EJ. Test-retest strength reliability: hand-held dynamometry in community-dwelling elderly fallers. *Arch Phys Med Rehabil.* 2002;83:811-815.

28. Bohannon RW. Manual muscle testing: does it meet the standards of an adequate screening test? *Clin Rehabil.* 2005;19:662-667.

29. Norkin CC, White DJ. *Measurement of Joint Motion: A Guide to Goniometry.* 3rd ed. Philadelphia, PA: FA Davis; 2003.

30. Hilz MJ, Dütsch M. Quantitative studies of autonomic function. *Muscle Nerve.* 2006;33:6-20.

31. Nelson ME, Rejeski WJ, Blair SN, et al. Physical activity and public health in older adults: recommendation from the American College of Sports Medicine and the American Heart Association. *Med Sci Sports Exerc.* 2007;39:1435-1445.

32. Freeman R. Assessment of cardiovascular autonomic function. *Clin Neurophysiol.* 2006;117:716-730.

33. Thiele BL, Strandness DE. Disorders of the vascular system: peripheral vascular disease. In: Andress R, Bierman EL, Hazzard WR, eds. *Principles in Geriatric Medicine.* 4th ed. New York, NY: McGraw-Hill; 1998:527-535.

34. Al-Ashkar F, Mehra R, Mazzone PJ. Interpreting pulmonary function tests: recognize the pattern, and the diagnosis will follow. *Cleve Clin J Med.* 2003;70:866,868,871-873.

35. Kaasalainen S, Crook J. A comparison of pain-assessment tools for use with elderly long-term-care residents. *Can J Nurs Res.* 2003;35:58-71.

36. Hølen JC, Hjermstad MJ, Loge JH, et al. Pain assessment tools: is the content appropriate for use in palliative care? *J Pain Symptom Manage.* 2006;32:567-580.

37. Hammond EJ. Electrodiagnosis of the neuromuscular system. In: Van Deusen J, Brunt D, eds. *Assessment in Occupational Therapy and Physical Therapy.* Philadelphia, PA: WB Saunders; 1997:175-197.

38. Ada L, O'Dwyer N, O'Neill E. Relation between spasticity, weakness and contracture of the elbow flexors and upper limb activity after stroke: an observational study. *Disabil Rehab.* 2006;28:891-897.

39. Bohannon RW, Smith MB. Inter-rater reliability of a modified Ashworth scale of muscle spasticity. *Phys Ther.* 1987;67:206-207.

40. Bonnet AM. Rating scales for Parkinson's disease: when and how to use them. *Rev Neurol.* 2000;156(suppl 2):70-75.

41. Goetz CG, Fahn S, Martinez-Martin P, et al. Movement Disorder Society-sponsored revision of the Unified Parkinson's Disease Rating Scale (MDS-UPDRS): process, format, and clinimetric testing plan. *Mov Disord.* 2007;22:41-47.

42. Greffard S, Verny M, Bonnet AM, et al. Motor score of the Unified Parkinson Disease Rating Scale as a good predictor of Lewy body-associated neuronal loss in the substantia nigra. *Arch Neurol.* 2006;63:584-588.

43. Greenberg DA, Aminoff MJ, Simon RP. *Clinical Neurology.* 2nd ed. Norwalk, CT: Appleton & Lange; 1993.

44. Milanov IG. Flexor reflex for assessment of common interneuron activity in spasticity. *Electromyography Clin Neurophys.* 1992;32:621-629.

45. Duncan PW, Badke MB. *Stroke Rehabilitation: The Recovery of Motor Control.* St. Louis, MO: Year Book Medical; 1987.

46. Ashburn A. A physical assessment for stroke patients. *Physiotherapy.* 1982;68:109-113.

47. Ansari NN, Naghdi S, Moammeri H, Jalaie S. Ashworth Scales are unreliable for the assessment of muscle spasticity. *Physiother Theory Pract.* 2006;22:119-125.

48. Corriveau H, Guarna F, Dutil E. An evaluation of the hemiplegic subject based on the Bobath approach. Part II: the evaluation protocol. *Scand J Rehabil Med.* 1998;20:5-11.

49. Chen IC, Cheng PT, Hu AL, et al. Evaluation in hemiplegic stroke patients. *Chang Gung Med J.* 2000;23:339-347.

50. DeSouza LH, Langton Hewer RL, Miller S. Assessment of recovery of arm control in hemiplegic stroke patients: arm function tests. *International Rehabil Med.* 1980;2:3-9.

51. Fugl-Meyer AR. Post-stroke hemiplegia: assessment of physical properties. *Scand J Rehabil Med.* 1980;7(suppl):83-93.

52. Lewis CB, Shaw K. The Fugl-Meyer Assessment after stroke. *Advance for PTs PTAs.* 2007;9:45.

53. Guarna F, Corriveau H, Chamberland J. An evaluation of the hemiplegic subject based on the Bobath approach. Part I: the model. *Scand J Rehabil Med.* 1988;20:1-4.

54. Benton A, Sivan A, des Hamsher K, Varney N, Spreen O. *Contributions of Neuropsychological Assessment.* 4th ed. New York, NY: Oxford University Press; 2004.

55. Van Deusen J, Jackson Foss J. Sensory deficits. In: Van Deusen J, Brunt D, eds. *Assessment in Occupational Therapy and Physical Therapy.* 2nd ed. Philadelphia, PA: WB Saunders; 2007:295-301.

56. Allison LK, Kiemel T, Jeka JJ. Multisensory reweighting of vision and touch is intact in healthy and fall prone older adults. *Exp Brain Res.* 2006;175:342-352.

57. Dellon AL. A numerical grading scale for peripheral nerve function. *J Hand Ther.* 1993;6:152-160.

58. Birke JA, Brandsma JW, Schreuders TA, Piefer A. Sensory testing with monofilaments in Hansen's disease and normal control subjects. *Int J Lepr Other Mycobact Dis.* 2000;68:291-298.

59. Morin A. Levels of consciousness and self-awareness: a comparison and integration of various neurocognitive views. *Conscious Cogn.* 2006;15:358-371.

60. Allen CK, Allen R. Cognitive disabilities: measuring the social consequences of mental disorders. *J Clin Psychiatry.* 1987;48:185-190.

61. Purser JL, Fillenbaum GG, Wallace RB. Memory complaint is not necessary for diagnosis of mild cognitive impairment and does not predict 10-year trajectories of functional disability, word recall, or short portable mental status questionnaire limitations. *J Am Geriatr Soc.* 2006;54:335-338.

62. Folstein MF, Folstein SE, McHugh PR. Mini-Mental State: a practical method for grading the cognitive state of patients for the clinician. *J Psychiatric Res.* 1975;12:189-198.

63. Gallagher D. The Beck depression inventory and older adults review of its development and utility. In: Brink T, ed. *Clinical Gerontology: A Guide to Assessment and Intervention.* New York, NY: Haworth Press; 1986:149-163.

64. Kørner A, Lauritzen L, Abelskov K, et al. The Geriatric Depression Scale and the Cornell Scale for Depression in Dementia. A validity study. *Nord J Psychiatry.* 2006;60:360-364.

65. Popoff S. A simple method for diagnosis of depression in geriatric medical patients. *Clin Med.* 1969;76:24-29.

66. Zung W, Richard D, Shrot M. Self-rating depression scale in an outpatient clinic. *Archives of Geriatric Psychiatry.* 1965;13:508-515.

67. Osborne RH, Hawthorne G, Lew EA, Gray LC. Quality of life assessment in the community-dwelling elderly: validation of the Assessment of Quality of Life (AQoL) Instrument and comparison with the SF-36. *J Clin Epidemiol.* 2003;56:138-147.

68. Muji-Skiki E, Trebinjac S, Avdi D, Dzumhur-Sari A. Measuring outcomes in acute neurorehabilitation in general hospital setting—our experience. *Bosn J Basic Med Sci.* 2006;6:61-67.

69. Sangha H, Lipson D, Foley N, et al. A comparison of the Barthel Index and the Functional Independence Measure as outcome measures in stroke rehabilitation: patterns of disability scale usage in clinical trials. *Int J Rehabil Res.* 2005;28:135-139.

70. Jette AM. Functional status index: reliability of a chronic disease evaluation instrument. *Arch Phys Med Rehab.* 1980;61:395-401.

71. Katz S, Downs TD, Cash HR. Progress in the development of the Index of ADL. *Gerontologist.* 1970;10:20-29.

72. Lum TY, Lin WC, Kane RL. Use of proxy respondents and accuracy of minimum data set assessments of activities of daily living. *J Gerontol A Biol Sci Med Sci.* 2005;60:654-659.

73. Landi F, Tua E, Onder G, et al. Minimum data set for home care: a valid instrument to assess frail older people living in the community. *Med Care.* 2000;38:1184-1190.

74. Kinatukara S, Rosati RJ, Huang L. Assessment of OASIS reliability and validity using several methodological approaches. *Home Health Care Serv Q.* 2005;24:23-38.

75. Williams JH, Drinka TJ, Greenberg JR. Development and testing of the assessment of living skills and resources (ALSAR) in elderly community-dwelling veterans. *Gerontologist.* 1991;31:84-91.

76. Pickens S, Naik AD, Burnett J, Kelly PA, Gleason M, Dyer CB. The utility of the Kohlman evaluation of living skills test is associated with substantiated cases of elder self-neglect. *J Am Acad Nurse Pract.* 2007;19:137-142.

77. Schibye B, Hansen AF, Søgaard K, Christensen H. Aerobic power and muscle strength among young and elderly workers with and without physically demanding work tasks. *Appl Ergon.* 2001;32:425-431.

78. Zamagni S. The elderly and work: the third age as vocation. *Radiol Med.* 2003;106(suppl 1):3-6.

79. Lindqvist K, Timpka T, Schelp L. Evaluation of an inter-organizational prevention program against injuries among the elderly in a WHO Safe Community. *Public Health.* 2001;115:308-316.

80. Nelson A, Powell-Cope G, Gavin-Dreschnack D, et al. Technology to promote safe mobility in the elderly. *Nurs Clin North Am.* 2004;39:649-671.

81. Clemson L, Cumming RG, Kendig H, Swann M, Heard R, Taylor K. The effectiveness of a community-based program for reducing the incidence of falls in the elderly: a randomized trial. *J Am Geriatr Soc.* 2004;52:1487-1494.

82. Tideiksaar R. Fall prevention in the home. *Topics in Geriatric Rehabil.* 1986;3:59.

83. Curtis KA, Newman PD. *The PTA Handbook: Keys to Success in School and Career for the Physical Therapist Assistant.* Thorofare, NJ: SLACK Incorporated; 2005:167-174.

84. Crosier J. A problem-solving algorithm: a tool for decision-making responsibilities for PTAs. *PT Magazine.* 2007;4:50-51.

85. Solomon D, Sue Brown A, Brummel-Smith K, et al. Best paper of the 1980s: National Institutes of Health Consensus Development Conference Statement: geriatric assessment methods for clinical decision-making. 1988. *J Am Geriatr Soc.* 2003;51:1490-1494.

86. Solano Jaurrieta JJ, López Alvarez E, Melón Lozano O, Virgós Soriano MJ. Making clinical decisions and functional situation in geriatrics. Is there a relationship? *Rev Esp Salud Pulica.* 1999;73:407-411.

87. Silverman M, McDowell BJ, Musa D, Rodriguez E, Martin D. To treat or not to treat: issues in decisions not to treat older persons with cognitive impairment, depression, and incontinence. *J Am Geriatr Soc.* 1997;45:1094-1101.

88. Grill E, Hermes R, Swoboda W, Uzarewicz C, Kostanjsek N, Stucki G. ICF Core Set for geriatric patients in early post-acute rehabilitation facilities. *Disabil Rehabil.* 2005;27:411-417.

89. Abrahams R, Macko P, Grais MJ. Across the great divide. Integrating acute, post-acute and long-term care. *J Case Manag.* 1992;1:124-134.

10

Interventions and Treatment in the Elderly

THERAPEUTIC EXERCISE PRESCRIPTION AND PROGRESSION

The treatment procedures established will follow the information gathered from the assessment and evaluation of each older individual. There is never a specific recipe or "cookie-cutter" treatment approach for a diagnostic situation due to the medical complexity often encountered in the elderly. This chapter reviews interventions and treatment guidelines for management of various conditions in the elderly population. It is not intended to be a cookbook but a guide for the effective, evidence-based provision of physical therapy care in the older adult.

Although treatment strategies parallel those in younger patients, appropriate care must be taken with some treatment techniques so that undue stress is not imposed on older, frailer individuals. For instance, less aggressive strengthening therapies may be desirable if an older individual has osteoporosis; it may be important to stress extension rather than flexion exercises in the presence of decreased bone mass and more time should to be allowed for learning and practicing skills and exercises. The treatment procedures may be much more comprehensive and holistic than those often employed with a younger client. For example, with an acute ankle sprain, the history taking would be no different but the treatment prescribed should take into account a more complex medical history,

such as history of falls, cardiovascular problems, presence of vestibular or cognitive problems, and preinjury status, to name just a few considerations. The PTA might still treat an ankle sprain initially with rest, ice, compression, and elevation, but the PTA would need to pay close attention to the elder's skin status related to the use of ice and compression techniques. Limiting the time of "rest" would also be crucial as the older individual will lose functional abilities much faster than a younger, fitter person. The PTA needs to frequently reassess variables (eg, length of the hamstrings) to make sure that the person does not lose flexibility as a result of the imposed rest. Determining *how* the ankle sprain occurred (eg, a result of a save from a fall on a stable surface; walking on rugged terrain; fear of falling; poor eyesight and/or other perceptual motor deficits; dizziness caused by drugs, dehydration, or vestibular complications) helps in establishing the need balance and gait training procedures to add to the typical ankle sprain protocol or determining the need to refer to other disciplines for reassessment of drugs or nutritional or medical status.

Gait Training

In geriatric practice, one of the primary functions of physical therapy in most conditions is to return an older individual to his or her previous ambulatory status. After an illness or surgical intervention for acute or chronic pathologies, especially when

Bottomley J. *Geriatric Rehabilitation: A Textbook for the Physical Therapist Assistant* (pp 267-302).
© 2010 SLACK Incorporated

bed rest and medical status have limited function, physical therapy intervention invariably includes gait training. In fact, gait training is paramount in regaining functional independence. Gait training is one of the most frequently prescribed rehabilitation techniques for older adults because gait is the most common of all human movements affected by many pathologies (as discussed in Chapter 4).

In the elder adult, the previous method of ambulation must be incorporated into gait training. For example, if an older person was using a standard walker prior to the current illness, return to independence walker ambulation would be a reasonable goal. However, if the older individual was ambulating independently without assistive devices, the use of a walker may be a step in the progression toward returning to the previous functional level of activity.

When assessing ambulatory abilities, safety is a primary consideration. The disease or medical condition, prognosis, and comorbidities, as well as overall level of fitness, will interact in determining the functional outcomes of an older adult. Many disease states may alter the efficiency and safety of ambulation. Current medical situations may prohibit recovery of previous functional levels attainable in rehabilitation, and the elderly patient may not be able to return to his or her prior level of independence.

Findings from the gait analysis tools described in Chapter 9 will guide the appropriate treatment design and assist in prioritizing needed interventions. Box 10-1 provides attributes that may lead to gait difficulties in older adults.

Multiple or single impairments could potentially lead to gait deviations in older adults. The effects of aging may lead to changes in gait as described in Table 10-1, which presents parameters that are considered *normal* versus *age-related* changes in gait. Walking speed is defined as the rate of walking measured by distance over a specific time interval. Speed of walking has been shown to impact safety. A slightly faster pace of walking, approximately 1.6 miles per hour, has been deemed to be a safe ambulatory speed. With slower or faster rates, endurance and the stability of gait are challenged, increasing the risk of falling.[1] The speed of walking ultimately can be a factor for predicting functional outcomes in older adults.[2] Intervention is often employed to speed up or slow down gait in order to improve safety and independence. Using auditory signals, such as a metronome or music with a beat, is helpful in keeping a specific pace and gradually increasing that speed. Treadmills are ideal for improving many parameters of gait, including walking speed.

Stride length is the distance of the heel strike of one foot to the heel strike of the same foot. Stride

Box 10-1: **Attributes of Gait Problems in the Elderly**

- Impaired motor control and vision
- Abnormal joint angle or range of motion
- Decreased or increased sensation
- Pain
- Instability or difficulty rising from the seated position
- Tendency to lean backward
- Flexed (forward-leaning trunk) posture
- Sideways lean in either direction
- Decreased rotation of pelvis and trunk
- Absence of heel strike during walking cycle
- Poor foot clearance (shuffling tendency)
- Decreased or absent push-off during walking cycle
- Poor endurance
- Balance problems

length progressively declines with advanced age or inactivity. Speed of walking will affect the stride length. As the stride length increases, the cadence (ie, number of steps per minute) of ambulation will become faster.

Stride length and width are variables that also determine safety and functional outcomes in older adults. Interventions that intentionally seek to control stride length are fundamental to the ability to adapt stride, walking cycle duration, swing and stance phases of gait, and cadence to environmental changes or constraints (eg, the ability to negotiate or avoid an obstacle). The ability to have power over moving forward during the stance phase and control of the movement of the body over the weight-bearing leg and the swinging leg will predict both speed and stride length. With concentration, all of these parameters of gait can be intentionally controlled.[3]

Walking cycle duration decreases with faster cadences and due to slower walking rates in the elderly (slower cadence) tends to be longer in the elderly. The stance phase is when the foot is in contact with the floor. The swing phase is when the foot is swinging forward to take the next step. Duration of both the stance and swing phases of gait relate to the durations of the total walking cycle and are shorter for the more rapid cycles of faster walking. Decreases in stance phase time are more pronounced than decreases in swing phases for faster walking.

Changes in the parameters presented in Table 10-1 will often affect endurance and balance, as will the

Table 10-1

NORMAL VERSUS AGE-RELATED PARAMETERS OF GAIT WITH AGING AND PATHOLOGY

GAIT PARAMETER	NORMAL GAIT	GAIT CHANGES WITH AGING AND PATHOLOGY
Walking speed	140 to 160 cm/sec free walking 195 to 220 cm/sec fast walking	118 to 125 cm/sec free walking 160 to 162 cm/sec fast walking
Stride length	150 to 160 cm free walking	126 to 140 cm free walking
Stride width	8 to 10 cm	Tends to be wider in older adults for balance
Swing-to-stance ratio	40:60	30:70—Progressively more time spent in stance
Walking cycle duration	1 sec free walking	1.25 sec free walking
Cadence	110 steps/min free walking 132 steps/min fast walking	Decreases dependent on pathology; slower cadence with aging and pathology
Foot clearance	1 to 2 cm	Decreases or increases dependent on pathology; creates a shuffling or a high-stepping gait pattern
Heel strike and push-off	Present	Frequently decreased

inability to smoothly get to a standing position from sitting; the tendency to lean forward, backward, or to the side; or changes in perceptual-motor abilities due to poor eye sight, sensory changes, or cognitive changes affecting judgment and safety. As discussed in Chapter 9, it is important that the PTA look at the patient holistically, screening for and incorporating interventions that adequately address deficits that might impact an older adult's safety during ambulation.

Other gait alterations that may be observed and require intervention include the lack of trunk or extremity flexibility, mobility, or strength. Trunk and pelvic rotation, for instance, is characterized by a clockwise and counterclockwise movement at the pelvis to assist in bringing the leg forward during the swing phase. Normal pelvic rotation would be about 10 degrees. As one side of the pelvis moves forward, the opposite arm moves forward, creating trunk rotation and assisting in balancing during gait. A decrease or absence of rotation of the pelvic girdle will result in decreased stride length and a diminished swing phase during gait. The decreased or lack of arm swing will destabilize the individual. The absence of trunk rotation makes it difficult for anyone to accommodate to changing environment demands.

The lack of rotation of the pelvis and trunk, diminished arm swing, and the decreased excursion at any of the lower extremity joints results in slower, less

stable, and energy-consuming ambulation. Additionally, changes in tone or motor control may compound the gait changes normally seen in aging. For example, a person who has had a stroke may have tone changes, perceptual-motor changes, muscle imbalances, and visual deficits (eg, hemianopsia), leading to significant changes in gait speed, stability, and energy cost. A hip fracture results in muscle weakness and imbalances as well as a leg length discrepancy leading to more lateral displacement during the stance phase and less time spent in stance. The classic Parkinsonian gait leads to short, shuffling, gradually accelerating gait patterns with the tendency to lean forward. Table 10-2 provides examples of potential problems encountered in the geriatric patient without pathology and suggested treatment approaches. Specific interventions for diagnoses such as hip fracture, cerebrovascular disease, and Parkinson's will be discussed in greater detail later in this chapter.

Interventions during gait should focus on reducing deviations, improving gait efficiency and safety, and increasing endurance. In summary, gait training involves a combination of mobility activities, standing and weight shifting, transfer activities, pre-gait strengthening, interventions during gait to normalize the gait pattern, instruction in assistive equipment utilization, and, in some cases, modification of the environment to provide safety and independence for

Table 10-2

SUGGESTED TREATMENT STRATEGIES FOR GAIT DEVIATIONS IN THE ELDERLY

GAIT DEVIATION	RECOMMENDED STRATEGY FOR INTERVENTION
Decreased endurance	Progressive ambulation program; gradually increasing distance and time
	Cardiovascular conditioning program; overall strengthening program
	Consider assistive devices that require less energy (eg, switch from standard to wheeled walker)
	Energy conservation techniques very helpful (refer to occupational therapy)
Difficulty with sit to stand	Quadriceps, hip, and trunk extensor strengthening
	Stretch potentially tight flexor muscles and focus on postural exercises (extension exercises are essential)
	Teach how to come forward in the chair and get weight over his or her feet before standing
	Strengthen shoulder musculature, latissimus dorsi, and triceps to assist in rising from the chair
	Provide right height chair with arm rests (may need to improve firmness of chair)
Decreased balance	Provide assistive devices as needed, though keep to minimum to promote self-accommodation
	Work on posture and motor control during all functional activities
	Balance protocol for improving strength, endurance, flexibility, adaptability, etc
	Safety-proof the environment with proper lighting, clear transitions, and uncluttered pathways
	Check wear and tear of shoes and provide with appropriate footgear as needed
Flexed posture (forward lean)	Extension, extension, extension
	Stretch hip flexion contractures and strengthen hip extensors
	Postural exercises with plenty of feedback for learning the correct posture
	Use a reverse walker or increase the height of walkers, canes, or crutches to discourage flexion
Sideways leaning posture	Strengthening hip abductors
	Provide with a heel or shoe lift to correct leg length discrepancy
	Proprioception and ample feedback for learning correct posture
Backward lean	Provide feedback for normalizing posture
	Stretch hip extensors and strengthen hip flexors
	Practice isolating trunk from pelvic motions
Lacks trunk/pelvic rotation	Practice trunk rotation exercise on mat, in sitting, and in standing
	Incorporate arm swing into gait training to facilitate trunk rotation
	Alternately resist forward pelvic motion to enhance proprioceptive input
	Use proprioceptive neuromuscular facilitation to integrate trunk, pelvic, and arm motions
	Visual feedback during gait using mirror or real-time video
Absent heel strike	Strengthen dorsiflexors of the ankle
	Isolate and practice heel strike

(Continued)

Table 10-2 continued

SUGGESTED TREATMENT STRATEGIES FOR GAIT DEVIATIONS IN THE ELDERLY

GAIT DEVIATION	RECOMMENDED STRATEGY FOR INTERVENTION
Decreased foot clearance	Strengthen and facilitate dorsiflexors of the ankle
	Strengthen hip and knee flexors
	Exaggerate flexion during gait (marching) to normalized
	If pathological muscle weakness, may consider an ankle-foot orthosis (AFO)
Decreased push-off	Strengthen plantarflexors of the ankle
	Isolate and practice push-off

ADL. Independent ambulation is frequently the most important goal for an older adult.

Mobility and Transfer Training

Mobility and transfer activities require flexibility and strength, coordination and integration of sensory information with environmental conditions and demands, and cognition or guidance that ensures the older adult's safety. Tasks might include such activities of rising from sitting to standing, standing to sitting in a controlled fashion, turning to transfer weight from one surface to another, or transferring to a lower or higher surface (eg, getting into a tub or transferring into a car seat).

One thing is clear in an older healthy adult compared to younger individuals: Despite similar movement patterns, the lack of joint flexibility and strength translates to a greater expenditure of energy for any given task. For example, in rising from a seated position or returning to sitting, older individuals tend to have difficulty transferring their weight forward over their feet and minimize the forward displacement during the rising or lowering process. As a result, they have trouble initiating movement due to the poor positioning. During treatment, therefore, it is important that the PTA work to reteach the elder to get his or her weight over his or her feet, transfer the weight forward, and standing smoothly and with control, rather than descending back into the chair in rapid and uncontrolled movements. Activities to facilitate safe chair rising and sitting might include instruction in upper extremity assistance and enhancing the individual's awareness of his or her body position relative to the chair. Armchairs that assist in rising from a seated position are also helpful. Examples include higher chairs that decrease the work of the lower extremities for standing, chairs with sturdy arm rests, or, in extreme cases, electric "ejection" chairs

that actually extend to bring the individual to a near-standing position.

Transfer and mobility exercises should also include training in floor-to-standing activities. These are high level activities but wonderful tools for facilitation of strength, flexibility, and confidence. Difficulty rising from the floor after a fall is common in older adults and is associated with substantial requirements for morbidity.[4] This tends to be an underappreciated problem and one that is rarely addressed when working with the elderly. Most falls associated with the inability to get up without help (85%) were not associated with serious injury.[4] The inability to get up after a fall is common and not simply a consequence of a fall-related injury. Fallers who remain on the floor for 1 hour or more are at risk for dehydration, pressure sores, and joint and muscle injury. Fear of falling appears to be increased in previous fallers, particularly those with a history of difficulty rising alone after a fall.[5] The Section on Geriatrics of the American Physical Therapy Association (www. geriatricspt.org) has developed a poster that provides a 9-step protocol for getting up from the floor; this is a helpful tool for teaching an older adult a step-by-step way of rising after a fall.

Pre-Gait Exercises

Pre-gait exercises are designed to improve trunk and extremity strength in addition to motor control. Strength training is directed toward increasing lower extremity strength, particularly the extensors of each lower extremity joint. Strengthening exercises should include those muscles and activities listed in Box 10-2. Strengthening is directed toward stabilizing the entire kinetic chain while attaining full extension. The intensity of exercise needs to be sufficient to result in improvement of one maximal repetition in the good (4/5) muscle range. Upper extremity strengthening should also be included to assist with

Box 10-2: Pre-Gait Exercises for the Elderly

- Back extension (erector spinae)
- Hip extension (gluteus maximus)
- Hip abduction (gluteus medius)
- Knee extension (quadriceps)
- Knee flexion (hamstrings and gastroc)
- Plantarflexors
- Dorsiflexors
- Shoulder stabilization/sitting pushup (latissimus dorsi)
- Elbow extension (triceps)
- Pelvic tilts
- Hip rises (bridging)
- Trunk twisting
- Sit to stand
- One leg stance
- Weight shifting (side walking, weave walking)
- Toe rises
- Hip hiking and leg swinging
- Swing-to to swing-through activities in gait
- Sideways and backwards ambulation

pushing up from the chair as well as lowering the body back into the seated position from standing. The other exercises listed are to facilitate trunk strength and mobility and enhance weight shifting and balance management during varying gait conditions, terrains, and environments (see Box 10-2).

Initial treatment may start in the parallel bars and progress to using an assistive device to independent movement. Encourage proper postural alignment throughout functional activities.

Balance Activities for Gait Training

Static and dynamic balance activities for gait training should be performed in sitting and standing positions. Each balance assessment tool (discussed in Chapter 9) can be used as an exercise to facilitate balance. Balance activities might include those tasks listed in Box 10-3.

Because attentional demands may affect the gait of an older client, training for gait safety during challenging or distracting situations may be appropriate.[6]

Assistive Devices for Locomotion

The prescription of an appropriate assistive device may help the older adult improve balance and mobility without loss of stability, as well as reduce problems of limb loading with painful joints. Table 10-3 provides the advantages and disadvantages of commonly used assistive devices for gait training in the elderly patient.

Gait training needs to focus on achieving mobility and stability and increasing the velocity of gait for ambulation to become functional. Older people generally do not have as much endurance as their younger peers and lack the aerobic reserves. Gait disorders, the use of assistive devices, and slower walking paces all increase the energy expenditure required for walking. It is important that vital signs be monitored during gait training activities. Endurance training using other modes of aerobic exercise (eg, biking, elliptical, swimming) demonstrates a positive impact on improving gait and balance in older individuals.[7] The environment may greatly influence the safety of an older person during gait, transfers, and other ADL. Environmental concerns include assessment of the distances and velocities that need to be covered during functional activities (eg, walking from the bathroom to the bedroom, walking to the car in the rain); the surfaces on which walking occurs; the safety of walkways, stairs, and other obstacles; and the need for transfers at

Box 10-3: Static and Dynamic Balance Activities

- Controlled reaching in sitting and standing
- Leaning in all directions in sitting and standing
  - Side-to-side
  - Forward
  - Backward
- Sitting posture control with external disturbances (gentle pushes)
- Weight shifting activities in all directions
- Stooping and bending activities
- Reaching and lifting
- Standing on high density foam pads
- Walking in sturdy shoes
- Walking barefoot
- Varying ambulation surfaces for walking
- Ramps up and down
- Stairs with and without railing
  - Motor control during ascension and descension
- Directional changes

Table 10-3

ASSISTIVE DEVICES FOR WALKING

ASSISTIVE DEVICE	WHY PRESCRIBE?	ADVANTAGES AND DISADVANTAGES OF PRESCRIPTION
Walkers	Greater stability Shifts weight bearing to arms Unweights painful lower extremities Assists weak lower extremities	More weight bearing with arms than other devices More stable than crutches or canes Difficult to maneuver on stairs
Standard	Need for stability	Greatest stability Difficult to maneuver Requires more attention Greater destabilizing with distraction
Rolling	Decrease energy costs	Less stable than standard walker Easier to propel with upper extremity weakness Reduces energy costs of walking
Hemi	Standard walker for stability Hemiplegia	Maneuvers with one upper extremity following stroke Centrally located hand rail for easier maneuverability Large base of support Provides mobility for individuals with one functional arm
Platform	Rheumatoid arthritis Wrist and hand pathology	Weight bearing on forearms Reduces stress through wrists/hands Heavy and tend to increase energy costs Permit weight shift through humerus
Rollators	Any pathology with low endurance	Rolling walking with brakes for downhill and transfers Comes with a seat for resting
Crutches	Shift of weight bearing to arms Need to unweight lower extremity	Permits more joint unloading than cane Less stable than walker Requires more coordination, greater upper extremity strength, and good balance Contraindicated if brachial plexus injuries present Loftstrand crutches permit hand use and reaching
Canes	Enhances stability Weight shift off painful extremity Compensates for visual losses Assists with proprioception	Appropriate for balance and stability assistance Minimal unloading of joint Need coordination Inappropriate with cognitive or coordination problems Quad cane helps for greater stability and poor upper extremity strength

home or in the community. Safety proofing the environment may be one task in which the PTA is involved when addressing gait training.

Wheelchair locomotion may be required to provide increased independence. Mobility is not defined by ambulation alone. The ability to move from one point to the next may involve wheelchair propulsion, use of a power wheelchair, short bouts of steps or ambulation, or a combination of these methods of locomotion.

Therapeutic Exercises

Many therapeutic interventions or components of therapeutic exercises are performed by the PTA under the direction and supervision of the PT and indicated in the physical therapy plan of care. Table 10-4 provides a listing of possible therapeutic exercises employed in the treatment of elderly individuals. The benefits of exercise are numerous. Therapeutic

Table 10-4

THERAPEUTIC EXERCISES PERFORMED BY PHYSICAL THERAPIST ASSISTANTS

THERAPEUTIC EXERCISE AND ACTIVITY	EXAMPLES OF PRESCRIBED EXERCISES AND ACTIVITIES	BENEFITS FOR ELDERS
Aerobic capacity/ endurance training	Increased workload over time	Increase aerobic capacity
Conditioning/reconditioning	Aquatic programs Graded gait and locomotion training Movement efficiency and energy conservation training Walking and wheelchair propulsion programs Aerobic equipment (eg, bike, elliptical, treadmill) Functional activities for conditioning	Improve maximum oxygen consumption Increase cardiac output Increase stroke volume Increase speed of muscle contraction Increase strength Increase endurance
Balance and coordination training	Motor function training or retraining Vestibular training Motor control and motor learning activities Neuromuscular education or re-education Perceptual training Posture awareness training Sensory training or retraining Complementary exercise programs (Tai chi, Qigong) Task-specific balance training	Increase trunk/extremity strength Decrease fear of falling Increase coordination Improve motor control Enhanced perceptual awareness Increase reaction time Improve rate of mental processing Modify vestibular parameters Improved balance strategies Improve awareness of posture Stability during functional activities
Postural stabilization/ body mechanics	Postural stabilization exercises and activities Posture awareness training Postural control training Body mechanics training	Increase trunk/extremity strength Decrease fear of falling Postural control Awareness of center of gravity Increase balance/coordination Increased endurance Increase reaction time Improve bone mass

(Continued)

Table 10-4 continued

THERAPEUTIC EXERCISES PERFORMED BY PHYSICAL THERAPIST ASSISTANTS

THERAPEUTIC EXERCISE AND ACTIVITY	EXAMPLES OF PRESCRIBED EXERCISES AND ACTIVITIES	BENEFITS FOR ELDERS
Agility and flexibility exercises	Range of motion exercises Muscle lengthening Stretching positions and exercises	Improve postural alignment Enhance functional independence Decrease stress on joints Decrease pain Increase joint mobility
Strength and endurance training	Active-assistive, active, and resistive exercises Concentric exercises Dynamic/isotonic exercises Eccentric exercises Isokinetic exercises Plyometric exercises	Increase muscle strength Improve quality of muscle contraction Increase muscle endurance Increase muscle control/coordination Increase weight bearing/bone mass Improve circulation/oxidative capacity Increase muscle force production Improve muscle metabolism Increase speed of muscle contraction Improve postural alignment
Gait and locomotion training	Pathology-specific gait training Assistive device training Perceptual training Wheelchair training	Increase gait efficiency Increase gait speed and safety Improve perception Increase independence
Relaxation training	Breathing strategies Movement strategies Relaxation techniques (eg, Jacobson) Complementary exercises Biofeedback training	Decrease stress Increase flexibility/agility Improve muscle strength and coordination Re-educate for muscle awareness Improve ability to relax tense muscle Improve respiratory pattern/efficiency

exercises have the potential of maximizing functional independence by improving overall fitness, balance and coordination, strength and flexibility; changing lipid levels; improving glucose metabolism; increasing bone mineral content; improving emotional states and cognitive abilities; enhancing chest wall mobility, circulation, overall homeostasis, and physiological efficiency. Box 10-4 summarizes the general benefits of exercise. Exercise prescription might include therapeutic exercises to address aerobic and endurance training, balance and coordination, postural stabilization and body mechanics, flexibility and joint mobility, strength training, gait training, and relaxation techniques for managing a variety of physiological, pathological, and physical conditions. Therapeutic exercise is one of the primary modes of physical therapy intervention.

Modalities

The PTA is often the clinician who will administer electrotherapeutic, mechanical modalities, and physical agents prescribed by the PT as part of the treatment plan. Older individuals benefit from the use of heat, cold, biofeedback, muscle re-education, compression therapies, mechanical motion

Box 10-4: **Benefits of Exercise**

Overall fitness	Strength	Flexibility	Endurance
Lipid levels	Glucose metabolism	Bone mineral	Chest wall mobility
Circulation	Emotional well being	Cognition	Reaction time
Mental processing	Aerobic capacity	Oxygenation	Vascular compliance
Coordination	Motor control	Gait speed	Muscle quality
Posture	Balance	Core stability	Independence

machines, and other physical modalities used to enhance manual and therapeutic interventions. As noted in Chapters 3 and 4, the normal aging changes of the skin, sensory changes, and pathologies that may affect the health of the skin and sensory integrity need to be considered in managing modalities with older patients. The risk of burns, frost bite, or other injury to the skin are important precautions to consider when employing any mechanical, electrical, or physical agent for treatment. Table 10-5 lists the electrotherapeutic modalities, physical agents, and mechanical modalities that may be used in the treatment of many conditions seen in geriatric care.

Manual Therapy Techniques

The PTA is trained in massage, both therapeutic and connective tissue massage techniques. Box 10-5 lists the manual therapy techniques that the PTA needs to be proficient at in order to manage older patients.

Box 10-5: **Manual Therapy Techniques**

- Massage
  - o Therapeutic massage
  - o Connective tissue massage
  - o Friction massage
- Tissue mobilization techniques
- Passive range of motion
- Stretching techniques
- Positioning for stretching

Functional Activities

One of the primary interventions that PTAs are involved in is re-teaching functional activities in self-care and home management. Table 10-6 provides a list of probable teaching and training areas that the PTA needs to be familiar with in the management of the older, frailer patient. To discharge a person home, his or her ability to care for him- or herself is

very important for safety and independence. Many factors, such as the use of a walker, and difficulty or inability to rise from a chair or get out of bed, may impede an older individual's ability to go home alone. Factors such as chronic illness, environmental barriers, sensory changes, cognitive problems, depression, or poor motivation may limit the older adult's ability to be discharged home. Therefore, it is very important that functional activities be a central therapeutic approach in the management of the elderly person. Poor functional status predicts poor functional outcomes. Typically the individual who is unable to manage basic ADL will extensively utilize health care services and require more family, community, and medical resources in order to stay at home (please refer to Chapter 1 for a review of functional status).

Assistive Devices and Equipment

Table 10-7 lists the potential assistive devices and therapeutic equipment that the PTA may use as part of the prescribed treatment protocol. The PTA needs to familiarize him- or herself with each of these item's application and proper use in the therapeutic setting.

SPECIAL PROGRAMS FOR SPECIFIC DIAGNOSIS

It is important that the PTA be able to treat pathology-specific conditions. In addition to strategies already discussed earlier in this chapter (which also are included for providing holistic intervention), many of the treatment strategies deal with specific pathologies and conditions. As reviewed in Chapter 4, it is crucial that PTAs be able to explain their role in the management of commonly seen pathologies. PTAs, in providing treatment, also are required to understand and recognize common diagnostic tests and procedures and their values and implications on treatment (eg, blood values, pulse oximetry, vital signs, x-rays). For example, the understanding of the outcomes of a cardiac stress test will assist in determining the range of cardiac response safely allowable during exercise and

Table 10-5

MODALITIES—ADJUNCT THERAPEUTIC INTERVENTIONS IN THE ELDERLY

ELECTROTHERAPEUTIC MODALITIES	BIOFEEDBACK
Iontophoresis (electrotherapeutic delivery of medications)	**Electrical Stimulation** • Transcutaneous electrical nerve stimulation (TENS) • Neuromuscular electrical stimulation (NMES) • High voltage pulsed current (HVPC) • Functional electrical stimulation (FES) • Electrical stimulation for tissue repair (ESTR) • Electrical muscle stimulation (EMS)
Physical agents	**Thermotherapy/Heat Agents** • Moist hot packs • Dry heat • Paraffin baths **Cryotherapy** • Cold packs • Ice massage • Vasocoolant spray **Athermal Agents** • Pulsed electromagnetic fields (diathermy) **Hydrotherapy** • Whirlpool baths/tanks • Contrast baths • Aquatic therapy (pools) • Pulsed lavage (wound care) **Sound Agents** • Ultrasound thermotherapy • Phonophoresis **Light Agents** • Infrared • Ultraviolet light • Laser

(Continued)

Table 10-5 continued

MODALITIES—ADJUNCT THERAPEUTIC INTERVENTIONS IN THE ELDERLY

ELECTROTHERAPEUTIC MODALITIES	BIOFEEDBACK
Mechanical modalities	**Compression Therapies** • Compression bandaging • Compression garments • Taping • Vasopneumatic compression devices **Gravity-Assisted Compression Devices** • Tilt table • Standing frame **Mechanical Motion Devices** • Continuous passive motion (CPM) **Traction Devices** • Intermittent traction • Positional traction • Sustained traction

functional interventions. Knowledge of indications and contraindications for exercise is central and will be considered below.

Aging is a normal physiological process. It lies outside the domain of disease. Nonetheless, the time-dependent loss of structure and function can be exacerbated when functional and physical losses associated with pathology are introduced. Additionally, disease may be a reaction to lifelong inactivity, nutrition, hydration, and lifestyle behaviors. As a result, PTAs need to look at the whole person not just the pathology presented at the clinic. PTAs will play a major role in stimulating, motivating, and encouraging an older individual when he or she views his or her diagnosis as the *beginning of the end*. Care, compassion, and active listening are often the most essential therapeutic skills the PTA might develop through experience in a variety of clinical settings (see Chapter 11).

This chapter will summarize the clinical signs and symptoms of specific systems and, where applicable, diseases. The functional changes associated with each system changes, and pathologies of that system will be presented in summary format for user-friendly access. Last, the rehabilitation interventions will be summarized. Where appropriate, specific disease states, such as osteoarthritis, Parkinson's, cerebrovascular disease, PVD,

diabetes, and the like will be singled out and presented in greater detail. (*Note: The symbol ** indicates intervention must only by done by a PT or specialized health care professional.*)

The Musculoskeletal System

I. Myopathy, Myositis, Fibromyalgia, and Myofibralgia

- *Physical signs and symptoms of muscular diseases*
  - Hip and shoulder weakness
  - Muscle girdle weakness in hip or shoulder in myopathy
  - Muscle tenderness or soreness
  - Diffuse musculoskeletal aching
  - Multiple tender trigger points (particularly in fibromyalgia)
  - Postural changes related to pain and weakness
  - Gait changes related to pain and weakness
  - Balance problems
  - Decreased endurance
  - Physical deconditioning associated with inactivity
- *Functional changes with muscular diseases*
  - Difficulty rising from a chair
  - Waddling analgesic gait

Table 10-6

FUNCTIONAL TRAINING: SELF-CARE AND HOME MANAGEMENT

Basic ADL training (Managing Self)

- All self-care activities
- Bathing
- Dressing
- Ambulation and walking indoors
- Eating and the ability to feed self
- Personal hygiene and toileting
- Transfers

Instrumental ADL (Managing Self Within Home)

- Household cleaning and/or doing light housework
- Cooking
- Management of community-based tasks
- Washing dishes
- Getting in and out of a tub
- Yard work
- Shopping
- Laundry
- Personal management of all home-specific tasks
- Climbing up and down stairs

Mobility Training (Managing Self Outside the Home)

- Combining basic ADL with IADL
- Use of walking aid in community settings
- Ability to use public transportation
- Ability to do sit-to-stand-to-sit in all settings

Functional Abilities of the Caregiver

- Training caregiver in all above areas
- Physical status of caregiver determines discharge safety

Barrier Accommodations or Modification

- Environment condition
- Determination of safety
- Modifications as warranted

Device and Equipment Training

- Assistive and adaptive device or equipment training during ADL
- Orthotic, protective, or supportive device or equipment training during self-care and home management
- Prosthetic device or equipment training during ADL

Functional Training Programs

- Back schools
- Task adaptation
- Travel training
- Simulated environments and tasks (eg, Easy Street)

Injury Prevention or Reduction

- Injury prevention education during self-care and home management
- Injury prevention or reduction with use of assistive devices and equipment
- Safety awareness training during self-care and home management

---

- o Difficulty with ambulation on varying surfaces and in changing environments
- o Instability and problems with balance loss
- o Frequent falls
- o Inability to lift things over head
- o Difficulty with bending, stooping, mobility during ADL
- o Difficulty carrying or lifting things

- o Self-imposed restriction of ADL
- o Poor functional mobility and endurance
- o Poor energy reserve
- o Decreased aerobic capacity
- o Postural instability during ADL
- o Depression
- o Lack of motivation

Table 10-7

THERAPEUTIC DEVICES AND EQUIPMENT IN THE ELDERLY POPULATION

Assistive Devices
- Canes
- Crutches
- Walkers
- Wheelchairs
- Long-handled reachers
- Power devices (eg, standing "ejection" chairs)
- Static and dynamic splints

Adaptive Devices
- Hospital beds
- Specialized chairs for positioning; raised chairs for joint protection
- Environmental controls
- Bed mobility and transfer training (eg, Hoyer Lifts)
- Dressing aids (eg, velcro closures, loops on clothes)
- Raised toilet seats
- Custom seating systems

Prosthetic Devices
- Lower extremity prosthetics
- Upper extremity prosthetics

Supportive Devices
- Neck collars
- Slings
- Supplemental oxygen
- Elastic wraps
- Compression garments
- Corsets and back braces

Orthotic Devices
- Shoe inserts
- Casts
- Braces
- Splints

Protective Devices
- Cushions
- Helmets
- Padded protective clothing
- Protective taping techniques
- Braces

- ***Physical therapy interventions with muscular diseases***
  - Pain management
  - Modalities as warranted
    - Biofeedback
    - Electrical stimulation (TENS, ESTR)
    - Thermotherapy
    - Cryotherapy
  - Manual therapies
    - Massage
    - Myofascial and soft tissue mobilitation
  - Muscle strengthening exercise
  - Flexibility and stretching exercises
  - Soft tissue mobilization
  - Joint mobilization as warranted**
  - Aerobic exercises
  - Postural and balance exercises
  - Stress management
  - Functional training to reduce stresses
  - Energy conservation training
  - Patient and family education as needed

II. Osteoporosis
- ***Physical signs and symptoms of osteoporosis***
  - Pain due to microfractures and postural stresses
    - Particularly in spine and hips
  - Stress fractures
  - Postural kyphosis with forward head, kyphotic spine, hip and knee flexion
    - Scoliosis also may occur with functional posturing
  - Balance problems due to postural problems and structural instability
  - Leg length discrepancy due to microfractures or fractures

o Gait changes (center of gravity forward)

o Cardiopulmonary problems associated with inactivity

o Poor nutritional status

o Muscle weakness due to position and lack of activity

o Muscle imbalances/tightness/weakness

- *Functional changes with osteoporosis*

  o Limited ambulation

  o Difficulty rising from a chair

  o Analgesic gait

  o Difficulty with ambulation on varying surfaces and in changing environments

  o Instability and problems with balance loss

    • Frequent fallers

    • Poor balance reactions

    • Fear of falling

  o Difficulty with reaching due to posture (eg, poor functional reach)

  o Difficulty with ADL

  o Difficulty carrying or lifting things

  o Self-imposed restriction of ADL

  o Poor functional mobility and endurance and cardiovascular reserve

  o Decreased aerobic capacity

  o Postural instability during ADL

  o Depression

  o Falling/fracture risk

- *Physical therapy interventions in osteoporosis*

  o Pain management

    • Modalities as warranted

      o Electrical stimulation (NMES, HVPC, FES, EMS)

      o Thermotherapy

      o Cryotherapy

      o Aquatic therapy

      o Taping

      o Compression bandaging

    • Manual therapies

      o Massage

      o Myofascial and soft tissue mobilization

  o Muscle strengthening exercises—particularly extension muscle groups

o Flexibility and stretching exercises

o Soft tissue mobilization

o Joint mobilization** (grades I and II)

o Aerobic exercises

o General conditioning, strengthening, and flexibility exercises

o Postural and balance exercises

o Early weight-bearing activities

  • Tilt table

o Gait training with assistive devices

o Safety and protective techniques/strategies during ADL

o Functional mobility and ADL

o Provision of adaptive environmental aids as needed

o Patient and family education

o Postoperative intervention as required

III. Osteoarthritis, Degenerative Joint Disease, and Rheumatoid Arthritis

- *Physical signs and symptoms of arthritic conditions*

  o Joint pain and stiffness

  o Decreased flexibility and range of motion

  o Soft tissue restrictions

  o Muscle tenderness/soreness

  o Diffuse musculoskeletal weakness and atrophy

  o Tender trigger points in muscles

  o Postural changes related to pain, joint restrictions, and weakness

  o Gait changes related to pain and weakness; analgesic gait

  o Balance problems

  o Decreased endurance

  o Physical deconditioning associated with inactivity

  o Poor nutrition

- *Functional changes with arthritic conditions*

  o Limited ambulation

  o Restricted ADL

  o Period of inactivity due to inflammatory states

  o Difficulty rising from a chair

  o Waddling analgesic gait patterns

  o Difficulty with ambulation on varying surfaces and in changing environments

o Instability and problems with balance loss
  • Fear of falling
o Difficulty with ADL due to joint restrictions and deformities and muscle weakness
o Pain with functional activities
o Self-imposed restriction of ADL
o Poor functional mobility and endurance
o Poor energy reserved
o Decreased aerobic capacity
o Postural instability during ADL
o Balance problems/risk of falls
o Depression
  • Lack of motivation

• *Physical therapy interventions with arthritic conditions*
  o Pain management
    • Modalities as warranted
      o Biofeedback
      o Electrical stimulation (TENS, ESTR, HVPC, FES)
      o Thermotherapy
      o Cryotherapy
      o Hydrotherapy (whirlpool baths, aquatic therapy)
    • Manual therapies
      o Massage
      o Myofascial and soft tissue mobilization
  o Muscle strengthening exercise
  o Flexibility and stretching exercises
  o Soft tissue mobilization
  o Aerobic exercises; general conditioning exercises
  o Gait training with assistive device as warranted
  o Postural and balance exercises
  o Joint protection techniques
  o Joint mobilization** (grades I and II)
  o Splinting to protect joints**
  o Provision of adaptive environmental aids
  o Proper shoes and orthotic fabrication to protect feet
  o Feeding and swallowing programs
  o Functional mobility and ADL activities
  o Patient and family education
  o Presurgical and postsurgical interventions with joint replacements

The Cardiovascular System

• *Physical signs and symptoms of cardiovascular conditions*
  o Poor cardiovascular accommodation to increased activity
  o Angina or shortness of breath at rest
  o Angina or shortness of breath with exertion
  o Decreased overall strength and endurance
  o Diffuse musculoskeletal weakness and atrophy
  o Skin color changes
  o Poor skin integrity with increased risk for breakdown
  o Claudication with walking
  o Nighttime leg cramps
  o Decreased endurance
  o Physical deconditioning with inactivity
  o Dementia related to poor profusion of oxygen in brain
  o Orthostatic hypotension

• *Functional changes with cardiovascular conditions*
  o Decreased energy reserve
  o Limited ambulation due to deconditioning
  o Restricted ADL
  o Period of inactivity due to cardiovascular symptoms
  o Decreased mobility due to poor cardiovascular or cardiopulmonary condition
  o Instability and problems with balance loss
    • Fear of falling
  o Difficulty with ADL due to joint restrictions and deformities and muscle weakness
  o Angina or claudication with functional activities
  o Self-imposed restriction of ADL; fear of activity-induced symptoms
  o Poor functional mobility and endurance
  o Poor energy reserve
  o Decreased aerobic capacity
  o Poor quality sleep
  o Decreased nutrition
  o Balance problems/risk of falls due to inactivity
  o Depression
    • Lack of motivation
  o Decrease in all aerobic activities

- **Physical therapy interventions with cardiovascular conditions**
  - Staged progressive conditioning exercises
  - Aerobic conditioning
  - Muscle strengthening exercises in all muscle groups
  - Flexibility exercises
  - Breathing and relaxation exercises
  - Patient and family education
  - Stress reduction
  - Referral for nutritional counseling
- **Physical signs and symptoms of peripheral vascular conditions**
  - Poor cardiovascular accommodation to increased activity
  - Increased blood pressure at rest and during activity or exercise
  - Diminished or bounding pulses
  - Claudication or night cramps
  - Skin color changes
  - Poor skin integrity at risk for breakdown
    - Increased risk of ulcerations and wounds
  - Decreased endurance
  - Symptoms associated with deconditioning
  - Physical deconditioning associated with inactivity
  - Poor nutrition
  - Dizziness, orthostatic hypotension, or systemic hypertension
- **Functional changes with peripheral vascular conditions**
  - Poor energy reserve
  - Limited ambulation
    - Inability to ambulate functional distances
  - Restricted ADL
  - Period of inactivity due to deconditioning and leg pain
  - Difficulty rising from a chair
  - Loss of proprioception and kinesthesia with unsafe ambulation
  - Difficulty with ADL due to lower extremity muscle weakness and pain
  - Claudication or angina with functional activities
  - Self-imposed restriction of ADL

- Poor functional mobility and endurance
- Poor energy reserve
- Decreased aerobic capacity
- Decreased ambulation during periods of lower extremity ulceration
- Diminished or absent ability to perform instrumental ADL
- Decreased functional mobility due to poor cardiovascular response

- **Physical therapy interventions with peripheral vascular conditions**
  - Buerger-Allen exercises
  - Wound care as warranted
  - Staged progressive conditioning exercises/aerobics
  - Progressive ambulation
  - Breathing and relaxation exercises
  - Strengthening and flexibility exercises
  - Provision of protective foot gear or orthotics
  - Total contact casting as needed for wound care
  - Patient and family education

Box 10-6: **Cardiovascular Manifestations**
- Atherosclerosis
- Ischemic heart disease
- Cardiomyopathy/congestive heart disease
- Conductive system diseases
- Valvular diseases of the heart
- Hypertension
- Peripheral vascular disease

The Pulmonary System

- **Physical signs and symptoms of respiratory conditions**
  - Chest congestion and productive cough
  - Axillary muscle use or pursed lip breathing
  - Labored breathing at rest
  - Shortness of breath with minimal exertion
  - Decreased chest cage mobility
  - Skin color changes; poor skin integrity
  - Decreased overall muscle strength and endurance

- o Decreased cardiopulmonary response to increasing activity levels
- o Balance problems
- o Decreased endurance
- o Physical deconditioning due to inactivity
- o Poor nutrition
- o Dementia due to poor oxygenation

- *Functional changes with respiratory conditions*
  - o Decreased energy reserve
  - o Limited ambulation
  - o Restricted ADL
  - o Period of inactivity due to respiratory distress
  - o Difficulty rising from a chair
  - o Difficulty with ADL due to respiratory stress and muscle weakness
  - o Self-imposed restriction of ADL
  - o Poor functional mobility and endurance
  - o Poor energy reserve
  - o Decreased aerobic capacity
  - o Postural instability during ADL
  - o Balance problems/risk of falls
  - o Poor nutritional status
  - o Decreased ability to sleep
  - o Depression
    - Lack of motivation

- *Physical therapy interventions with respiratory conditions*
  - o Chest physical therapy and respiratory drainage techniques
  - o Postural drainage
  - o Relaxation and breathing exercises
    - Segmental expansion exercises
    - Diaphragmatic excursion exercises
  - o Flexibility and strengthening exercises
  - o Conditioning and endurance exercises
  - o Instruction in energy conservation
  - o Patient and family education
  - o Referral for nutritional counseling

Box 10-7: Pulmonary Manifestations

- Pneumonia
- Chronic obstructive pulmonary disease
- Asthma and resistive pulmonary diseases

Box 10-8: Airway Clearance Techniques

Breathing Strategies

- Active cycle of breathing or forced expiratory techniques
- Assisted cough/huff techniques
- Autogenic drainage
- Paced breathing
- Pursed lip breathing

Manual and Mechanical Techniques

- Chest percussion
- Chest vibration and shaking

Positioning

- Positioning to alter work of breathing
- Positioning to maximize ventilation and perfusion
- Pulmonary postural drainage

The Neuromuscular System

I. Alzheimer's disease

- *Physical signs and symptoms of Alzheimer's disease*
  - o Insidious and slowly progressive loss of cognitive functions
  - o Functional capacity is initially maintained
  - o ADL limited by cognitive losses
  - o Loss of integration of movement
  - o Progressive loss in all areas of function
  - o Tone changes
    - Gegenhalten tone
    - Myoclonic jerks
  - o Joint contractures
  - o Orthostatic hypotension
  - o Malnutrition; become cachectic
  - o Progresses to bedridden status

- *Functional changes with Alzheimer's disease*
  - o Decreased energy reserve

o Gradual loss in all self-care capabilities

- Inability to care for self leads to institutionalization

o Instability and problems with balance loss

- Fear of falling

o Restricted functional mobility due to safety

o Poor functional mobility and endurance

o Poor energy reserve

o Decreased aerobic capacity

o Poor quality sleep

o Decreased nutrition

o Depression

- Lack of motivation

o End stage disease—bedridden

- ***Physical therapy interventions with Alzheimer's disease***

o Sensory integration techniques

o Balance and coordination exercises

o Gait and transfer training

o Endurance and conditioning exercises

o Tone modification techniques

o Strengthening using tone to facilitiate

o Validation therapy

o Patient and family education and support

o ADL

o Modification of environment for safety

o Referral for nutritional counseling

II. Cerebrovascular Accidents

- ***Physical signs and symptoms of cerebrovascular accidents***

o Hemiplegia

o Tone changes—flexor or extensor synergies; flaccidity or spasticity

o Perceptual-motor problems

o Gait disturbances

o Balance and coordination problems

o Poor cardiovascular accommodation to increased activity

o Decreased overall strength and endurance

o Diffuse musculoskeletal weakness and atrophy in addition to hemiplegia

o Speech, language, and feeding problems

o Multi-infarct dementia

- Dementia related to poor profusion of oxygen in brain

o Postural and positioning problems

o Physical deconditioning associated with inactivity

o Poor cardiovascular response to increasing levels of activity

- ***Functional changes with cerebrovascular accidents***

o Cognitive changes

o Decreased energy reserve

o Limited ambulation due to physical deficits

o Restricted ADL

o Period of inactivity due to cardiovascular symptoms

o Decreased mobility due to poor cardiovascular/cardiopulmonary condition

o Instability and problems with balance loss; balance disturbances

- Fear of falling

o Difficulty with ADL due to one-side restrictions or neglect of muscles and muscle weakness

- Perceptual-motor deficits

o Restricted self-feeding and dressing

o Self-imposed restriction of ADL; fear of activity-induced symptoms

o Poor bed mobility

o Diminished transfer ability

o Poor functional mobility and endurance

o Difficulty with communication and speech

o Poor quality sleep

o Decreased nutrition

o Balance problems; risk of falls due to inactivity

o Depression

- Lack of motivation

o Decrease in all aerobic activities

- ***Physical therapy interventions with cerebrovascular accidents***

o Pre-gait training and gait activities

- Normalization of gait

o Provision of assistive devices as warranted

o Positioning and posturing in chair and bed

o Provision of appropriate shoes and orthotics or bracing as warranted

o Range of motion and joint mobilization

o Strengthening and endurance exercises

o PNF, Bobath, Brunnstrom, and other sensory integration techniques

o Feeding and swallowing programs

o Speech therapy

o Training in all basic ADL

  • Adaptive equipment training as needed

o Patient and family education

III. Parkinson's Disease

- ***Physical signs and symptoms of Parkinson's disease***

  o Tone changes; increasing rigidity

  o Perceptual-motor problems

  o Gait disturbances

    • Shuffling, gradually accelerating gait

    • Tendency to lean forward at waist

  o Balance and coordination problems; absence of balance reactions

  o Loss of spontaneous response to balance loss

    • Disappearance of protective extension

  o Difficulty initiating movement

  o Poor cardiovascular accommodation to increased activity

  o Decreased overall strength and endurance

  o Diffuse musculoskeletal weakness and atrophy in addition to rigidity

  o Facial masking with absence of spontaneous facial expressions

  o Speech and language and feeding problems

  o Postural and positioning problems

  o Physical deconditioning associated with inactivity

  o Poor cardiovascular response to increasing levels of activity

  o Decreased mental acuity

  o Tremors at rest

  o Loss of bowel and bladder function

  o Knee and hip flexion contractures

- ***Functional changes with Parkinson's disease***

  o Cognitive changes limiting safety

  o Restricted ambulation due to physical deficits

  o Gradual loss of abilities in ADL

  o Instability and problems with balance loss; balance disturbances

    • Fear of falling

  o Difficulty with ADL due to one-side restrictions and neglect of mucles and muscle weakness

    • Perceptual-motor deficits

  o Restricted self-feeding and dressing

  o Self-imposed restriction of ADL due to difficulty

  o Poor bed mobility

  o Diminished transfer ability

  o Poor functional mobility and endurance with poor energy reserve

  o Difficulty with communication and speech

  o Poor quality sleep

  o Decreased nutrition

  o Balance problems; risk of falls due to inactivity

  o Depression

    • Lack of motivation

  o Decreased in all aerobic activities

- ***Physical therapy interventions with Parkinson's disease***

  o PNF and sensory integration techniques

  o Gait training and assistive devices and balance training

    • Provision of assistive devices as warranted

  o Bed mobility and transfer training

  o Functional mobility exercises

  o Provision of appropriate shoes and orthotics or bracing as warranted

  o Range of motion and joint mobilization

  o Strengthening and endurance exercises

  o Deep breathing and relaxation exercises

  o Feeding and swallowing programs

o Speech therapy

o Training in all basic ADL

  • Adaptive equipment training as needed

o General conditioning, strengthening, and flexibility exercises

o Fine motor coordination exercises

o Patient and family education

Box 10-9: **Neuromuscular Manifestations**

• Confusion and delirium

• Dementias

• Alzheimer's disease

• Cerebrovascular disease

• Parkinson's disease

• Huntington's disease

• Amyotrophic lateral sclerosis

• Normal pressure hydrocephalus

• Orthopedic nerve root compression

• Spinal cord injury

• Peripheral neuropathy

Vestibular System

• **See Table 10-8 and Box 10-10.**

Urinary Incontinence

• ***Physical signs and symptoms of urinary incontinence***

o Decreased mobility and self-imposed restriction in activity

o Abdominal pain and cramping

o Dehydration and malnutrition

o Cognitive impairment, delirium

o Depression

o Restlessness or agitation

o Poor posture in standing, transfers, and ambulation with guarding postures and behaviors

o Poor appetite with resulting poor nutritional status

o Physical problems associated with bed rest and inactivity

o Skin problems associated with incontinence

Table 10-8

DISEASES AND INTERVENTIONS: VESTIBULAR CONDITIONS IN THE ELDERLY

Infections of the Inner Ear

• Usually viral (less commonly bacterial)
  o Although symptoms similar with viral and bacterial infections, treatments very different
  o Proper diagnosis is essential
• Inner ear infections are not the same as middle ear (bacterial infections) affecting the area around the eardrum
• Typically results from a systemic viral illness (eg, mononucleosis or measles)

Unlocalized Vertigo in the Elderly

• Dizziness or ataxia without localizing signs are often designated as *disequilibrium of the elderly*
• Attributed to the ravages of age
• *Presbyastasis,* a term synonymous with disequilibrium of aging
  o Gradual attrition of neural and sensory cells
    • Reduction in hair cell and nerve fiber numbers
  o Cerebellar Purkinje cells gradually reduce over life

(Continued)

Table 10-8 continued

DISEASES AND INTERVENTIONS: VESTIBULAR CONDITIONS IN THE ELDERLY

- Neuronal and fiber loss also occurs in the extrapyramidal system
  - Leads to movement disorders
- Vision and position sense also show gradual deteriorations with age
- Reaction time is reduced with age
- Age-related ataxia

Labyrinthitis and Vestibular Neuronitis (or Neuritis)

Causes of Labyrinthitis

- Inflammation of labyrinth
- Infections of the inner ear affecting both branches of the vestibulocochlear nerve
- Usually only affects one ear

Causes of Neuritis

- Inflammation of vestibular nerve
- Affects the vestibular branch of the vestibulocochlear nerve

Symptoms

- Labyrinthitis
  - Hearing loss
  - Tinnitus
  - Dizziness or vertigo
  - Nausea, vomiting
  - Unsteadiness and imbalance
  - Can affect ability to sit up, stand, or walk
  - Difficulty with vision
  - Impaired concentration
- Neuronitis
  - No hearing loss
  - Dizziness or vertigo
  - Can be mild or severe
  - Subtle dizziness or violent spinning sensation (vertigo)
  - Nausea, vomiting
  - Unsteadiness and imbalance
  - Can affect ability to sit up, stand, or walk
  - Difficulty with vision
  - Impaired concentration

Characteristics of Symptoms

- Onset is usually sudden
- Severe dizziness develops abruptly during routine daily activities
- In some cases, symptoms present upon awakening in the morning

(Continued)

Table 10-8 continued

DISEASES AND INTERVENTIONS: VESTIBULAR CONDITIONS IN THE ELDERLY

- Gradually resolves and recovery may last several weeks
  o Some people are completely free of symptoms
  o Others have chronic dizziness (if virus has damaged the vestibular nerve)

Treatment: Labyrinthitis/Neuritis

- If treated promptly, inner ear infections cause no permanent damage
- In some cases, permanent loss of hearing or damage to vestibular system
  o Medications
    - Control of nausea and suppress dizziness during acute phase
    - *Benadryl* (diphenhydramine)
    - *Antivert* (meclizine)
    - *Phenergen* (promethazine hydrochloride)
    - *Ativan* (lorazepam)
    - *Valium* (diazepam)
    - Reduction of inflammation; steroids often used (eg, prednisone)
    - Anti-viral drugs (eg, *Acyclovir*)
    - Antibiotics (eg, amoxicillin) if middle ear infection present

Vestibular Rehabilitation Exercises

- Physical therapy
- Habituation exercises to retrain the brain's ability to adjust to vestibular imbalance
- Known as compensation
- Key component = keep moving despite dizziness and imbalance

Otitis Media

- An inflammation of the middle ear
- Cause: blockage of the eustachian tube during a cold, allergy, or upper respiratory infection
- Presence of bacteria or viruses lead to the accumulation of fluid (a buildup of pus and mucus) behind the eardrum
- Occurs most often in children
- Symptoms: dizziness, vertigo, nausea, imbalance during ADL

Allergies

- An allergy can lead to fluid buildup in inner ear, creating instability, vertigo, and dizziness
- Drugs used to treat allergies may dehydrate and lead to vestibular symptoms

Exposure to Ototoxin

- Ototoxicity = "ear poisoning" due to drugs or chemicals
- Damages the inner ear or vestibulocochlear nerve
- Results in temporary or permanent disturbances of hearing, balance, or both
- Many chemicals have ototoxic potential such as over-the-counter drugs, prescription meds, environmental chemicals

(Continued)

Table 10-8 continued

DISEASES AND INTERVENTIONS: VESTIBULAR CONDITIONS IN THE ELDERLY

Symptoms of Ototoxicity

- Vary from drug to drug
- Range from mild imbalance to total incapacitation
- Tinnitus to total hearing loss
- Bilateral vestibular loss
- Usually does not produce intense vertigo, vomiting, and nystagmus
- Headache, a feeling of fullness, imbalance producing intolerance to head movement, wide-based gait, difficulty walking in dark, bouncing and blurring of vision (oscillopsia)
- Constant feeling of unsteadiness at rest and during movement
- Light-headedness and severe fatigue

Treatment for Ototoxicity

- No treatment reverses damage
- Treatment aimed at reducing effects of damage and rehabilitation of function
- Hearing aids for those with hearing loss
- Medications; removal of offending ototoxin
- Surgery
- Cochlear implants with profound hearing loss
- Vestibular rehabilitation exercises
- Habituation to assist in developing strategies for maintaining balance

Head Trauma

- Post-traumatic vertigo refers to dizziness that follows a neck or head injury
- Positional vertigo
- Post-traumatic Meniere's syndrome
- Labyrinthine "concussion"
- Post-traumatic migraine
- Cervical vertigo
- Temporal bone fracture
- Perilymph fistula
- Psychogenic vertigo
- Epileptic vertigo
- Diffuse axonal injury (DAI)
- Postconcussion syndrome
- Whiplash injury syndrome

Treatment of Post-Traumatic Vertigo

- Treatment is individualized to the diagnosis. Treatment usually includes a combination of medication, changes in lifestyle, and possibly physical therapy. Occasionally, surgery may be recommended.

(Continued)

Table 10-8 continued

DISEASES AND INTERVENTIONS: VESTIBULAR CONDITIONS IN THE ELDERLY

Benign Paroxysmal Positional Vertigo (BPPV)

- Debris collected within inner ear
- Debris called *otoconia* are small crystals of calcium carbonate (called "ear rocks")
- With head movement, displaced otoconia shift sending false signals to brain

Symptoms of BPPV

- Vertigo, dizziness, and nausea
- Dizziness with position change or any head movement
- Sensation of unsteadiness with turning of head or looking up
- Intermittent pattern of symptoms is usual
  - o Often associated with state of hydration, environmental circumstances, etc

Vestibular Rehabilitation

- Particle-repositioning maneuvers
  - o Epley maneuver
  - o Semont-Liberatory maneuver
  - o Log roll for lateral canal BPPV
- Effective in treating BPPV
- Vestibular physical therapy
- Retraining the brain
  - o Brandt-Daroff habituation exercises
  - o Canalinth rolling and habituation exercises
  - o Liberatory maneuvers

Surgery for BPPV

- Canal plugging
  - o Canal plugging blocks most of the posterior canal's function without affecting the functions of the other canals or parts of the ear
  - o Poses a small risk to hearing
  - o Effective in about 90% of individuals
  - o Should not be considered until all 3 maneuvers/exercises have been attempted and failed

Meniere's Disease

Vestibular disorder that produces recurring set of symptoms as a result of abnormally large amounts of fluid called *endolymph* collecting in the inner ear

Symptoms of Meniere's

- Main symptoms are spontaneous
- Violent vertigo
- Fluctuating hearing loss
- Ear fullness
- Tinnitus
- Exhaustion often occurs; need for sleep

(Continued)

Table 10-8 continued

DISEASES AND INTERVENTIONS: VESTIBULAR CONDITIONS IN THE ELDERLY

Treatment

- Aimed at reducing severity and number of attacks
- Involves adhering to reduced-sodium diet
- Use of diuretics
- Goal of reducing inner ear fluid pressure
- Potential efficacy of using betahistine HCl (Serc) as a vestibular suppressant for
  - Medications—reduction of vertigo, nausea, vomiting
    - Diazepam (*Valium*)
    - Promethazine (*Phenergan*)
    - Dimenhydrinate (*Dramamine*)
    - Meclizine hydrochloride (*Antivert*)
  - Reduction of fluid
    - Diuretics
    - Anti-histamines
    - Ototoxic (ear-poisoning) medication
    - With intractable symptoms—hair cell structures of the inner ear are selectively destroyed

Vestibular Rehabilitation

- Helps with imbalance between attacks
- Helps retrain body and brain to process balance information
- Improve tolerance for activity
- Enhance overall energy level

Endolymphatic Hydrops

- Primary or secondary
- Primary idiopathic endolymphatic hydrops
  - Known as Meniere's disease
- Secondary endolymphatic hydrops (SEH)
  - Underlying causes
    - Following head trauma
    - Following ear surgery
    - Can occur with other inner ear disorders, allergies, or systemic disorders (diabetes or autoimmune disorders)

Symptoms of Hydrops

- Characteristic of Meniere's disease
  - Sudden, violent attacks or episodes of vertigo
  - Pressure or fullness in the ears
  - Tinnitus
  - Hearing loss
  - Dizziness
  - Postural imbalance

(Continued)

Table 10-8 continued

DISEASES AND INTERVENTIONS: VESTIBULAR CONDITIONS IN THE ELDERLY

Symptoms of Secondary Endolymphatic Hydrops

- Symptoms tends to be present more continuously (rather than spontaneous)
- Less violent
- SEH may cause less damage to hearing and balance than Meniere's disease

Treatment for Hydrops

- Hydrops diet regimen
- Medications
- Treat persistent dizziness, nausea, or vomiting
- Vestibular rehabilitation
- Surgery—very rare

Cervicogenic Dizziness

- Controversial diagnosis though often used
- Causes—neck pain accompanies dizziness
- Clinical syndrome of *disequilibrium*
- Cervical spondylosis, trauma, and arthritis
- Trauma—whiplash or head injury
- Symptoms—vertigo called *cervicogenic dizziness* (does not involve a sense of spinning); imbalance increasing with head movements

Treatment for Cervicogenic Dizziness

- Majority improve with treatment of the cervical problem
- Anti-inflammatory drugs
- Gentle mobilization
- Exercise and instruction in proper posture
- Vestibular therapy and important adjunct

Box 10-10: The Vestibular System and Balance in Elderly

Aging of the Inner Ear

- Inner ear provides information to brain regarding changes in head position
- Decrease mobility of parts and particle accumulation results in improper functioning of vestibular system
- Leads to dizziness, vertigo, imbalance, spatial disorientation, and other symptoms

Inner Ear Changes with Age

- Increases susceptibility to infection
- Decrease in immune system responsiveness
- Viral infections in labyrinth (labyrinthitis)
- Viral infections of vestibular nerve (neuronitis)

- Bacterial infections in inner ear (otitis media)
- Bacterial infections of neural sheaths of brain (meningitis) may spread to inner ear
- Allergies lead to production of inner ear fluid or swelling of eustachian tube
- Imbalance of fluid and blood balance due to dehydration and other medical conditions

Postural Disturbances

- Longer response latencies
- Delayed reaction times
- Diminished sensory acuity
- Impaired signal detection
- Postural response patterns disordered

- *Functional changes with urinary incontinence*
  - Restricted ADL, diminished functional mobility
  - Restricted ambulation due to physical deficits
  - Self-imposed restrictions on hydration
  - Decreased energy reserve
- *Physical therapy interventions with urinary incontinence (Table 10-9)*
  - PNF and sensory integration techniques to facilitate pelvic floor muscles
  - Visceral mobilization techniques
  - Conditioning and strengthening exercise
  - Monitor dietary intake and hydrate
  - Biofeedback; neuromuscular re-education
  - Behavioral interventions
  - Training for functional activities that facilitate toileting

Wound Care

- *See Table 10-10*

Balance and Falls

- Teach falling and rising from the floor strategies
- Teach to accommodate for impaired visual cues (simulate environments they may encounter)
- Teach safety with varying surfaces with and without movement
- Create obstacle courses for training in equilibrium/balance
- Teach strategies for accommodating to hypotension problems
- Restore confidence if the patient has experienced previous falls

Table 10-9

THERAPEUTIC INTERVENTIONS FOR URINARY INCONTINENCE IN THE ELDERLY

INTERVENTIONS FOR URINARY INCONTINENCE	OTHER INTERVENTIONS FOR URINARY INCONTINENCE IN THE ELDERLY

• Muscle re-education
• Biofeedback techniques
• Re-innervation and electrical stimulation
• Kegel exercises during activity
• Functional modifications
• Education
• Teach awareness
• Food and fluid modifications
• Behavioral changes
• Muscle contractions
  o Permeometer
  o Femina cones
	• Nursing home settings
	  o Prompted voiding for cognitively impaired
	  o Habit training
	  o Interdisciplinary involvement
	  o Monitoring nutrition and hydration
	  o Remodeling and safety proofing the environment
	  o Providing cues/reminders
	• Home settings
	  o Revamping home
	  o Safety proofing
	  o Improving accessibility
	• Improving physical condition
	  o Endurance exercises
	  o Pelvic floor exercises
	  o Functional exercises
	• Modification of nutritional intake and output
	  o Avoiding coffee, tea, and other irritants
	  o Consuming 2.0 L of water per day
	  o Weight loss as needed
	• Bowel/bladder program

Table 10-10

INTEGUMENTARY REPAIR AND PROTECTION TECHNIQUES

- Debridement—nonselective
  - Enzymatic debridement
  - Wet dressings
  - Wet-to-dry dressings
- Debridement—selective
  - Debridement with other agents (eg, autolysis)
  - Enzymatic debridement
- Dressings
  - Hydrogels
  - Wound covering
  - Total contact casts
- Topical agents
  - Cleansers
  - Creams
  - Moisturizers
  - Ointments
  - Sealants

- Education should include the following:
  - Risk for falls
  - Home safety assessment
  - Compensation techniques
- Strengthening to Prevent Falls
  - Stress extension
  - Back extensors
  - Anterior tibialis
  - Hip abductors and extensors
  - Quadriceps
- Joint Mobilization to Prevent Falls
  - Mobilization of the ankle
    - Heel rocking techniques
    - Tibial and fibular splay
  - Cervical mobilization
  - Thoracic spinal mobilization
  - Extremity mobilization
- Endurance Training to Prevent Falls
  - Conditioning exercises

  - Aerobic exercises
  - Graded walking and progressive exercises
  - Functional activities
    - Instrumental exercises to increase aerobic capacity
- Stretching and Flexibility to Prevent Falls
  - Heel cord stretching
  - Hip and knee flexor stretching
  - Trunk and spinal flexor stretching
  - Alternative forms of stretching (eg, yoga, T'ai Chi, Qigong, etc)
- Respiratory Exercises for the Prevention of Falls
  - Proper fitting and unworn shoes and orthotics enhance stability
  - Teach stepping strategies
  - Change in visual input/lighting to challenge gait
  - Vestibular stimulation
  - Obstacle courses to challenge balance and simulate environmental challenges
  - Stress balance activities
- Balance Organization and Movement Strategies
1. *Ankle Strategy: Displacing the Center of Gravity*
  - Correction around the ankles the focus
  - Slow, small corrective movements
  - Support surface firm and larger than feet
  - Head, hips, and ankles move in phase
  - Muscle activation opposite hip strategy; backward sway: anterior tibula, hamstrings, and paraspinious
2. *Hip Strategy: Displacing the Center of Gravity*
  - Correction around the hips
  - Large and fast corrective movements
  - Support surfaces shorter than feet
  - Head, hips, and ankles move out of phase
    - Muscle activation
    - Backward sway: hip abductors, quadriceps, anterior tibula
    - Forward sway: paraspinious, hamstrings, gastrocnemius
3. *Step or Suspensory Strategy*
  - When movement exceeds limits of stability and prevents ankle or hip strategies

- Sensory Organization
  - Moving in low or fluctuating light sources
  - Walking with head movements
  - Walking on various surfaces and terrains
  - Practice functional activities in everyday environments
  - Make use of visual, vestibular, somatosensory, and proprioceptive input for posture control
  - Suppress each of these senses and inputs when they provide inaccurate information for orientation
- Challenge Center of Gravity Location
  - Flashlight for visual feedback
  - Weight shifts with boundaries and limits of stability
  - Standing tolerance activities
  - Reaching and bending tasks
- *Balance Activities: Using Tests for Treatment*
  - Static sitting and standing
  - Standing with eyes closed
  - Sit-to-stand-to-sit
  - Sternal nudge in standing
  - Directional changes
  - Turning in a 360-degree circle
  - One-legged stance; controlled stand-to-sit
  - Stair climbing (forward, sideways, backward)
  - Ambulating with weights for displacement
  - Sharpened Romberg positioning
  - Duncan's functional reach
  - Mini-squat
  - Fancy balance equipment (eg, Balance Master System, Kinematic System, NeuroCom, etc)
  - Gaze stabilization and visual motor exercises
  - Vary posture (sit, stand, walk)
  - Vary speed and duration
- *Alternative Therapies*
  - Balls, hammocks, rocking chairs
  - The fitter, BAPS boards
  - Swimming and aquatics programs
  - T'ai Chi
  - Modified yoga
  - Dancing
  - Biofeedback

HEALTH PROMOTION AND WELLNESS PROGRAMS

The following recommendation for older adults describes the amounts and types of physical activity that promote health and prevent disease. The recommendation applies to all adults aged 65 years and older and to adults aged 50 to 64 with clinically significant chronic conditions or functional limitations that affect movement ability, fitness, or physical activity. For the purposes of this recommendation, a chronic condition is *clinically significant* if a person receives (or should receive) regular medical care and treatment for it. A functional limitation is *clinically significant* if it impairs the ability to engage in physical activity. Thus, adults age 50 to 64 with chronic conditions that do not affect their ability to be active (eg, controlled hypertension) would follow the adult recommendation.[8] The parts of the recommendation that follow that are not italicized repeat the recommendation for adults, meaning these parts apply to all adults; the italicized parts are specific for older adults.

It is always important to keep in mind that regular physical activity, including aerobic activity and muscle-strengthening activity, is essential for healthy aging. This preventive recommendation specifies how older adults, by engaging in each recommended type of physical activity, can reduce the risk of chronic disease, premature mortality, functional limitations, and disability.

Aerobic Activity

To promote and maintain health, older adults need moderate-intensity aerobic physical activity for a minimum of 30 minutes 5 days each week or vigorous-intensity aerobic activity for a minimum of 20 minutes 3 days each week. Also, combinations of moderate-intensity and vigorous-intensity activity can be performed to meet this recommendation. *Moderate-intensity aerobic activity involves a moderate level of effort relative to an individual's aerobic fitness. On a 10-point scale, where sitting is 0 and all-out effort is 10, moderate-intensity activity is a 5 or 6 and produces noticeable increases in heart rate and breathing. On the same scale, vigorous-intensity activity is a 7 or 8 and produces large increases in heart rate and breathing. For example, given the heterogeneity of fitness levels in older adults, for some older adults a moderate-intensity walk is a slow walk, and for others it is a brisk walk.* This recommended amount of aerobic activity is in addition to routine ADL of light-intensity (eg, self-care, cooking, casual walking, or shopping) or moderate-intensity activities lasting less than 10 minutes in duration (eg, walking around home or office, walking from the parking lot).

Muscle-Strengthening Activity

To promote and maintain health and physical independence, older adults will benefit from performing activities that maintain or increase muscular strength and endurance for a minimum of 2 days each week. It is recommended that 8 to 10 exercises be performed on 2 or more nonconsecutive days per week using the major muscle groups. *To maximize strength development, a resistance (weight) should be used that allows 10 to 15 repetitions for each exercise. The level of effort for muscle-strengthening activities should be moderate to high. On a 10-point scale, where no movement is 0 and maximal effort of a muscle group is 10, moderate-intensity effort is a 5 or 6 and high-intensity effort is a 7 or 8.* Muscle-strengthening activities include a progressive weight training program, weight-bearing calisthenics, and similar resistance exercises that use the major muscle groups.

Benefits of Greater Amounts of Activity

Participation in aerobic and muscle-strengthening activities above minimum recommended amounts provides additional health benefits and results in higher levels of physical fitness. *Older adults should exceed the minimum recommended amounts of physical activity if they have no conditions that preclude higher amounts of physical activity and they wish to do one or more of the following: (a) improve their personal fitness, (b) improve management of an existing disease where it is known that higher levels of physical activity have greater therapeutic benefits for the disease, and (c) further reduce their risk for premature chronic health conditions and mortality related to physical inactivity.* In addition, to further promote and maintain skeletal health, older adults should engage in extra muscle-strengthening activity and higher-impact weight-bearing activities, as tolerated. To help prevent unhealthy weight gain, some older adults may need to exceed minimum recommended amounts of physical activity to a point that is individually effective in achieving energy balance, while considering diet and other factors that affect body weight.

Flexibility Activity

To maintain the flexibility necessary for regular physical activity and daily life, older adults should perform activities that maintain or increase flexibility at least 2 days each week for at least 10 minutes each day.

Balance Exercise

To reduce risk of injury from falls, community-dwelling older adults with substantial risk of falls (eg, with frequent falls or mobility problems) should perform exercises that maintain or improve balance.

Integration of Preventive and Therapeutic Recommendations

Older adults with 1 or more medical conditions for which physical activity is therapeutic should perform physical activity in the manner that effectively and safely treats the conditions. So as to prevent other conditions from developing, older adults should also perform physical activity in the manner recommended for prevention as described herein. When chronic conditions preclude activity at minimum recommended levels for prevention, older adults should engage in regular physical activity according to their abilities and conditions so as to avoid sedentary behavior.

Activity Plan

Older adults should have a plan for obtaining sufficient physical activity that addresses each recommended type of activity. In addition to specifying each type of activity, care should be taken to identify, how, when, and where each activity will be performed. Those with chronic conditions for which activity is therapeutic should have a single plan that integrates prevention and treatment. For older adults who are not active at recommended levels, plans should include a gradual (or stepwise) approach to increase physical activity over time using multiple bouts of physical activity ($\geq$10 minutes) as opposed to continuous bouts when appropriate. Many months of activity at less than recommended levels is appropriate for some older adults (eg, those with low fitness) as they increase activity in a stepwise manner. Older adults should also be encouraged to self-monitor their physical activity on a regular basis and to re-evaluate plans as their abilities improve or as their health status changes.

The benefits of regular physical activity in older adults are extensive. As noted in the adult recommendation, regular physical activity reduces risk of cardiovascular disease, thromboembolic stroke, hypertension, type II diabetes mellitus, osteoporosis, obesity, colon cancer, breast cancer, anxiety, and depression. Of particular importance to older adults, there is substantial evidence that physical activity reduces the risk of falls and injuries from falls,[9] prevents or mitigates functional limitations,[10-13] and is effective therapy for many chronic diseases. Clinical practice guidelines identify a substantial therapeutic role for physical activity in coronary heart disease,[14-16] hypertension,[17,18] peripheral vascular disease,[19] type 2 diabetes,[20] obesity,[21] elevated cholesterol,[22] osteoporosis,[23,24] osteoarthritis,[25,26] claudication,[27] and chronic obstructive pulmonary disease.[28] Clinical practice guidelines identify a role for physical activity in the management of depression and anxiety disorders,[29] dementia,[30] pain,[31] congestive heart failure,[32] syncope,[33] stroke, prophylaxis of venous thromboembolism,[34] back pain,[35] and constipation.[36] There is some evidence that physical activity prevents or delays cognitive impairment[37-39] and disability,[40-42] and improves sleep.[43,44]

The 2001 consensus statement on the dose-response relationship between physical activity and health applies to all adults (although the statement notes that the effect of age on dose-response relationships has not been carefully studied).[45] As an example of studies providing evidence of a dose-response relationship in older adults, at least 33 of 44 papers that provided data on the dose-response relationship between physical activity and health either recruited adults age 65 and over, or followed cohorts of adults over time until a substantial percentage were age 65 and over at the end of follow-up.[46,47]

The recommendation for older adults states that greater volumes of aerobic activity help prevent unhealthy weight gain. The dose-response consensus panel found evidence that increased levels of physical activity are associated with prevention of weight gain, but the nature of the dose-response relationship was unclear and, in general, there was insufficient information on whether age modified dose-response relationships.[45] The recommendation in the 2005 dietary guidelines that additional physical activity helps prevent unhealthy weight gain applies to older adults.[48]

With sufficient skill, experience, fitness, and training, older adults can achieve high levels of physical activity. The promotion of physical activity in older adults should avoid ageism that discourages older adults from reaching their potential. At the same time, it is difficult or impossible for some older adults to attain high levels of activity. Several areas should be emphasized in promoting physical activity in older adults as described below.

Reducing Sedentary Behavior

There is substantial evidence that older adults who do less activity than recommended still achieve some health benefits. Such evidence is consistent with the scientific consensus for a continuous dose-response relationship between physical activity and health benefits.[49] For example, lower risks of cardiovascular disease have been observed with just 45 to 75 minutes of walking per week.[50]

Increasing Moderate Activity and Giving Less Emphasis to Attaining High Levels of Activity

Realistic goals for aerobic activity will commonly be in the range of 30 to 60 minutes of moderate-intensity activity a day, as illustrated by the Health Canada recommendation for older adults.[51] Vigorous activity has higher risk of injury and lower adherence.[52] Age-related loss of fitness, chronic diseases, and functional limitations act as barriers to attaining high levels of activity. Vigorous activity and high levels of activity are appropriate for selected older adults with sufficient fitness, experience, and motivation.

Taking a Gradual or Stepwise Approach

The standard advice to increase physical activity gradually over time is highly appropriate and particularly important for older adults. This advice minimizes risk of overuse injury, makes increasing activity more pleasant, and allows positive reinforcement for small steps that lead to attainment of intermediate goals. It can be appropriate for older adults to spend a long time at one level (eg, attending exercise classes 2 or 3 days a week) so as to gain experience, fitness, and self-confidence. Very deconditioned older adults may need to exercise initially at less effort than a 5 on a 10-point scale and may need to perform activity in multiple bouts ($\geq$10 minutes) rather than in a single continuous bout.[52] In addition, activity plans need to be re-evaluated when there are changes in health status.

Performing Muscle-Strengthening Activity and Engaging in All Recommended Types of Activity

Muscle-strengthening activity is particularly important in older adults given its role in preventing age-related loss of muscle mass[53] and bone[54] and its beneficial effects on functional limitations.[55-58] Currently, only about 12% of older adults perform muscle-strengthening activities at least twice a week.[59]

Sustaining Emphasis on Individual-Level and Community-Level Approaches

As with younger adults, promotion of physical activity in older adults relies upon both individual and community approaches that are evidence based and reflect theory and research on behavior change. For example, the Task Force on Community Preventive Services has recommended or strongly recommended several community-level interventions as effective in promoting physical activity, such as interventions to increase access to places of physical activity combined with informational outreach.[60]

Using Risk Management Strategies to Prevent Injury

Chronic conditions increase risk of activity-related adverse events (eg, heart disease increases risk of sudden death and osteoporosis increases risk of activity-related fractures). Activity-related musculoskeletal injuries act as a major barrier to regular physical activity.[61] While these considerations lead to more emphasis on risk management, there is insufficient research on effective strategies to prevent injuries. Risk management strategies mainly reflect clinical experience, expert opinion, and legal liability concerns. Evidence that risk management strategies can be effective comes from the observation that published exercise studies routinely implement risk management and serious adverse events in these studies are rare.[62,63] However, research studies presumably exclude adults at high risk of injury.

CONCLUSION

Physical activity improves the quality of life in many ways for people of all ages. Physical benefits include improved and increased balance, strength, coordination, flexibility, and endurance. Physical activity has also been shown to improve mental health, motor control, and cognitive function. Active lifestyles provide older persons with regular occasions to make new friendships, maintain social networks, and interact with other people of all ages. Improved flexibility, balance, and muscle tone can help prevent falls, a major cause of disability among older people. It has been found that the prevalence of mental illness is lower among people who are physically active. Therefore, it is inherent in physical therapy interventions that the highest level of physical activity and independence be the goal in geriatric rehabilitation.

The benefits of physical activity can be enjoyed even if regular practice starts late in life. Throughout this text, common diseases among older people have been discussed, including cardiovascular disease, arthritis, osteoporosis, stroke, and hypertension. Being active starting at an early age can help prevent many of these diseases, and regular movement and activity can also help relieve the disability and pain associated with many pathological conditions. Physical activity can also contribute greatly to the management of diseases such as depression and Alzheimer's disease.

Organized exercise sessions, appropriately suited to an individual's fitness level, or leisure walks can provide the opportunity for making new friends and maintaining ties with the community, reducing feelings of loneliness and social exclusion. Physical activity improves self-confidence and self-sufficiency—qualities that are the foundation to psychological well-being and improve the quality of life. Physical therapy is the foundation of interventions towards maintaining and improving functional status. Every older adult has the potential of benefiting from physical therapy assessment, examination, and interventions.

PEARLS

- Therapeutic treatment procedures need to be individualized to meet the specific needs of the older adult.
- A primary function of physical therapy is to return an older individual to his or her previous functional status (or better).
- Changes in gait occur with aging and pathology.
- The speed of walking determines safety. A slower gait actually increases the fall risk by challenging endurance and balance.
- Gait training involves a combination of mobility activities, standing and weight shifting, transfer activities, pre-gait strengthening, and normalizing gait patterns.
- Gait disorders, the use of assistive devices, and slower paces all increase the energy expenditure required for walking.
- Therapeutic exercises have the potential of maximizing functional independence by improving fitness, balance, coordination, strength, flexibility, and endurance.
- Skin status needs to be checked frequently when managing modalities with older patients.
- Functional activities should be a central therapeutic approach in the management of an elderly person.

- A functional limitation is clinically significant if it impairs the ability to engage in physical activity.

- Physical therapy is the foundation of intervention toward maintaining and improving functional status.

References

1. Hardy SE, Perera S, Roumani YF, Chandler JM, Studenski SA. Improvement in usual gait speed predicts better survival in older adults. *J Am Geriatr Soc.* 2007;55:1727-1734.

2. Cesari M, Kritchevsky SB, Penninx BWJ, et al. Prognostic value of usual gait speed in well-functioning older people: results from the Health, Aging and Body Composition Study. *J Am Geriatr Soc.* 2005;53:1675-1680.

3. Varraine E, Bonnard M, Pailhous J. Intentional on-line adaptation of stride length in human walking. *Exp Brain Res.* 2000;130:248-257.

4. Tinetti ME, Liu WL, Claus EB. Predictors and prognosis of inability to get up after falls among elderly persons. *JAMA.* 1993;269:65-70.

5. Van Sant AF. Rising from a supine to erect stance: description of adult movement and a developmental hypothesis. *Phys Ther.* 1988;68:185-192.

6. Jaffe DL, Brown DA, Pierson-Carey CD. Stepping over obstacles to improve walking in individuals with poststroke hemiplegia. *J Rehabil Res Dev.* 2004;41:283-292.

7. Buchner DM, Cress ME, de Lateur BJ. A comparison of the effects of three types of endurance training on balance and other fall risk factors in older adults. *Aging.* 1997;9:112-119.

8. Haskell WL, Lee IM, Pate RM, et al. Physical activity and public health: updated recommendation for adults from the American College of Sports Medicine and the American Heart Association. *Med Sci Sports Exerc.* 2007;39:1423-1434.

9. American Geriatrics Society, British Geriatrics Society, and American Academy of Orthopaedic Surgeons Panel on Falls Prevention. Guideline for the prevention of falls in older persons. *J Am Geriatr Soc.* 2001;49:664-672.

10. Kesaniemi Y, Danforth Jr E, Jensen M, Kopelman P, Lefebvre P, Reeder B. Dose-response issues concerning physical activity and health: an evidence-based symposium. *Med Sci Sports Exerc.* 2001;33(6 suppl):S351-S358.

11. Keysor J. Does late-life physical activity or exercise prevent or minimize disablement? A critical review of the scientific evidence. *Am J Prev Med.* 2003;25(suppl 2):129-136.

12. LIFE Study Investigators. Effects of a physical activity intervention on measures of physical performance: results of the Lifestyle Interventions and Independence for Elders Pilot (LIFE-P) Study. *J Gerontol A Biol Sci Med Sci.* 2006;61A:1157-1165.

13. Nelson M, Layne J, Bernstein M. The effects of multidimensional home-based exercise on functional performance in elderly people. *J Gerontol A Biol Sci Med Sci.* 2004;59A:154-160.

14. Fletcher G, Balady G, Amsterdam E. Exercise standards for testing and training: a statement for healthcare professionals from the American Heart Association. *Circulation.* 2001;104:1694-1740.

15. Pollock M, Franklin B, Balady G. AHA Science Advisory. Resistance exercise in individuals with and without cardiovascular disease: benefits, rationale, safety, and prescription: an advisory from the Committee on Exercise, Rehabilitation, and Prevention, Council on Clinical Cardiology, American Heart Association; position paper endorsed by the American College of Sports Medicine. *Circulation.* 2000;101:828-833.

16. Thompson P, Buchner D, Piña IL. Exercise and physical activity in the prevention and treatment of atherosclerotic cardiovascular disease: a statement from the Council on Clinical Cardiology (Subcommittee on Exercise, Rehabilitation, and Prevention) and the Council on Nutrition, Physical Activity, and Metabolism (Subcommittee on Physical Activity). *Circulation.* 2003;107:3109-3116.

17. American College of Sports Medicine. Position stand: exercise and hypertension. *Med Sci Sports Exerc.* 2004;36:533-553.

18. Chobanian A, Bakris G, Black H. The Seventh Report of the Joint National Committee on Prevention, Detection, Evaluation, and Treatment of High Blood Pressure: the JNC 7 report. *JAMA.* 2003;289:2560-2572.

19. McDermott M, Liu K, Ferrucci L. Physical performance in peripheral arterial disease: a slower rate of decline in patients who walk more. *Ann Intern Med.* 2006;144:10-20.

20. Sigal R, Kenny G, Wasserman D, Castaneda-Sceppa C. Physical activity/exercise and type 2 diabetes. *Diabetes Care.* 2004;27:2518-2539.

21. US Preventive Services Task Force. Screening for obesity in adults: recommendations and rationale. *Ann Intern Med.* 2003;139:930-932.

22. Geliebter A, Maher M, Gerace L, Gutin G, Heymsfield SE, Hashim EL. Effects of strength or aerobic training on body composition, resting metabolic rate, and peak oxygen consumption in obese dieting subjects. *Amer J Clin Nutr.* 1997;66:557-563.

23. Going S, Lohman T, Houtkooper L. Effects of exercise on bone mineral density in calcium-replete postmenopausal women with and without hormone replacement therapy. *Osteoporos Int.* 2003;14:637-643.

24. US Department of Health and Human Services. *Bone Health and Osteoporosis: A Report of the Surgeon General.* Rockville, MD: 2004.

25. American College of Rheumatology. Recommendations for the medical management of osteoarthritis of the hip and knee: 2000 update. American College of Rheumatology Subcommittee on Osteoarthritis Guidelines. *Arthritis Rheum.* 2000;43:1905-1915.

26. American Geriatrics Society. Exercise prescription for older adults with osteoarthritis pain: consensus practice recommendations. A supplement to the AGS Clinical Practice Guidelines on the management of chronic pain in older adults. *J Am Geriatr Soc.* 2001;49:808-823.

27. Stewart K, Hiatt W, Regensteiner J, Hirsch A. Exercise training for claudication. *N Engl J Med.* 2002;347:1941-1951.

28. Pauwels RA, Buist AS, Calverley PM, Jenkins CR, Hurd SS. GOLD Scientific Committee. Global Strategy for the Diagnosis, Management, and Prevention of Chronic Obstructive Pulmonary Disease. NHLBI/WHO Global Initiative for Chronic Obstructive Lung Disease (GOLD) Workshop summary. *Am J Respir Crit Care Med.* 2001;163:1256-1276.

29. Brosse A, Sheets E, Lett H, Blumenthal J. Exercise and the treatment of clinical depression in adults: recent findings and future directions. *Sports Med.* 2002;32:741-760.

30. Doody R, Stevens J, Beck C, et al. Practice parameter: management of dementia (an evidence-based review). Report of the Quality Standards Subcommittee of the American Academy of Neurology. *Neurology.* 2001;56:1154-1166.

31. American Geriatrics Society Panel on Persistent Pain in Older Persons. The management of persistent pain in older persons. *J Am Geriatr Soc.* 2002;50(6 suppl):S205-S224.

32. Remme W, Swedberg K. Guidelines for the diagnosis and treatment of chronic heart failure. *Eur Heart J.* 2001;22:1527-1560.

33. Brignole M, Alboni P, Benditt D, et al. Guidelines on management (diagnosis and treatment) of syncope. *Eur Heart J.* 2001;22:1256-1306.

34. Scottish Intercollegiate Guidelines Network (SIGN). *Prophylaxis of venous thromboembolism: a national clinical guideline.* Edinburgh, Scotland. Publication no. 62; 2002.

35. Hagen K, Hilde G, Jamtvedt G, Winnem M. The Cochrane review of advice to stay active as a single treatment for low back pain and sciatica. *Spine.* 2002;27:1736-1741.

36. Pemberton J, Phillips S. American Gastroenterological Association Medical Position Statement: guidelines on constipation. *Gastroenterology.* 2001;119:1761-1766.

37. Abbott R, White L, Ross G, Masaki K, Curb J, Petrovitch H. Walking and dementia in physically capable elderly men. *JAMA.* 2004;292(12):1447-1453.

38. Larson E, Wang L, Bowen J, et al. Exercise is associated with reduced risk for incident dementia among persons 65 years of age and older. *Ann Inter Med.* 2006;144:73-81.

39. Weuve J, Kang J, Manson J, Breteler M, Ware J, Grodstein F. Physical activity, including walking, and cognitive function in older women. *JAMA.* 2004;292:1454-1461.

40. Penninx B, Messier S, Rejeski W, et al. Physical exercise and the prevention of disability in activities of daily living in older persons with osteoarthritis. *Arch Intern Med.* 2001;161:2309-2316.

41. Singh M. Exercise to prevent and treat functional disability. *Clin Geriatr Med.* 2002;18:431-462,vi-vii.

42. Tseng B, Marsh, D Hamilton M, Booth F. Strength and aerobic training attenuate muscle wasting and improve resistance to the development of disability with aging. *J Gerontol A Biol Sci Med Sci.* 1995;50(special issue):113-119.

43. King A, Oman R, Brassington G, Bliwise D, Haskell W. Moderate-intensity exercise and self-rated quality of sleep in older adults. a randomized controlled trial. *JAMA.* 1997;277:32-37.

44. Singh N, Clements K, Fiatarone M. A randomized controlled trial of the effect of exercise on sleep. *Sleep.* 1997;20:95-101.

45. Kahn E, Ramsey L, Brownson R, et al. The effectiveness of interventions to increase physical activity: a systematic review. *Am J Prev Med.* 2002;22(4 suppl):73-107.

46. Janssen I, Jolliffe C. Influence of physical activity on mortality in elderly with coronary artery disease. *Med Sci Sports Exerc.* 2006;38:418-423.

47. Lee I, Skerrett P. Physical activity and all-cause mortality: what is the dose-response relation? *Med Sci Sports Exerc.* 2001;33(6 suppl):S459-S471; discussion:S93-S94.

48. US Department of Health and Human Services and US Department of Agriculture. *Dietary Guidelines for Americans, 2005.* 6th ed. Washington, DC: US Government Printing Office; 2005.

49. Loucks A, Verdun M, Heath E. Low energy availability, not stress of exercise, alters LH pulsatility in exercising women. *J Appl Physiol.* 1998;84:37-46.

50. Manson J, Greenland P, LaCroix A, et al. Walking compared with vigorous exercise for the prevention of cardiovascular events in women. *N Engl J Med.* 2002;347:716-725.

51. Health Canada. *Canada's Physical Activity Guide to Healthy Active Living for Older Adults.* Ottawa, Ontario, Canada; 1999.

52. Franklin B, Whaley M, Howley E. *ACSM's Guidelines for Exercise Testing and Prescription.* 6th ed. Champaign, IL: Human Kinetics Publishers; 2000:137-164.

53. US Department of Health and Human Services. *Physical Activity and Health: A Report of the Surgeon General.* Atlanta, GA: US Dept of Health and Human Services, Centers for Disease Control and Prevention, National Center for Chronic Disease Prevention and Health Promotion; 1996.

54. Martinson B, Crain A, Pronk N, O'Connor P, Maciosek M. Changes in physical activity and short-term changes in health care charges: a prospective cohort study of older adults. *Prev Med.* 2003;37:319-326.

55. King A, Pruit L, Phillips W, Oka R, Rodenburg A, Haskell W. Comparative effects of two physical activity programs on measured and perceived physical functioning and other health-related quality of life outcomes in older adults. *J Gerontol A Biol Sci Med Sci.* 2000;55(A):M74-M83.

56. Latham N, Anderson C, Bennett D, Stretton C. Progressive resistance strength training for physical disability in older people. *Cochrane Database Syst Rev.* 2003;(2):CD002759.

57. Gordon N, Gulanick M, Costa F, et al. Physical activity and exercise recommendations for stroke survivors: an American Heart Association scientific statement from the Council on Clinical Cardiology, Subcommittee on Exercise, Cardiac Rehabilitation, and Prevention; the Council on Cardiovascular Nursing; the Council on Nutrition, Physical Activity, and Metabolism; and the Stroke Council. *Circulation.* 2004;109:2031-2041.

58. American College of Cardiology/American Heart Association. *Methodology Manual for ACC/AHA Guideline Writing Committees.* American College of Cardiology Foundation and the American Heart Association; 2006.

59. US Department of Health and Human Services. Strength training among adults aged >65 years—United States 2001. *MMWR.* 2004;53:25-28.

60. Federal Interagency Forum on Aging-Related Statistics. *Older Americans 2004: Key Indicators of Well-Being. Federal Interagency Forum on Aging-Related Statistics,* Washington, DC: US Government Printing Office; 2004.

61. Hootman J, Macera C, Ainsworth B, Addy C, Martin M, Blair S. Epidemiology of musculoskeletal injuries among sedentary and physically active adults. *Med Sci Sports Exerc.* 2002;34:838-844.

62. Buchner D, Coleman E. Exercise considerations in older adults: intensity, fall prevention, and safety. *Phys Med Rehabil Clin N Am.* 1994;5:357-375.

63. Ory MG, Resnick B, Jordan P, et al. Screening, safety, and adverse events in physical activity interventions: collaborative experiences from the behavior change consortium. *Ann Behav Med.* 2005;29(suppl):20-28.

Section III

Special Considerations in Geriatric Rehabilitation Therapies

11

Communication, Education, and Learning

Communication is the exchange of information between individuals through a common set of symbols, signs, or behaviors. Communication, whether verbal, through touch, gestures, or in written form, is essential for effectively interacting with the world around us. This chapter addresses changes in learning abilities and theories and styles of learning that can enhance communication with the elderly individual. Barriers that affect communication and learning, such as sensory or cognitive deficits, and approaches to dealing with these obstacles are also presented. Patient motivation and participation in treatment as well as desired outcomes are an important part of rehabilitation; their roles in facilitating effective communication are discussed

Rehabilitation provides many teaching and learning components as part of any therapeutic intervention, and education is an integral part of practice in rehabilitation. PTs and PTAs educate patients, consumers, caregivers, health care providers, students, policymakers, among many others. It is important that PTAs, as part of the health care team, are able to express themselves and openly listen in a culturally competent manner with the patients and all others involved in the care of the older person.

DEFINING LEARNING AND CHANGES IN LEARNING WITH AGING

Cultural stereotypes and myths foster the notion that learning abilities and memory capabilities decline with age.[1] On the contrary, in our society, elderly individuals must learn new skills as new technology alters basic systems of communication, transportation, finance, and recreation on nearly a daily basis. As values change, societal rewards change, and new learning is required.

Learning is the acquisition of information or skills. It is usually measured by looking for improvements in task performance. When someone improves his or her performance at a given intellectual or physical task, that is learning (see Box 11-1).

Cognitive functioning in elderly individuals shows a slight decline in learning ability with age. The question is, is there a change in the brain that affects acquisition of information or are there other factors involved? Physiological responses, physical health status, pathology, vision or hearing problems, depression, and motivation all might influence learning. It is hard to separate the elements of functioning that may influence learning ability, although a number of studies have tried. Although other factors contribute to the decline in task performance, most researchers still attribute this decline to a diminished ability to learn new tasks or acquire new information with age.[2,3]

Attention is the ability to focus; *selective attention* is the ability to distinguish relevant from irrelevant information. Older adults appear to perform tasks requiring sustained or selective attention extremely well into old age. All age groups can learn; however, older individuals may just require more time. Tasks that use familiar symbols or objects, with simple responses required

Bottomely J. *Geriatric Rehabilitation: A Textbook for the Physical Therapist Assistant* (pp 305-328).
© 2010 SLACK Incorporated

Box 11-1: **Definitions: Memory and Learning**

Learning	Gaining knowledge, understanding, and mastery of skills
Cognition	Mental ability or process of acquiring knowledge; knowledge gained through perception, reasoning, intuition
Memory	Mental ability of retaining and recalling information and past experiences
Intelligence	Capacity to acquire and apply knowledge
Attention span	Ability to concentrate and stay focused for a length of time without distraction
Selective attention	Ability to strain out extraneous distractions and tend to a specific task
Language	Verbal sounds, gestures, and/or written symbols that represent organized communication used by people with shared history, traditions, and culture
Semantic knowledge	Word retrieval associated with naming people and things
Phonologic knowledge	Word and sound recognition through hearing
Lexical knowledge	Ability to name an item and understand the meaning of a word or symbol
Syntactic knowledge	Ability to combine words in a meaningful way
Visual-spatial learning	Ability to identify incomplete figures, recognize fixed objects, or arrange objects to match a design
Procedural learning	Ability to acquire motor or cognitive skills through practice
Problem solving	Ability to find a solution to a question or situation that presents or poses a challenge

and low interference from prior learning are favorable to new learning by older individuals.[4]

Language is one important aspect of learning. Within language is the aspect of *semantic knowledge*, which involves word retrieval and is tested by having respondents name common objects. Semantic knowledge appears to decline with age, although significant differences are not found until relatively late in the lifespan, especially over the age of 75. Linguistic abilities that are not affected with age include *phonologic knowledge* (ie, use of sounds of language), *lexical knowledge* (ie, the name of an item and the meaning of a word), and *syntactic knowledge* (ie, ability to combine words correctly).[5]

Visual-spatial ability, a part of informational processing, shows a decline with age. This affects visual tasks such as identifying incomplete figures, recognizing fixed objects, or arranging blocks into a design. Aging also appears to affect both the ability to perceive and the ability to reproduce figures in 3 dimensions.[6]

Procedural learning is a form of *implicit* (embedded or inherent) memory, which refers to the ability to acquire motor or cognitive skills gradually through practice.[7] Acquisition of such skills is visible by increased accuracy or speed of performance as a result of repeated exposure to a specific procedure, without conscious recollection of the prior learning episode or the rules underlying the task. For example, someone may have learned how to play the piano when

he or she was quite young, and despite limited lessons or practice, still be able to sit down at a piano and read sheet music and play a song never practiced.

In measures of *general intelligence* (ie, their intelligence quotient, or IQ), older adults display what is called the *classic aging pattern*. The most frequently used test in studies of adult intelligence and age-related changes is the Wechsler Adult Intelligence Scale (WAIS). IQ is a test score that is compared with the normal or average score of 100. When the WAIS is used for adults aged 20 and over, there is an age factor built into the determination of what is normal. Measured IQ performance peaks about age 25 and only slightly declines thereafter. Because of the built-in age factor, there could be a 40-point difference between the score at age 25 and the score at age 75, and yet the IQ score would be the same.[8]

Performance scores that measure *problem-solving* ability tend to decline with age. Verbal scores that measure learning knowledge, such as comprehension, arithmetic, and vocabulary, tend to remain stable. Relatively little decline in performance occurs prior to age 50. Substantial declines in intelligence measures appear to occur after age 70 in a small percentage of older adults.[9] The majority of older individuals not only maintain their cognitive abilities but also have the ability to learn new material (eg, a new language) and skills (eg, golf).

Many abilities in which declines occur can be improved through training and practice in memory techniques, problem-solving skills, and other cognitive strategies. Short-term memory loss is common and determining whether forgetfulness is benign or a precursor of dementia is often difficult. The average 70 year old can take up to 4 times longer than a 20 year old in tests involving memory. Older adults are also slower in reaction time than younger adults, which is evidenced through both delays in physical response and the speed of information processing. For example, an older driver may respond more slowly to the changing of a green traffic light to yellow to red; as a result of not responding as rapidly to the visual information, processing this sensory stimulus and integrating it to the physical action of applying the brake takes a longer period of time. Older individuals have some difficulty developing logical strategies spontaneously but given practice, are able to execute complex predetermined plans.[10]

THEORIES AND STYLES OF LEARNING

Learning and memory are closely related concepts. Simply, people must learn before they can remember. Learning without memory is not very helpful. Memory tasks are often used to assess learning. "How much you have learned?" is translated to, "How much do you remember?" While *learning* is acquisition of a new skill or information through practice and experience, *remembering* is the retrieval of information that has been stored in memory.[11] General learning and memory involve 3 processes: encoding (acquisition, or getting information into the system), storage (retrieving information), and retrieval (recalling information) (Box 11-2).

There are several different theories that dominate the study of learning and memory. The *associative* view of learning suggests that one learns by linking new information to previous knowledge. Theories on *information processing* or *conceptual learning* as a mode for learning and memory suggest that imagination and mental flexibility, rather than concrete information, play a role in learning. In these theories, memory is often discussed in terms of information: how information is put into the system, how it is

stored, and how it is retrieved. Other theories concern *contextual learning* (ie, when learners connect information to their own frame of reference). Thus, learning is part of memory (ie, the acquisition, registration, or encoding of information).

Associative learning and memory involve the linking of ideas or events that occur together in time; this type of learning involves a stimulus-response bond. The incorporation of a word task into memory occurs by learning an association between 2 commonly unrelated items, such as basket and orange, where in this example the association lies perhaps in picking oranges and placing them in a basket. The ability to recall a paired stimulus represents the contents of memory. Several factors influence the amount of information that can be processed with increasing age, such as the pace of learning and the environment in which learning occurs.

The pace of learning is the speed with which a task is performed and is one variable known to affect older learners. Older subjects perform poorly when the learning interval is short but do much better when they are given more time to respond.[11] If a method called *self-pacing* is permitted (ie, if the learner is allowed as much time as he or she wants), older subjects improve in the number of correct responses they are capable of giving.[12]

Contextual learning is linked to associative learning and is often supported by the individual placing some situational meaning to lists of words, activities, or other learning endeavors. For example, if an important piece of information is presented in bold type, it is more likely to be perceived as important because this has been stressed through visual intonation. Learning occurs because the information has been presented in context. There is no evidence of an age-related impairment in the encoding of perceptual-conceptual information.[13] This is an important finding for geriatric rehabilitation professionals. Much of the printed or spoken information we provide for elderly patients could conceivably be learned better if presented in a perceptual-contextual format.

The ability to perform associative learning tasks may be affected by variables such as cautiousness,

---

Box 11-2: Theories of Memory and Learning

Associative learning	Association of ideas or events that occur together in time
Information processing	The manner in which an individual receives, retains, and retrieves information
Conceptual learning	The mental flexibility and the capacity for abstract thinking
Contextual learning	Mental ability of retaining and recalling information in context from past experiences

anxiety, and interference. These factors are often associated with *errors of omission* (not responding) or *errors of commission* (responding incorrectly). Errors of omission occur most often in fast-paced associative learning situations (rather than errors of commission). Errors of omission are reflective of cautiousness or a reluctance to venture a response unless one is absolutely certain of its accuracy. Research suggests that the poorer performance of older adults, as reflected in omission errors, is a function of their being more cautious.[10]

Anxiety also affects performance. Eisendorfer and associates[14] tested this theory by introducing a drug that blocked physiological arousal. The result was significantly fewer errors in older subjects on associative learning tasks compared to elders given an inactive drug.

Associative learning in older adults is susceptible to the effects of interference from prior learning. When one word is frequently associated with another word in everyday situations, such as dark-light or water-ocean, the pair is said to have high associative strength. When one word is infrequently associated with another, such as dark-fast or water-book, the pair has low associative strength. If the associative habits of older individuals are more established through a greater number of years of experience, it follows that age-related differences should be least for high-associative pairs.[15] An older adult has more trouble when learning, and recall involves forming associations that are contrary, or in competition with, previously learned verbal associations.

Information processing determines how information is handled and has to do with the older adult's learning style. Information processing has to do with the typical manner in which an individual receives, retains, and retrieves information, as well as how the individual responds emotionally in a learning experience. This theory of learning grew from analogies with computer operations. Information processing has become a prominent theory in consideration of memory and perception. It involves associative, conceptual, and contextual learning. Information processing is the mechanism through which an individual processes, stores, and remembers events, tasks, lists, and the like. It involves the "wiring" of the human hard drive—the brain.

Conceptualization is mental flexibility and the capacity for abstraction. This appears to decline with age, with the greatest difference occurring in extreme old age.

Performance of *complex motor tasks*, such as rapid sequences of finger movements or lower extremity sequencing activities, can be improved in terms of speed and accuracy over several weeks by daily practice sessions. There is more graymatter activated by the practiced sequence task. There appears to be a slowly evolving, long-term, experience-dependent reorganization of brain tissue activated. This may underlie the acquisition and retention of the motor skill.[8]

Cortical functions concerned with the execution of skilled movements can also be studied through complex interactive tasks. Brain activity in elderly subjects trained for a long time to perform a highly skillful activity (ie, sequencing dancing steps) increased compared to electrophysiological brain activity in a group of elderly control subjects with no previous experience in the particular skilled-motor activities. Long-term practice seems to produce better control of performance, reducing the need to concentrate on the skilled activity.[8] In other words, practice makes perfect with less thought required.

In an interesting study, the authors[16] reviewed the evidence of age differences in episodic memory for content of a message and the context associated with it. Specifically, that memory for context is more vulnerable to aging than memory for content. The major clinical implication of these findings is that elderly humans overwhelmingly seek, create, or imagine context in order to provide meaning when presented with information.

HUMAN MEMORY AND AGING

Nearly half of people age 50 or older complain of mild, age-related memory problems. The good news is that studies show that 65% of aging affects are a result of lifestyle rather than genetics.[17] This means that lifestyle choices can prevent memory loss. The 4 effective ways of keeping the memory sharp include a brain-healthy diet, regular exercise, stress reduction, and memory-boosting techniques.[18]

There are many myths about the effects of aging on memory. For example, people are supposed to forget things recently learned, but memories from the distant past are supposed to be clear and vivid, sometimes startlingly so. Early learning also appears to have a significant impact on an elderly individual's resourcefulness for both verbal and physical skills in later life[19] (Box 11-3).

Sensory memory is considered to be sense specific. Two types of sensory modalities are defined within this context of memory. The visual memory store is called *iconic memory*. Facsimiles of auditory stimuli are termed *echoic memory*. Both are considered fleeting and the initial stage of information processing. Since visual abilities decline with age, it is possible that age differences in sensory store make some stimuli more difficult for older people to attend to and remember. If hearing is a problem, speech comprehension is more likely to cause problems with encoding information. However, minor deficits in sensory storage probably do not contribute significantly to the more severe memory problems in long-term storage experienced in the elderly.[20]

There are essentially 4 types of memory. *Short-term* or *immediate memory* involves recall after very little delay (as little as 5 seconds up to 30 seconds). *Recent memory* involves recall after a brief period (from 1 hour to several days). *Remote memory* refers to recall of events that took place a long time ago but that have been referred to frequently throughout the course of a lifetime. *Old memory* refers to recall of events that occurred a long time in the past and have not been thought of or rehearsed since.

It is commonly believed that all kinds of memory show a decline with advancing age; however, studies do not consistently support this idea. While it is true that there is an age-related deficit in recall of various types, it is not clear whether this deficit results from declining memory or declining ability to learn in the first place. If the focus on establishing memory problems is based on the ability to recall previously learned material, the evidence seems to point to an age deficit in the performance of both immediate and delayed recall.[21] The greater loss with age occurs in short-term and recent memory compared to remote or old memory. The decline with age in memory function is less for rote memory (ie, material that has been memorized) than for logical memory (ie, material requiring problem solving from past learning).[11]

People with higher intelligence appear to be less susceptible to memory loss with increasing age compared to their less intelligent counterparts. In fact, individuals who are continuously learning and curious have lower incidence of dementias and some escape memory loss altogether. This pattern suggests that memory losses are associated with inactivity of the brain more so than age. Older individuals who exercise their memories through reminiscence and learn new information regularly tend to maintain both remote and recent memory.[22]

In order to be remembered, something needs to be learned. Learning is often called *encoding*. Just as information must be translated into the proper code (or language) for a computer to process it further, information from the environment must be encoded for the human processing system to store, use, and later retrieve it. Encoding is the learning or acquisition phase of memory. It is storage that most people think of as memory. It is the laying away of encoded information in storehouses for later use. The sensory store is conceptualized as a "way station" for essentially unprocessed information from the environment. In order for information to be recalled, it must be processed and transferred to later stores (short term and long term). *Short-term* store is presumed to hold relatively small amounts of information for a slightly longer time than the sensory store (eg, a phone number from directory assistance), commonly on the order of a few seconds, whereas the *long-term* store is seen as having a very large capacity for storing information which can be retained over long periods of time. Figure 11-1 provides a schematic representation of the memory system.[23]

As Figure 11-1 demonstrates, acquired information is first perceived and processed (sensory store) for a second and then placed in temporary neuron hold, or what is called the *working* or *short-term memory*. Information in short-term memory is kept briefly and decays quickly unless it is rehearsed (eg, a phone number or e-mail address). We use short-term or working memory thousands of times per day.

If information is important or practiced, neuron pathways through the hippocampus, a central area in the brain where short-term memory is converted to long-term memory, strengthen and reinforce the

Box 11-3: **Types of Memory and Learning**	
Sensory memory	Memory established through specific senses (eg, smell, sight, sounds)
Iconic memory	Visually based memory (eg, recognizing a place or an object)
Echoic memory	Memory established by sounds and what is heard
Olfactory memory	Recall of smells (eg, aroma of turkey cooking)
Short-term memory	Also called immediate memory, mental ability or the process of recall after very little delay in instructions, experience, sensory input, etc
Recent memory	Recall after a brief period (eg, 1 hour, 1 day)
Memory	Mental ability of retaining and recalling information and past experiences
Remote memory	Recall of events that took place a long time ago
Old memory	Recall of events that occurred a long time in the past (eg, childhood memories)

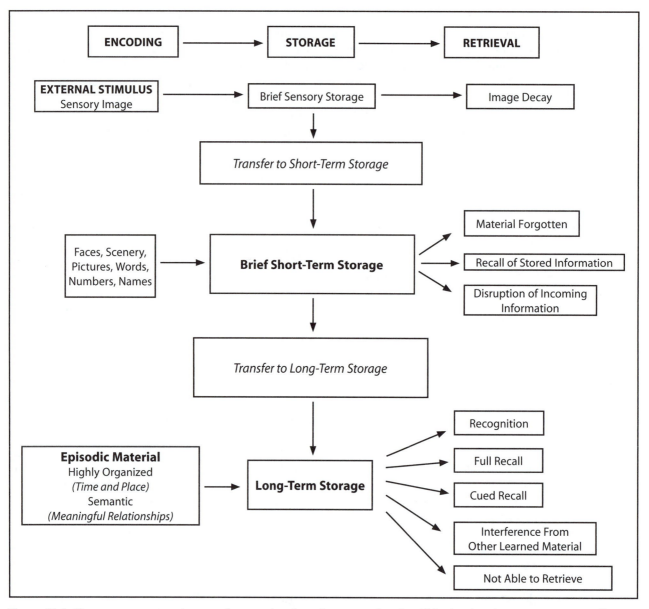

Figure 11-1. The memory system is a rough approximation of memory theories. This chart's primary purpose is to illustrate (1) the 3 phases of memory (encoding, storage, and retrieval), and (2) the 3 storage systems (sensory, short term, and long term). The additional material shows the differences in encoding, storage, and retrieval for the 3 stores.

connections so that information can be transferred to *long-term memory* for later retrieval. This process is called *consolidation*. The capacity of long-term memory in the human brain is enormous.

The recall of information stored in the long-term memory or *retrieval* of information is the next step demonstrated in this diagram. The retrieval of memories is like going through the mind's file cabinet and pulling the information needed to respond to the environment. Retrieval accuracy can be influenced by many things and may not always be entirely accurate. Retrieval of information may also be disrupted by environmental distractions, preconceived notions

of how things should be, or misinterpretation of cues that spurred the memory.

The final phase of memory is *retrieval*, which is the finding of the information when it is needed. The major age differences in memory performance are related to short-term and long-term store. There do not appear to be significant age differences in sensory storage, but there is evidence that some of the age differences in memory lie specifically in the retrieval phase. Older people may have the necessary information in storage, but they can not get to it as easily as younger people. One way to show that retrieval, rather than learning or storage, difficulties are involved is to compare 2 common methods of retrieval: recall and recognition. *Recall* is the remembrance of what has been learned or experienced, while *recognition* is the perception that an object or person has been encountered and learned before. What does it mean, then, that one can recognize material that one cannot recall? It means that the information was learned and stored, because it can be recognized as correct, but it also means that the individual could not retrieve it when asked for simple recall, although the individual can if presented with multiple choices. It means that the failure of recall was a failure in retrieval; that the search for the desired information in the storehouses of memory failed even though the information was there.

Memory Storage Related to Age

The second phase of memory, storage, involves retention or loss of information. Memory storage deals with how much and how long information can remain in storage before it is lost or displaced and forgotten. The 3 storage systems are outlined in Figure 11-1. Sensory and short-term *stores* are retained for only brief periods of time. Long-term stores are considered to have an unlimited capacity, and information is rarely lost from it.[24]

The short-term store is considered to be temporary memory with a limited capacity (ie, 6 to 9 items with acoustic encoding). Short-term storage is working on the information for proper storage in the long-term store. As a result, the short-term memory store is sometimes called *working memory*. If information is bumped out of short-term store before it is properly encoded, it probably will be lost forever.

Studies of *memory span* (the ability to recall the longest string of items, such as numbers, letters, words, that can be repeated after a single, brief presentation) show few age differences. An example would be hearing a phone number from directory assistance with no pen in hand. There is also a *recency effect*. Older individuals do best on the first (primary effect) and the last few words given (recent effect). The only age difference found is in regard to the pace with which the lists are presented. Older learners need more time.[25]

The long-term store is what people generally think of as memory. Since the probability of diseases that can affect brain tissue (ie, cardiovascular) or brain functions (ie, neurological) or psychological problems like depression is much greater in old people, this sort of loss may be a factor in age differences in memory. The biggest problem for older individuals is the ease or difficulty of accessing information in this vast repository of facts and ideas accumulated over a lifetime.

Memory Retrieval Related to Aging

Older adults also have more difficulty retrieving stored information. Difficulties in encoding and retrieval account for most of the overall age differences observed in memory experiments. Recall and recognition are key to the retrieval process.[26] An elderly individual might recognize words but cannot recall them. For example, older learners might not be able to recognize the word *basket*, but can recall seeing it when asked if *basket* was on the list. The use of efficient encoding strategies (such as organizing words by categories or alphabetically) may be especially important for recall. Word recognition shows modest gain until age 60 and only moderate decline thereafter. In contrast, the word recall shows marked age-related changes beginning in young adulthood and accelerating in old age. Older persons have a lot of information in memory storage—many files to rifle through during retrieval tasks that involve recall. Older learners benefit when retrieval cues are improved. *Cued recall* (ie, starts with..., or categories: animals, names, professions, vegetables) aids elderly individuals in better recall.[26]

Remote Memory and Aging

Recall of ancient memories is an interesting area in the study of memory and aging. One of the many myths of aging is that old people cannot remember recent events but can recall, with great clarity and detail, events in the distant past.[27] In the 19th century it was thought that information is forgotten in a sequence that is the reverse of the order in which it was acquired (Ribot's Law).[28] Memory for an event is greatest immediately following the event and then declines systematically; recognition memory declines less rapidly than recall. Evidence on age differences in remote memory suggests that such differences are very small. Even though remote memory holds up well with age, recall of recent events is usually superior. It is possible that remote memories are provided with greater detail and clarity as they have experienced enhancement and enrichment over many years of life. What is probably happening when people feel that ancient events are clearer in their mind is that a particularly sharp memory from the past is being compared with some vaguely encoded events of the last day or two.[29]

Remote memory is commonly evaluated by recall and recognition of public events (ie, World War II, President Kennedy's assassination). No age-related differences have been found in recall of recent events compared to remote events. Strong memory, called a *flashbulb memory*, occurs when a remote event had such personal significance that it has strong emotions associated with it and has been thought of (rehearsed) many times.[30]

Older people rehearse ancient memories more often (reminiscing). But the reversal of the strength of a memory is a natural phenomenon that occurs at all ages and is incorrectly viewed as a sign of aging. The truth is that memory is a notoriously leaky repository in humans of all ages.

Memory may also be affected by temporary or permanent changes in brain function or brain chemistry. Prescription drugs or voluntary use of alcohol or drugs can impede memory. These effects, fortunately, are usually transient.

Everyday memories may be a more relevant area of memory testing in older individuals. It may be difficult to encode word lists into memory and retrieve them later. However, older adults remember the time and place of an event and retrieve with ease information about income, education, or number of grandchildren. If it is practical, they have no difficulty encoding the instructions for exercise. Elders may not spontaneously organize word lists for effective recall, but ask an 80-year-old soap opera fan to recount the last 2 weeks of *The Young and the Restless* or *Days of Our Lives* and the response is likely to be confident, highly organized, and accurate.

Episodic memories concerning specific events (eg, weddings, graduations, prom) that occurred in an elder's life and *semantic memories*, which concern general context-free facts about the world, such as the meaning of words, rules of grammar and arithmetic, and personal beliefs, are often not affected by age. In contrast, *prospective memory,* which is remembering a future event (ie, a physical therapy appointment or what time to take dinner out of the oven) is where elders reported problems with forgetting. However, research indicates that this is not true. In fact older individuals remembered prospective information as well or better than younger subjects.[29] Time monitoring strategies, such as a calendar or a kitchen timer, were found to be important modalities for enhancing prospective memory for both young and older adults.

Age differences have been found to be small when written materials, texts, or novels were evaluated. A well-organized news item was retained more accurately by older readers. When there is prior knowledge about a topic and when the older individual has good verbal ability, written material was remembered well. Recalling the gist of a well-organized text passage proved to be strong in the older subjects as well as young adults. The older person may focus on the main idea, whereas the younger person may be more concerned about detail. What appears to be

inefficient processing in older people may actually reflect adaptive changes. As a result of life experiences or lower levels of energy, older individuals may focus on higher levels of meaning, devoting less attention to detail.

Self-reports of memory found that all age learners may present a distorted picture of what actually occurred. Older adults report more memory failures and are more likely to be upset when memory failure occurs. For instance, older adults reported that they forget names, routines, and objects more often than younger adults do. In unfamiliar situations, the self-reporting of memory problems was more common in the elderly.[31] External aids, such as visual cues, proved to be very helpful tools in assisting with recall, particularly with regard to prospective memory.

Problem solving is another type of cognitive activity. It is more complex and may involve aspects of learning and memory not previously discussed. *Twenty questions* is a frequently used method for testing problem-solving abilities. In this task, the individual is presented with an array of pictures or words, only one of which is the correct choice. The task is to determine the correct choice by asking less than 20 questions that can be answered with a yes-or-no response. The most efficient strategy is to ask questions that are limited (ie, "Is it a vegetable?"). Each question eliminates a set of possible answers. Through the process of elimination, the correct picture or word is selected. This test requires focus and deductions involved in solving the puzzle or problem.

Problem solving requires that a person assess the present state of a situation, define the desired state (or goal), and find a way to transform the present state to the desired state.[32] There are 4 main steps in the process of problem solving[33]: (1) understanding the problem (gathering information and identifying its important elements), (2) devising a plan (using past experiences for guidance, establishing relevant strategies, determining the efficiency of the plan), (3) carrying out the plan, and (4) reviewing what has been done (ie, was the problem solved?).

Problem solving is often the center of physical therapy interventions in all functional activities, so it is important that we pay attention to the older learner's ability to learn or relearn a functional task. Some difficulties encountered by older problem solvers include failure to ignore irrelevant information and a tendency to fixate on useless hunches. For instance, employing effective strategies with older learners determined that performance is improved with brief training procedures.

The ability to think logically about concrete or tangible problems, such as classification and conservation, develops during middle childhood. The ability to think logically about hypothetical situations or problems is achieved in adolescence. Do these abilities decline in old age? Studies of elderly individuals' performance on various tasks have yielded mixed results. Some show that the elderly do poorer than younger people; others find no age differences in formal operational tasks.[34] Success is positively correlated with higher levels of education and higher intelligence scores. Giving an older learner more time and training in a task has been shown to improve an older person's performance. The elderly possess the competence to perform a task but do not spontaneously employ the necessary strategies. After training, the elderly may not transfer the use of these strategies to the problems encountered in real life. It is important in providing physical therapy interventions that attempts be made to replicate as many possible situations and tasks that an older client might encounter upon discharge.

Memory Enhancement in Older Adults

One of the best ways for any aged individual to encode information for later retrieval is to organize it. Older subjects do not consistently organize information for later recall. In one investigation, lists of words with "clusters" based on similarity in meaning (ocean/sea) or relatedness (piano/music) were used to test age-related differences. These natural ways to organize and encode the list of words were rarely used by older learners.[35]

Another way to encode information for later retrieval is to use what are commonly called *mnemonic devices*. These techniques use verbal or visual associations to link pieces together that might not by themselves have clear relationships. For instance, many people use the name Roy G Biv (Red-Orange-Yellow-Green-Blue-Indigo-Violet) to remember the order of colors in the light spectrum or a rainbow. A common *verbal mnemonic*: "i before e, except after c," is often used when attempting to spell a word. An example of *visual mnemonics* might be "picturing" a shopping list (milk, mushrooms, and sun lotion) by visually imagining Elsie the cow under a mushroom to protect her from the sun. Encoding is facilitated by the use of imagery. Retrieval is facilitated by using cues to stimulate recall.[34]

Age differences in memory can be reduced or eliminated altogether if older adults are instructed in the use of encoding strategies and given additional time to complete memory tasks. Age differences in encoding and the use of organizational strategies are most evident in tasks that require constant attention or are new, unfamiliar tasks (eg, driving to a familiar place by a different route). Practiced tasks require little attention or conscious awareness (such as routine household chore, playing a familiar tune on a piano).

Exercising the mind by continuing to learn and being involved in challenging mental activities increases memory capacity and delays/prevents cognitive loss as previously discussed. Other important factors also are important in maintaining memory as one ages. Box 11-4 provides tips for maintaining memory.

Motor Learning in the Elderly

Beyond the cognitive components of learning (eg, memory, intelligence), motor learning is a very important part of therapeutic interventions with the elderly. Considerable age-related changes in the neuromuscular and sensory systems (described in Chapter 3) paint a picture of progressive decline. However, practicing movement patterns has been found to be very effective in re-establishing ease of movement patterns and postural control.[36] Motor learning can occur at any age. Many of the declines in functional capabilities are the result of compensation for muscle imbalances, postural changes, and pain. Rehabilitation efforts that address these compensatory problems will result in relearning of sequential movements.

Improvements in perceptual performance, as a function of activity training (ie, sensory learning), have provided new insights into the resiliency of the adult brain.[37] The acquisition and retention of skills may share many characteristics with the functional flexibility in early-life learning and development. In other words, if one method does not work, try another. This is what children are often seen doing as they learn new motor tasks along the developmental path.

The sensory distortions after a stroke or other neurological diseases, such as Parkinson's disease, may dramatically affect the approach a clinician employs for education and task training. Procedural learning impairment, however, is not an early feature of Parkinson's disease and emerges with progression of the disease.[38] For instance, patients with Parkinson's demonstrate less ability with learning sequential information and reaction or respond slower than an individual without the disease. One of the problems is that, if the sequence learning is a motor control task, difficulties that characterize Parkinson's disease (eg, tremor, impaired facility of movement, rigidity, and loss of postural reflexes) have a decrease in reaction time. Individuals with Parkinson's have difficulty initiating and performing complex, sequential movements. Practice generally leads to faster initiation and execution of movements. In one study, Parkinson's subjects improved

Box 11-4: Tips for Maintaining Memory

- Exercise your mind
  - Learn to play a new musical instrument or a new language; read, play Scrabble, take part in conversations, start new hobbies or careers
- Exercise your body
  - Aerobic exercise, stretching, and strengthening improve cognitive function
- Lower your blood pressure
  - A wonderful side effect of exercise
- Eat and drink healthy foods and beverages
  - Eat fruits, vegetables, whole grains, and omega-3 rich foods
  - Reduce alcohol intake
  - Drink sufficient water
- Stop smoking
  - Nonsmokers perform better on mental tests (reduced blood pressure, improved oxygenation, and better circulation to the brain)
- Use reminders and cues
  - Write things down
  - Follow habits for placing objects in certain places (like keys)
  - Establish cues that remind you of certain tasks and activities (eg, put books to be returned to library in a visible spot to remind you to take them back)
- Take your time to remember
  - Normal aging may slow thinking speed
- Experience compensates by establishing shortcuts
- Eliminate distractions to enhance concentration
- Slow down and pay full attention
- Learn relaxation techniques
  - Mild anxiety improves memory
  - Too much tension and anxiety impairs learning
- Maintain a positive attitude
  - Creates positive emotional states
  - Improve acquisition, consolidation, and retrieval of memories
- Reduce stress
  - Chronic stress results in significant memory dysfunction
- Get a good night's sleep
  - Reduces stress
  - Rapid eye movement (REM) sleep has been shown to help consolidate new memories
- Keep a rational perspective
  - Everyone forgets things even at younger ages
  - Do not focus on what you can not recall, focus on what you can remember
- Our total memory store comprises our wisdom
  - Use experience

speeded performance of sequential targeting tasks by practice and retained the improvement across test intervals. This learning effect for persons with Parkinson's disease supports practice as an effective rehabilitation strategy to improve motor performance of specific tasks.

Teaching Strategies in the Elderly

We spend our whole lives learning. The lifecycle is an educational process. Most learning occurs through everyday experiences. Adults of all ages benefit from formal educational experiences, such as learning about the role of exercise and heart disease, and these can assist the older adult in making lifestyle changes. Rehabilitation settings are excellent environments for learning how to compensate for deficits in sensory input, memory, and physical changes that may occur with aging or disease.

Although the misconception is that older adults may have more difficulty in the acquisition or encoding of information and in retrieving stored information, these age differences have been found to be quite minimal. Clearly, adults of all ages, in the absence of pathology, have no difficulty in learning.[39] Most of the studies on memory training involve encoding of information into long-term store and focus on training older learners in encoding strategies. When instructed in memory techniques, elderly learners utilize these strategies for motor tasks and remembering their exercise program (see Table 11-2).

Face-name recall (ie, remembering people's names) is one of the most common memory problems. Yesavage and Rose, in a series of studies, examined the effectiveness of imagery in face-name recall.[40] Elderly subjects were taught to form associations using visual imagery, and those subjects who learned this technique were found to have significantly improved face-name recall. In a subsequent study, pretraining in muscle relaxation techniques reduced performance anxiety and significantly improved learning in the same subjects using imagery.

It appears that memory performance of healthy elderly people can be improved through memory training. Whether the improvement is maintained over time has not been well documented. Rehearsal of encoding strategies is effective in keeping information in short-term memory, but organizational strategies, mnemonics, and imagery are more useful for encoding information into long-term memory. Likewise, in prospective memory (ie, remembering an appointment), use of time-monitoring strategies, like calendars or timing devices, has been shown to be particularly effective. Most of the research on memory focuses on the use of internal memory aids (encoding strategies). As most people, young or old, generally use external aids (such as making lists), it would be helpful for future research to examine external strategies for improving memory in the elderly.[41]

The elderly do just as well as younger people on recognition tasks but have more difficulty with verbatim recall. They are adept at retaining the general idea of a text but have difficulty remembering the details. These findings are important when developing a means of assessing learning in the elderly. For example, multiple-choice or true-or-false items may be more effective procedures since both involve recognition memory. Short-answer or fill-in-the-blank questions, on the other hand, would be difficult because they require recall of specific information. Providing sufficient time for recall is also important. It is important for the PTA to remember to give elder patients ample time to recall what they have been taught so they can accurately bring each step to mind and perform a task (eg, remembering to lock their wheelchair, put the foot pedals up, and get their weight forward in the chair prior to standing and subsequently taking a walk).

When teaching the elderly, it must be kept in mind that there may be some loss of vision or hearing. Compensation for these losses could facilitate processing of the information. Larger print, the avoidance of rapid speaking, seating the hearing impaired near the speaker to facilitate lip reading, and repetition of the main points are helpful in assisting the elderly in learning tasks and retaining information. The capacity to pay attention may decline with age, and repetition ensures that the learner may grasp a point even if inattentive when the information was first presented.

Many principles of learning amplify the information-processing model of learning: People learn best in pleasant surroundings, they are most likely to repeat activities that they experience as pleasant, overlearning allows task performance to be accomplished automatically, and people are most likely to remember those tasks in which they have been actively involved (ie, "doing" influences the depth of encoding and storage). In addition, if individuals "forget" something they once knew, they relearn it faster than if they had never learned it before.

Physical Fitness Relationship to Memory and Learning

Investigation reveals that a physically active lifestyle is directly linked with specific cognitive benefits in older men and women. There are benefits from physical activity beyond those attained through cognitive stimulation and extend to the oldest old regarding the relationship between physical activity and executive function, controlling for important sources of variability (eg, education, IQ).[42] This also supports the position of the 1996 report of the Surgeon General.[43] Moderate levels of activity and life-long physical activity benefit cognitive function as well as physical health. Therefore, a physically active lifestyle seems to maintain and enhance specific aspects of cognitive function in older men and women, and the benefits seem to increase with more vigorous activity participation.[44]

The Therapeutic Setting: Identifying Barriers to Memory and Learning

Memory complaints, depression, and drug use are important variables to consider when assessing memory loss. The extent of memory problems is probably exaggerated with age, especially when posited against depression, drug use, or both. There is a tendency for depressed persons to underestimate their abilities. Complaints of memory problems are not reflected in objective tests of memory performance. Drug side effects may affect cognitive function and memory (see Chapter 7 and refer to Table 11-1 for a summary of levels of mental impairment with aging). Significant correlations between depression and complaints of poor memory have been found.[45]

In the process of implementing treatment, PTs and PTAs consistently function in the role of teacher. It is important for each PTA to be aware of the content of the information he or she is conveying and the capability of the elderly individual for learning. Therapists must understand the developmental changes that occur in older persons that ultimately affect their

Table 11-1

LEVELS OF MENTAL IMPAIRMENT WITH AGING

Normal Forgetting

- Because of neuronal shrinkage and loss, information processing time increases and the effectiveness of memory decreases over time with age
- Memory is still in the average range for age, sex, and educational level and considered normal if cognitive scores are in the middle 50% or better of the comparable age group
- Shows as slight trouble remembering events and things (eg, misplacing keys from time to time or forgetting where one parked the car at the mall)

Age-Associated Memory Impairment

- When memory abilities fall below the average range (bottom 25%) for age, sex, and education
- May have significant trouble recalling recent events that may be noticeable to others
- Consistently forgets where one places things
- Has difficulty following written instructions (eg, recipes)
- Difficult to differentially diagnose from mild cognitive impairment

Mild Cognitive Impairment

- Difficult to diagnose
- Characterized by abnormal mental status scores on neuropsychological testing performance
- Deficits in abstract thinking, language, visual-spatial functioning, and problem solving
- Amnestic type of memory loss (forget the past); usually progresses to Alzheimer's disease
- Experience depression, apathy, or irritability
- Deficit recall of recent information
- Impaired performance on memory tests
- Essentially normal judgment, perception, and reasoning skills initially
- Normal functioning in ADL

Dementia

- Any disease that results in death or dysfunction of neurons with symptoms of memory loss and cognitive deficits
- Significant difficulties performing ADL
- Strongly correlated with advancing age
- Not reversible and progressive in nature

learning capabilities and adapt instructional sessions to enhance the learning process (Box 11-5).

Documented changes in sensory function can limit or distort reception, perception, monitoring, feedback, and transmission of incoming stimuli. A general slowing of neural processes seems to occur with age as demonstrated by decreased conduction over multisynaptic pathways. There is also a progressive age-related change in response to touch, proprioceptive, vestibular, and other stimuli. There are reported visual declines in acuity, accommodation, field luminance factors, color sensitivity, perception of ambiguous figures and illusions, figural aftereffects, serial learning, figure ground organization, closure, spatial abilities, and visual memory.[46]

Aging changes also occur in the outer ear, the inner ear, and central auditory processing that are reflected in a decreased ability to inhibit background noise and other irrelevant signals and decrease auditory acuity and perception of high frequency sounds. The older person's ability to hear and understand speech in less than ideal listening environments is particularly affected. Attention deficits further compromise the accuracy of input and registration

Box 11-5: **Primary Aging Changes That Affect Memory and Learning**

Hearing loss	Inability to accurately encode auditory information
Visual problems	Unable to accurately read instructions or see objects or materials presented for learning; inaccurately encodes visual information
Sensory loss	Poses difficulty in accurately perceiving sensory input from surroundings, the environment, situation, or activity; poor perception can lead to safety issues and create difficulty in learning new tasks
Proprioceptive changes	Inability to accurately assess positions for reproduction of attempted learning tasks; impacts awareness of limb or body affecting safety
Kinesthetic changes	Difficulty learning or relearning motor patterns needed for purposeful functional tasks
Vestibular problems	Unable to accurately monitor head position or detect head movement; any head movement causes dizziness and a feeling of instability during functional tasks; often results in fear of falling and self-restriction of activity

of stimuli. Inaccuracies in the first stage of learning (input and registration) affect the subsequent stages of information processing. Stimuli that is not adequately registered cannot be effectively encoded (stored) or retrieved.

A slowing in learning ability in the elderly is reported whether a simple motor movement or a complex cognitive process is involved. Older adults benefit from having longer periods of time for inspection and response. Self-paced learning leads to the best performance. The elderly tend to make more errors of omission than errors of commission. For example, they may lock their wheelchair and get the footrests out of the way, but neglect to position their feet directly under them prior to standing. Concrete information is learned more accurately and efficiently than abstract information, and concept learning is also better when information is conveyed in concrete (as opposed to abstract) language. When the opportunity to practice psychomotor tasks is given, learning and performance improve, regardless of the difficulty of the task. When unlimited numbers of attempts are given for the mastery of a task, the elderly can recall information as effectively as younger persons; however, the elderly need more attempts to attain this goal. Elderly who are given verbal feedback concerning their performance improve significantly on subsequent related problems. As a general rule, they perform best when instructions are given in a supportive manner. The factors that influence older adult learning need to be considered if learning is to be accomplished in the therapeutic setting.

In considering the age-related changes in learning, it becomes clear that health care professionals who interact with the elderly must be particularly sensitive to learner needs and diligent in structuring teaching settings to maximize and individualize

learning. For example, some people are auditory learners and some are visual learners, while others need kinesthetic input and learn by doing. Some tasks are better taught by demonstration and some by verbal instruction. Most adult learners develop a preference for learning that is based on childhood learning patterns.[47] An assessment of the patient's learning style is a fundamental step prior to beginning any educational activity. Determining the patient's learning style will help identify the preferred conditions under which instruction is likely to be most effective. The most frequently used method of delineating learning styles is in describing visual, auditory, and kinesthetic learners. Table 11-2 outlines the characteristics and suggested teaching strategies for these types of adult learners.

Visual learners prefer seeing what they are learning. Pictures and images help them understand ideas and information better than explanations. A phrase these learners may use is, "The way I see it is." The teacher needs to create a mental image for the visual learner as this will assist in the ease of holding onto the information. If a visual learner is to master a skill, written instructions must be provided. Visual learners will read and follow the directions as they work and will appreciate it even more when diagrams are included.

Auditory learners prefer to hear the message or instruction being given. These adults prefer to have someone talk them through a process rather than reading about it first. A phrase they may use is, "I hear what you are saying." Some of these learners may even talk themselves through a task and should be given the freedom to do so when possible. Adults with this learning style remember verbal instructions well and prefer someone else read the directions to them while they do the physical work or task.

Table 11-2

LEARNING STYLES IN THE ELDERLY

LEARNING STYLE	CHARACTERISTICS	SUGGESTED TEACHING STRATEGIES
Visual	Prefers written instructions Provide photographs Provide illustrations Prefers a timeline or calendar Sensitive to visual distractions Remembers visual materials Studies written material	Provide interesting visual material in different formats Provide organized visual presentations Provide handout material A variety of technologies (computer, videos, photos)
Auditory	Remembers what they say and what other people say to them Remembers through verbal repetition Repeats what they have heard aloud to confirm material to be learned Prefers to discuss ideas they do not immediately understand Remembers verbal instructions well Has difficulty working quietly for long Easily distracted by noise and silence Verbally expresses interest Enjoys group activities/discussions	Include multimedia applications utilizing sounds, music, video, or taped instructions Vary speed of material presented (slow down) Background music helps auditory learner to focus if environment is quiet Write down key points/words to enhance verbal message or instruction Verbally review written points to avoid confusion Vary pitch and volume to help create aural texture Rephrase points and questions in different ways Place in a position they can hear in, ensuring that hearing aids are in working order and room is not too noisy
Kinesthetic	Learns by doing Remembers best by getting actively/ physically involved in learning Writes notes but rarely refers to Enjoys computer learning Has trouble staying still for long Enjoys hands-on activities Tends to fiddle with things while listening to instruction/working Remembers what they do and experience through movement or sensory stimulation Enjoys using tools or lessons that involve active participation Motor memory occurs quickly Has good motor coordination	Encourage learner to take notes Permit frequent breaks in teaching session to allow learner to practice segments of movement Encourage the learner to verbalize each step Incorporate multimedia information into teaching Provide tactile-kinesthetic activities during sessions Have product samples available for practice Encourage the learner to demonstrate learned task

Kinesthetic learners want to sense the position and movement of the skill or task. These learners generally do not like lecture or discussion classes but prefer those that allow them to "do something." These adults do well learning a physical skill when there are materials available for hands-on practice.

Although it is important to determine what type of learner a patient is in order to facilitate learning, it is also a good idea to provide information in a variety of formats. It is easier for PTAs to educate an older individual in the style he or she prefers, yet, with the elderly, the PTA may have to step out of his or her comfort zone and match the patient's learning style.

The learning environment determines and influences the educational experience. An environment that is conducive to learning promotes the process, and as a general rule, an environment that is familiar to the learner is the preferred environment for learning new skills. Familiar settings induce a sense of security in which pertinent new information can be attended to. Learning in the natural environment (ie, the home or work environment) eliminates the need for the client to transfer or generalize information to a home or work setting. In unfamiliar settings, the learner is more likely to be attracted by, and responsive to, novel environmental stimuli. When unfamiliar treatment environments must be used, they should be structured to simulate the natural environment whenever possible and to diminish the number of competing stimuli. Once a new skill is learned, practice in a variety of environments will assist in generalizing its use.

Environments and procedures that are orderly and organized enhance the learner's ability to process information in an orderly and organized fashion. A cluttered or busy environment creates irrelevant, distracting stimuli in the learning environment and impedes the learning process.

Physical and psychological comfort is an important consideration in the treatment setting. Noise levels, color schemes, adequate lighting, ventilation, and comfortable room temperature should all be considered. Glossy, highly waxed floors and work surfaces that distort and reflect light should be avoided. Comfortable chairs and proper table heights are also recommended. Background noises (ie, computers, air conditioners, running water, appliances) should be eliminated so they do not interfere with foreground sound perception. Most kitchen and bathroom settings compromise hearing; the lack of carpeting, drapes, and padded furniture impose additional noise and reverberating sounds.

The personality of the therapist is also an important source of psychological comfort for the elderly learner. A calm, patient, unhurried, interested, knowledgeable, and assured health care provider can decrease situational stress and promote a climate of acceptance and reassurance. Conveying verbally and nonverbally that the elderly individual is a valued person with valuable ideas to contribute and that experimentation and failure are important processes in learning new skills enhances the environment. Positive reinforcement for good efforts, as well as good performance, is crucial in facilitating the learning process in an elderly person.

Teaching methods and techniques in the therapeutic setting include all those behaviors employed by instructors to communicate particular pieces of information to the learners. Variables that influence learning include the organization of material, the rate of presentation, the choice of task, the mode of presentation, and covert strategies.

New information needs to be presented in a highly organized fashion. Visual displays should be simple configurations that explicitly demonstrate a few salient points. Verbal instructions and directions must emphasize the most important information in a simple manner. Written instructions need to be clear with section headings, large print, and emphasis on major points. Only information relevant to the task at hand should be presented. Differences and similarities between new and old tasks need to be identified. Whole-part–whole learning is a recommended strategy with the elderly. With this technique, the entire task and anticipated goal are introduced, then the parts are identified, and each is related to the preceding steps and to the whole. For instance, the person whose end goal is independent meal preparation has to accomplish many component steps in the process of reaching that goal. It is important for the individual to understand the importance of each step (eg, mobilizing joints and strengthening particular muscle groups or increasing fine motor coordination and endurance) and how each step relates to the end objective.

Information should be presented at a rate compatible with the learner's ability to comprehend and respond. Generally, this rate will correspond with the complexity of concepts and tasks being taught. Simple, concrete tasks require less time to learn. When instructing the elderly, directions should be presented slowly and ample time for practice provided. If fatigue or confusion occurs, the instructional sessions should be shortened.

It is important that the choice of task be directed toward attainment of a pre-established, desirable goal. The task should allow the learner to express and fulfill his or her own personal needs (eg, creativity, socialization, mastery). Tasks that interest the learner should be selected, if possible. A preliminary development of an interest inventory will identify what is important to the individual learner. In other words, activities chosen need to be relevant and meaningful to the learner and the purpose for learning each task needs to be clear. Self-care tasks seem to have the greatest relevance for most elderly individuals. Goals, such as transfer training, eating, and dressing, are concrete and usually experienced as meaningful. Practice of self-care tasks in a familiar environment is best for obtaining follow through of the learned tasks. Activities, such as mat exercises or fine hand coordination exercises, may not seem relevant to the older learner. In these cases, it is important to relate the activities to the established treatment goals. Explain and demonstrate the mobility and strengthening components of mat activities as they relate to functional goals. This will help in making the activities more concrete and necessary for accomplishing the end goal.

Tasks should be sufficiently challenging but easy enough to ensure successful experiences. Building on past successes will promote advancing toward the treatment goals. A knowledgeable, enthusiastic therapist can also help to motivate learners to engage in the necessary tasks to be learned.

Presentation of information to an older learner is very important. Instructions to the older learner need to be concrete, simple, and clear. Information should be presented one step at a time. The learner should be given the opportunity to practice each step before subsequent steps are introduced. Carefully planned demonstrations are also helpful modes of education. With a good demonstration, the learner is given the opportunity to initiate the exact movement until each step has been completed. It is also advised that demonstrations be performed in the same position as the learner will be in for the task. For demonstration to be effective in influencing the learner, it requires skillful observation and visual memorization of the teacher's movements, followed by a transfer of the complex visual information to an opposite orientation, which can be frustrating for the older learner.

To accommodate for hearing loss, the instructor needs to be within 10 feet of the listener, use a low-pitched speaking voice with a moderate volume (shouting distorts sound in the presence of hearing losses), and position him- or herself so that the listener can see the speaker's mouth. Since much information is communicated by facial expression, gestures and body language are important facilitators for conveying information. Verbal and nonverbal language needs to be congruent because understanding is enhanced when nonconfusing visual stimuli accompany auditory information.

To compensate for some of the aging changes in vision, using a large, bold print on a solid background is helpful for printed material. The use of a visual aid, such as a magnifying glass, may be used when large print is not available. Lighting is also important; too much light can create glare, and too little light will diminish the older learner's ability to see anything.

Motor learning may be enhanced by physically guiding the learner's extremities through the desired patterns of movement. It is preferable for the teacher to stand behind the learner so that the learner can concentrate on the sensation of movement. Movements should be repeated several times without any alteration in the motion. The learner is eventually weaned from guided patterning and asked to perform the movement without the teacher's verbal, tactile, proprioceptive stimulus, and motor assistance.

There are several covert strategies for enhancing memory. Older adults tend not to spontaneously use organized methods or ploys to enhance learning and memory, as previously discussed; they do, however, benefit from instructions in memory strategies. The use of memory strategies is a means of compensating for real or anticipated deficits in memory.

It is important to optimize overall health status by implementing the concept of *independence*. The more one can do for oneself, the more one is capable of doing independently. The more that is done for an aged individual, the less capable he or she becomes of functioning on an optimal independent level and the more likely the progression of a disability. The advancing stages of disabilities increase the individual's vulnerability to illness, emotional stress, and injury. Aged persons' subjective appraisal of their health status influences how they react to their symptoms, how vulnerable they consider themselves, and when they decide they can or cannot accomplish an activity. Often an aged person's self-appraisal of her or his health is a good predictor of rehabilitation clinician's evaluation of health and functional status, but such assessments may also differ in many ways. In older persons, perceptions of their health may be determined in large part by their level of psychological well being and by whether or not they continue in rewarding roles and activities.[48]

As an aged individual's perception of his or her health status is an important motivator in compliance with a rehabilitation program, it is important to discuss this further. One notable study showed that even when age, sex, and health status (as evaluated by physicians) were controlled for, perceived health and mortality from heart disease were strongly related.[48] Those who rated their health as poor were 2 to 3 times as likely to die as those who rated their health as excellent. Despite awareness among older persons of their actual state of health, the aged are known to fail to report serious symptoms and wait longer than younger persons to seek help. It is with this in mind that rehabilitation professionals need to listen carefully to their aged clients. Older individuals are far from hypochondriacs and deserve serious attention when they bring complaints to their caregivers. Their perceived level of health will greatly impact the outcomes of functional goals in the geriatric rehabilitation setting, whether it is acute, subacute, rehabilitative, home, or chronic care. Poorly perceived health translates to problems with motivation and participation in the rehabilitation process.

Motivation may be a barrier to learning. Adults learn best when convinced of the need for knowing the information. Often a life experience or situation stimulates the motivation to learn.[49] Meaningful learning can be intrinsically motivating. The key to using adults' natural motivation to learn is tapping into their most teachable moments. For example, a patient concerned about how urinary incontinence is affecting her lifestyle might be motivated to learn about Kegel exercises more so than her counterpart who is not experiencing incontinence. The factors that serve as sources of motivation for adult learning are presented in Table 11-3. Health care providers involved in educating adults need to convey a desire to connect with the learner. Providing a challenge to the learner without causing frustration is additionally important. Above all, provide feedback and positive reinforcement about what has been learned.

Improvement in rehabilitation tasks correlated well with the patient's own appraisal of her or his potential for recovery but not very well with others' appraisal. Positive reinforcement (frequent positive feedback) for older persons in rehabilitation greatly improved their performance and feelings of success.[50] This indicates that aged persons can improve in their physical functioning when modifications in therapeutic interventions provide more frequent feedback. Some research indicates that older persons with chronic illness have low initial aspirations with regard to their ability to perform various tasks. As situations in which successes or failures occurred, their aspirations changed to more closely reflect their abilities. When subjects were given an unsolvable problem, younger subjects ascribed their failure to not trying hard enough, while older subjects ascribed their failure to inability. These age differences indicate a variation in the perceived locus of control. This holds extreme importance in the rehabilitation potential of an aged person. If the cause of failure is seen as an unbeatable obstacle by a person, future failure to succeed can be expected.

Aged individuals may have a higher anxiety level in rehabilitation situations because they fear failure or are afraid of looking bad in front of their family or therapist. If anxiety is high enough, then the behavior is redirected toward reducing the anxiety rather than accomplishing the task. Individuals set their own goals for task achievement even if they are directed toward meeting the therapist's goals.

Depression also plays a big role in learning and memory. Verbal learning and memory of elderly patients with major depression and nondepressed older people show a marked difference.[51] Except for verbal retention, the depressive group had deficits in most aspects of performance, including cued and uncued recall and delayed recognition memory. In depressed elders, performance declined more rapidly with age than did the performance of older adults without depression. The results indicate that the integrity of learning and memory are compromised in the presence of late-life depression. Depression in an elderly individual in a rehabilitation setting needs to be addressed as part of a comprehensive therapeutic intervention. Failure to do so will result in poor learning capabilities for new activities, and failure at a task could further exacerbate the depression.

Table 11-3

SOURCES OF MOTIVATION

- Social relationships
  - Motivated to learn to please family (especially grandchildren), friends, therapist; inspired to make progress because of association with others
- External expectations
  - Compliance with instructions from someone else; fulfills recommendations from someone in authority
- Social welfare
  - To return to productivity such as employment, improve participation in community and family activities
- Personal advancement
  - To return to previous level of independence or to learn new skills for advancement in life
- Stimulation or escape
  - To reduce boredom or to find a diversion for routine activities; to add excitement and stimulation to everyday life
- Cognitive interest
  - To learn for the sake of learning; to satisfy an inquiring mind or lifelong interest

CULTURE AND EDUCATION OF THE GERIATRIC PATIENT

Culture refers to integrated patterns of human behavior that include the language, thoughts, communications, actions, customs, beliefs, values, and institutions of racial, ethnic, religious, or social groups.[52]

PTs caring for older adults face challenges in the evaluation and intervention processes as they attempt to provide adequate educational programs. Developing effective strategies and skills that address the delivery of culturally competent care is critical in health care education and practice. These strategies and skills are driven by cultural factors, which can prove to be enhancements or impediments to favorable educational or health care outcomes.[53] When the distinctive cultural factor of race or ethnicity is combined with the unique features of age, the challenges are multiplied. It is imperative that rehabilitation professionals increase their knowledge, awareness, and sensitivity toward diverse patient populations.[53]

Understanding the sociocultural perspective of health, illness, and healing of the older adult and his or her social network is aided by knowledge of different styles of communication and previous experiences with allopathic and traditional health care providers. Beyond the surface structures of culture (eg, language, music, food, clothing), the culturally competent PT must be aware of the deep structure of culture, racial, and ethnic differences and the effect of social, environmental, and historical factors on health behaviors. The clinician needs to demonstrate culturally congruent behaviors and show appreciation and respect for cultural differences.[54]

Sensitivity to health beliefs and awareness of cultural concepts related to disease, as well as treatments used by various ethnicities, will create a culturally welcoming, nonjudgmental, flexible, and therapeutic environment. A therapist's response and adaptation to different cultural contexts and circumstances can set the stage for enhancing the rehabilitation outcomes.[55]

The environmental design should also be linguistically welcoming. Providing posters, written materials, instructions, and other informative visual media in the patient's language is fundamental for learning. It is important to provide a therapist, when possible, that is able to speak the same language if the patient does not speak English. If such a therapist is not available, having a family member or friend who understands both languages and can translate information is a crucial component for teaching and therapeutic intervention.

Educational approaches must be suitable for the populations being taught. Nonetheless, the same educational principles previously discussed can easily be applied regardless of cultural or ethnic background. Adults, regardless of culture or ethnicity, are self-directed. With this in mind, they do not need to be told everything. When rehabilitating older individuals, it is important to allow them to do their own problem solving and work through their own difficulties. Older adults have a wealth of experiences from which they can draw to enhance learning. It is important the PT tap into these experiences to discover the learning styles of the patients. Learning occurs more rapidly if the elder considers the task important. Therefore, it is essential that the older adult know why he or she needs to perform the task. For example, telling the older individual that a specialized balance exercise is directed at preventing falls will most likely result in his or her engagement in this exercise.

Patient educational goals focus on understanding of health status, care, and informed decision making; the ability to cope with disease and treatment; and the promotion of a healthful lifestyle as a standard of care. To address these goals requires that the practitioner teaching the patient, and his or her family, to assess the patient's current knowledge level, learning needs, and readiness to learn. The teaching plan is based on these assessments and is documented in the patient record. Learning objectives or expected outcomes are identified, and the teaching plan is developed. Throughout the teaching-learning process, the PTA evaluates learning outcomes and teaching strategies. Has the patient or family member truly learned? Demonstration of learning outcomes is more than simply repeating facts and information. Can the patient or family member accurately demonstrate skills or apply information taught? Strategies for evaluation include the following:

- Direct questioning

- Return demonstration by the patient

- Indirect questioning (ask what patients will tell their spouse/families that they have learned)

- Asking patients to assist in the ADL or other functional task ("I brought your clothes for the day. Do as much as you can, and I'll here to help and guide you.").

PTAs are teachers and have an obligation to facilitate learning for patients and families. Accurate assessment of learning needs and readiness includes assessment of cultural values and health practices as well as literacy issues. Every effort should be made to ensure that teaching plans incorporate patients' cultural values and beliefs. By addressing cultural and literacy issues, PTAs can facilitate successful learning outcomes for patients and families, enhancing their ability to cope with illness and improve overall health.

Cultural beliefs related to illness affect how and when health care is sought and what health practices will be followed. Often individuals will follow traditional health practices before seeking the medical professional, as a last resort. For example, when urinary incontinence is viewed as a normal part of aging and a doctor is viewed as providing help with a problem, an incontinent person may not see a doctor unless there is an additional problem. An understanding of cultural influences on health care practices enables the PTA to effectively individualize the teaching plan. Presenting the information in the learner's cultural context, and including certain folk practices, if not detrimental, will strengthen the plan of care for the patient.[56]

The individual's or family's past experience with health care providers influences the elder's adherence and continuation of use of health care services. Understanding these experiences from the patient's perspective can strengthen the relationship, and misconceptions and culturally offensive behaviors can be avoided.[56]

It should be stressed that the elder patient's perspective of his or her health is no less important than that of the PT's in negotiating a therapeutic plan. Comparison of the therapist's model with that of the patient can enable the clinician to identify major differences that can affect clinical management. In applying a culturally sensitive framework, it is important for health care professionals to recognize the influence that individual cultures have on their attitudes toward health.[57] It is equally important to emphasize the cross-cultural differences that exist and realize that our view of healing and rehabilitation is seen through the lens of the American and Western culture.[58] The PTA may be able to provide important and helpful insights to the PT—indeed, the rest of the team—about issues of cultural importance to the elder's care since he or she often spends the most time with him or her.

EDUCATING CAREGIVERS IN GERIATRIC SETTINGS

Caring for an elderly parent, relative, or friend can be satisfying and enjoyable, often resulting in an improved relationship for both parties. Most children help their parents willingly when needed and derive satisfaction from doing so. Caregiving can also serve as a substitute for a void in someone's life and enhance feelings of self-worth. For elderly spouses, the caregiver role may help to compensate for the loss of other roles as one ages, providing a new sense of usefulness. In some instances, accepting a caregiving role helps put other stresses in perspective.[59]

Comprehensive treatment for older individuals at home should include informational and instructional materials accompanied by complete and detailed directions for their caregivers and perhaps, interventions for their family caregivers, especially if the caregiver is also elderly. Caregivers need to know how to care for their loved one prior to discharge from any geriatric setting. Caregivers typically do not need, or want, detailed background information about the task to be accomplished. Rather, they usually want the most direct, basic, and practical information on "how to" strategies. The most frequently used intervention strategies focus on caregiver education related to managing ADL and also emotional support for the transition from care setting to home. Discharge planning should begin on admission. PTs should strive to establish a policy with their facility, whereby, they automatically receive a referral for evaluation fall-risk assessment, and discharge planning as a part of admission orders for anyone over the age of 65.

The results of educational interventions with caregivers are varied but generally result in an improved knowledge of the illness and how to care for their loved one.[60] It must be remembered, that the stress related to the discharge process may be overwhelming for caregivers; they are getting bombarded with information and education from every discipline involved with the elder's care and as a result, they may experience information overload. Therefore, it is important to provide verbal and written instructions, provide multiple sessions for demonstration and practice, and follow-up with a review to determine proficiency. Ideally, a home visit is helpful in transference of learning into the real-life environment, rather than the virtual environments that we attempt to provide in geriatric settings. It is imperative that caregiver education starts early, includes written and verbal informational and instructional materials, and be provided with instructions and practice of the skills he or she will need as a caregiver at home.

Caregiving responsibilities are usually assumed by a spouse, child, or another relative (ie, sibling, grandchild, niece, or nephew) or neighbors or friends. In addition, caregivers are usually female, over the age of 65, and may have health issues of their own. Education strategies are similar to those already presented for the elderly patient in rehabilitation.

Caregiver roles traditionally include performing basic physical tasks, such as transferring, bathing, positioning, toileting, feeding, managing medications, as well as providing transportation, cooking, housecleaning, and shopping. With older individuals spending shorter times in formal care settings, caregiver roles are often expanded to include technical tasks, such as changing a colostomy bag, cleaning and redressing wounds, caring for and using a feeding tube, or administering injections.

Caregivers need clear and consistent instructions in how to provide proper and safe care for their family member. Effective caregiver education that addresses all aspects of the patient's care as well as self-care for the caregiver enhances physical, medical, and emotional outcomes of the recipient of care and reduces the stress and burden experience by the caregiver. All too often, caregiver instruction is brief, provided only verbally and often delivered within a few hours of the elder's discharge from the formal care setting. This leaves little time for questions, problem solving, or time to practice the skills and activities that are expected. The caregiver goes home frightened that he or she will make a mistake, forget to do something, or injure his or her loved one. Meanwhile, the recipient of care is also overwhelmed with information and instruction and goes home feeling insecure about the abilities of his or her caregiver. This can easily lead to frustration and conflict in "how to" accomplish a functional task.

One educational strategy is helpful for optimizing the success in the acquisition of caregiving skills. Teaching *concrete problem-solving* skills can be empowering. Instead of focusing on the problems and challenges that a caregiver may have, this approach is based on posing situations that might occur in the home setting. Caregivers learn methods that will assist them in defining the problems, setting goals, constructing knowledge, identifying resources, and building the capacity through the skill development for problem solving. Learning the skill of problem solving will lead to the use of logic for overcoming any situation that may occur. Concrete problem-solving practice has the potential of assisting the caregiver to calmly approach a problem that may be encountered at home.

The goal of physical therapy in caregiver education will be to instruct the caregiver in the physical management for ADL for their loved one but also determine any physical limitations and stresses that the caregiver may experience. Caregiving brings added stress to daily routines. It is important that the caregiver learn to identify the sources of the stress, recognize when he or she is stressed, and identify ways of controlling it. Some suggestions include the following:

- Setting realistic goals and expectations
- Establishing caregiver's own physical limits
- Knowing when to ask for and accept help
- Talking to caregiver about taking care of him- or herself by
  - Expressing his or her feelings
  - Maintaining his or her health
  - Taking time for him- or herself
- Involving other people by:
  - Holding a family conference
  - Seeking professional assistance
  - Using community resources.

Caregivers will be most responsive to educational programs that meet their immediate and specific needs and provide skills and tools they need to solve problems. Caregivers need to identify their learning needs and help to develop the learning plan. Caregivers—especially older caregivers—may need help in overcoming inhibitions, fears, and beliefs about their abilities to carry out unfamiliar tasks. They must also establish knowledge for how to access family and community resources and learn to ask for help.

Caregiving should not be based solely on the needs of the receiver. The caregiver must attend to his or her needs and the needs of other family members.[61] Although providing care to a family member can be a rewarding experience, it can lead to significant stress, both psychologically and physically. Therefore, it is important that the PT and PTA recognize and identify possible stressors and implement strategies that minimize caregiver stress. By educating the caregiver to be a critical thinker when assessing problems, developing solutions, and mobilizing resources to overcome the problem, caregiver stresses are significantly reduced.[54] It is important to give positive feedback to caregiver learning, compliment a task done correctly, and set up practice sessions to allow success to increase the confidence of both the caregiver and the elderly patient.

CONCLUSION

As rehabilitation professionals, providing education is a large portion of our physical therapy interventions. PTs and PTAs educate patients, consumers, caregivers, health care providers, students, legislators, and others. This chapter has discussed the aging changes that may result in difficulty with communication, learning, and memory in the older adult. This changes the teaching strategies often used in providing information and instructional material to the older adult.

With aging comes a gradual decline in cognitive function. How much cognition function remains intact depends on lifestyle choices. Cognitive learning and memory abilities, particularly those involving speed and problem solving, show some decline related to aging. An elderly individual's competence may decline, and environmental influences may also be a prominent impediment to learning. If the elderly patient is to maximize the outcomes from therapeutic interactions, therapists must pay attention to communication, learning style, sensory changes, motivation, the environments in which they teach older adults, as well as to the methods used to teach.

PEARLS

- Learning is defined as the acquisition of a new skill or information through practice and experience, whereas remembering is the retrieval of information that has been stored in memory.

- Encoding and retrieval problems are the cause of memory difficulties in older adults, and instruction in organizing, slower pacing, and verbal and visual associations can improve performance.

- Sensory and short-term stores of memory are limited in capacity, whereas long-term stores have unlimited storage capacity.

- Problem-solving ability appears to decline with age and may be due to education level and fluid intelligence. Training can improve older people's problem-solving ability but they may not transfer these strategies to problems encountered in real life.

- Memory performance of the healthy elderly can be improved through memory training.

- Orderly environments enhance an older person's ability to process information, whereas a cluttered and busy environment creates distracting stimuli and impedes learning.

- Variables that positively influence learning for the older person are:

  o A supportive approach by the therapist with much positive reinforcement

  o A highly organized presentation of material that is simple, concrete, and step-by-step

  o An appropriate rate of presentation of information

  o Self-chosen meaningful tasks

  o Using memory strategies

  o Having ample time for repetition and practice

- An elderly person's perception of his or her health status will impact the progress he or she makes in rehabilitation

- Depression, anxiety, and motivation will influence learning and memory abilities

- Caregiver education is an integral part of comprehensive education and teaching

- One is never too old to learn.

A good resource for enhancing education, learning, and memory is provided by the National Institute on Aging. *Toolkit for Trainers* is a free downloadable training curriculum that teaches older adults how to find reliable health information online at www.nih-seniorhealth.gov/toolkit, from the NIH Senior Health Web site. The toolkit comes with lesson plans, student worksheets, health-oriented Web-searching exercises, and glossaries. An introductory online video gives an overview, and trainer tips help with creating a senior-friendly classroom environment.

REFERENCES

1. Hess TM. Memory and aging in context. *Psychol Bull.* 2005;131:383-406.
2. Zauszniewski JA, Martin MH. Developmental task achievement and learned resourcefulness in healthy older adults. *Arch Psychiatr Nurs.* 1999;13:41-47.
3. D'Eredita MA, Hoyer WJ. An examination of the effects of adult age on explicit and implicit learning of figural sequences. *Mem Cognit.* 1999;27:890-895.
4. Vakil E, Agmon-Ashkenazi D. Baseline performance and learning rate of procedural and declarative memory tasks: younger versus older adults. *J Gerontol B Psychol Sci Soc Sci.* 1997;52:P229-P234.
5. Spitzer M, Bellemann ME, Kammer T, et al. Functional MR imaging of semantic information processing and learning-related effects using psychometrically controlled stimulation paradigms. *Brain Res Cogn Brain Res.* 1996;4:149-161.
6. Karni A, Meyer G, Jezzard P, Adams MM, Turner R, Ungerleider LG. Functional MRI evidence for adult motor cortex plasticity during motor skill learning. *Nature.* 1995;377:155-158.
7. Cohen NJ, Squire LR. Preserved learning and retention of pattern analyzing skills in amnesia: dissociation of knowing how and knowing that. *Science.* 1980;210:207-210.
8. Deary IJ, Bastin ME, Pattie A, et al. White matter integrity and cognition in childhood and old age. *Neurology.* 2006;66:505-512.
9. Crawford S, Channon S. Dissociation between performance on abstract tests of executive function and problem solving in real-life-type situations in normal aging. *Aging Mental Health.* 2002;6:12-21.
10. Allain P, Nicoleau S, Pinon K, et al. Executive functioning in normal aging: a study of action planning using the Zoo Map Test. *Brain Cogn.* 2005;57:4-7.
11. Norman GR. The adult learner: a mythical species. *Acad Med.* 1999;74:886-889.

12. Vakil E, Agmon-Ashkenazi D. Baseline performance and learning rate of procedural and declarative memory tasks: younger versus older adults. *J Gerontol B Psychol Sci Soc Sci.* 1997;52:P229-P234.

13. Schwartz BS, Glass TA, Bolla KI, et al. Disparities in cognitive functioning by race/ethnicity in the Baltimore memory study. *Environ Health Perspect.* 2004;112:314-320.

14. Eisendorfer D, Nowlin J, Wilkie F. Improvement of learning in the aged by modification of autonomic nervous system activity. *Science.* 2000;170:1327-1329.

15. Royall DR, Palmer R, Chiodo LK, Polk MJ. Executive control mediates memory's association with change in instrumental activities of daily living: the Freedom House Study. *J Am Geriatr Soc.* 2005;53:11-17.

16. Sekiya H, Magill RA, Sidaway B, Anderson DI. The contextual interference effect for skill variations from the same and different generalized motor programs. *Res Q Exerc Sport.* 1994;65:330-338.

17. Bennett DA, Schneider JA, Buchman AS, Mendes de Leon C, Bienias JL, Wilson RS. The Rush Memory and Aging Project: study design and baseline characteristics of the study cohort. *Neuroepidemiology.* 2005;25:163-175.

18. Hohaus L. Remembering to age successfully: evaluation of a successful aging approach to memory enhancement. *Int Psychogeriatr.* 2007;19:137-150.

19. Sekuler R, McLaughlin C, Kahana MJ, Wingfield A, Yotsumoto Y. Short-term visual recognition and temporal order memory are both well-preserved in aging. *Psychol Aging.* 2006;21:632-637.

20. Weaver CJ, Maruff P, Collie A, Masters C. Mild memory impairment in healthy older adults is distinct from normal aging. *Brain Cognition.* 2006;60:146-155.

21. Buckner RL. Memory and executive function in aging and AD: multiple factors that cause decline and reserve factors that compensate *Neuron.* 2004;44:195-208.

22. Morasco BJ, Gfeller JD, Chibnall JT. The relationship between measures of psychopathology, intelligence, and memory among adults seen for psychoeducational assessment. *Arch Clin Neuropsychol.* 2006;21:297-301.

23. de Fockert JW. Keeping priorities: the role of working memory and selective attention in cognitive aging. *Sci Aging Knowledge Environ.* 2005;34.

24. Friedman D, Nessler D, Johnson R. Memory encoding and retrieval in the aging brain. *Clin EEG Neurosci.* 2007;38:2-7.

25. Nilsson LG. Memory function in normal aging. *Acta Neurol Scand Suppl.* 2003;179:7-13.

26. Dodson CS, Bawa S, Slotnick SD. Aging, source memory, and misrecollections. *J Exp Psychol Learn Mem Cogn.* 2007;33:169-181.

27. McKinnon MC, Black SE, Miller B, Moscovitch M, Levine B. Autobiographical memory in semantic dementia: implication for theories of limbic-neocortical interaction in remote memory. *Neuropsychologia.* 2006;44:2421-2129.

28. Nilson A. The relativity of abnormity. *Sven Med Tidskr.* 2006;10:101-118.

29. Piolino P, Desgranges B, Benali K, Eustache F. Episodic and semantic remote autobiographical memory in ageing. *Memory.* 2002;10:239-257.

30. Cohen G, Conway MA, Maylor EA. Flashbulb memories in older adults. *Psychol Aging.* 1994;9:454-463.

31. Schmutte T, Harris S, Levin R, Zweig R, Katz M, Lipton R. The relation between cognitive functioning and self-reported sleep complaints in nondemented older adults: results from the Bronx aging study. *Behav Sleep Med.* 2007;5:39-56.

32. Blanchard-Fields F, Mienaltowski A, Seay RB. Age differences in everyday problem-solving effectiveness: older adults select more effective strategies for interpersonal problems. *J Gerontol B Psychol Sci Soc Sci.* 2007;62:P61-P64.

33. Hartley AA. Adult age differences in deductive reasoning processes. *J Gerontol.* 1981;36:700-706

34. Macdonald SW, Stigsdotter-Neely A, Derwinger A, Bäckman L. Rate of acquisition, adult age, and basic cognitive abilities predict forgetting: new views on a classic problem. *J Exp Psychol Gen.* 2006;13:369-390.

35. Schacter D. *The Seven Sins of Memory: How the Mind Forgets and Remembers.* New York, NY: Houghton Mifflin; 2001.

36. Seidler RD. Aging affects motor learning but not savings at transfer of learning. *Learn Mem.* 2007;14:17-21.

37. Walker MP, Stickgold R. Sleep, memory, and plasticity. *Ann Rev Psychol.* 2006;57:139-166.

38. Muslimović D, Post B, Speelman JD, Schmand B. Motor procedural learning in Parkinson's disease. *Brain.* 2007;130:2887-2897.

39. Thomas CM. Bulletin boards: a teaching strategy for older audiences. *J Gerontol Nurs.* 2007;33:45-52.

40. Yesavage JA, Rose T. The effects of a face-name mnemonic in young, middle aged, and elderly adults. *Exp Aging Res.* 1984;10:55-57.

41. Colodny A. Teaching for life: integrating aging into the rehabilitation education program. *SCI Nurs.* 2002;19:67-70.

42. Kramer AF, Hahn S, Cohen NJ. Aging, fitness and neurocognitive function. *Nature.* 1999;400:418-419.

43. US Department of Health and Human Services. *Physical Activity and Health: A Report of the Surgeon General, Executive Summary.* Atlanta, GA: US Dept of Health and Human Services; 2006. Publication HE 20.7602:56.

44. Bixby WR, Spalding TW, Haufler AJ, et al. The unique relation of physical activity to executive function in older men and women. *Med Sci Sports Exerc.* 2007;39:1408-1416.

45. Wilson RS, Mendes de Leon CF, Bennett DA, Bienias JL, Evans DA. Depressive symptoms and cognitive decline in community population of older people. *J Neurol Neurosurg Psychiatry.* 2004;75:126-129.

46. Mahncke HW, Bronstone A, Merzenich MM. Brain plasticity and functional losses in the aged: scientific bases for a novel intervention. *Prog Brain Res.* 2006;157:81-109.

47. Van Wynen EA. A key to successful aging: learning-style patterns of older adults. *J Gerontol Nurs.* 2001;27:6-15.

48. Bayliss EA, Ellis JL, Steiner JF. Barriers to self-management and quality-of-life outcomes in seniors with multimorbidities. *Ann Fam Med.* 2007;5:395-402.

49. O'Brien G. Principles of adult learning. Melbourne, Australia: Southern Health Organization. 2004. www.southern-health.org.au/cpme/articles/adult_learning.htm. Accessed December 12, 2007.

50. Stoedefalke KG. Motivating and sustaining the older adult in an exercise program. *Top Geriatr Rehab.* 1985;1:78-83.

51. Barnes DE, Alexopoulos GS, Lopez OL, Williamson JD, Yaffe K. Depressive symptoms, vascular disease and mild cognitive impairment: findings from the Cardiovascular Health Study. *Arch Gen Psychiatry.* 2006;63:273-279.

52. Boutin-Foster C, Foster JC, Konopasek L. Physician, know thyself: the professional culture of medicine as a framework for teaching cultural competence. *Acad Med.* 2008;83:106-111.

53. Office of Minority Health, US Department of Health and Human Services. *Teaching Cultrual Competence in Health Care: A Review of Current Concepts, Policies, and Practices.* Washington, DC: US Dept of Health and Human Services; 2002.

54. Wilson, SH, Dorne R. Impact of culture on the education of the geriatric patient. *Top Geriatr Rehab.* 2005;21:282-294.

55. Chang M, Kelly AE. Patient education: addressing cultural diversity and health literacy issues. *Urol Nurs.* 2007;27:411-417.

56. Rankin SH, Stallings KD, London F. *Patient Education in Health and Illness.* 5th ed. Philadelphia, PA: Lippincott, Williams & Wilkins; 2005.

57. Kleinman A, Eisenberg L, Good B. Culture, illness, and care: clinical lessons from anthropologic and cross-cultural research. *Ann Intern Med.* 1978;88:251-258.

58. Anderson LM, Scrimshaw SC, Fullilove MT, Fielding JE, Normand J. Culturally competent healthcare systems. a systematic review. *Am J Prev Med.* 2003;24(3 suppl):68-79.

59. Madden CM; Fetterman E. Caregiver connections: a caregiver support and continuing education system. *J Nutr Educ Behav.* 2002;34 (suppl 1):S65-S66.

60. Gitlin LN, Hauck WW, Dennis MP, Winter L. Maintenance of effects of the home environmental skill-building program for family caregivers and individuals with Alzheimer's disease and related disorders. *J Gerontol A Biol Sci Med Sci.* 2005;60:368-374.

61. Smith J, Forster A, Young J. A randomized trial to evaluate an education programme for patients and carers after stroke. *Clin Rehabil.* 2004;18:726-736.

Index

Bottomley J. *Geriatric Rehabilitation: A Textbook
for the Physical Therapist Assistant* (pp 329-350).
© 2010 SLACK Incorporated

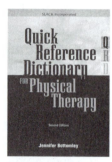
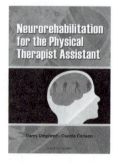